FOODS THAT LIE

HOW TO STOP OVEREATING AND EAT LIKE A NORMAL PERSON

LIBBY MARAMA GRACE

This book is not a medical manual. The information is provided to help readers make informed behavioral decisions and is not a substitute for medical treatment. If you suspect you have a medical condition, please seek competent medical help from a doctor.

Printed by KDP, Amazon

Published by Final Quit

www.finalquit.com

First Edition

ISBN 978-1-0670206-0-6 (Paperback)

ISBN 978-1-0670206-1-3 (Hardback)

ISBN 978-1-0670206-2-0 (Ebook)

ACKNOWLEDGMENTS

This material builds upon the work of numerous brilliant minds, including Mark Schatzker, whose work illuminates the crucial role of flavor in shaping food preferences; Fred Provenza, whose research offers critical insights into feeding behavior; B.F. Skinner, whose intermittent reinforcement experiments expose the mechanism at the heart of overeating; and Allen Carr, whose understanding of addiction reveals the path to escape.

I am deeply grateful to all of those whose work is referenced within.

CONTENTS

1

BEHAVIOR CHANGE REQUIRES A CHANGE OF MIND

I SPENT YEARS DIETING, losing weight, gaining weight, restricting, binge eating, and everything in between. Then I spent years trying to *stop* dieting, yet somehow failed at this, too. Through it all, I became fatter, sicker, and more and more ashamed. At last, drowning in a pit of despair and feeling as though the situation might very well be hopeless, a sequence of ideas slotted together in my mind, and I suddenly saw the way out. As a consequence, returning to a healthy weight became not only achievable but *easy*.

The method did not involve resisting cravings or suffering feelings of deprivation. It did not involve restricting calories, carbohydrates, fats, or proteins. Nor did it involve exercise routines, nutritional supplements, or forced 'habit change.' Instead, something quite simple happened: what I thought about certain foods changed. And as a consequence, *I no longer wanted them.*

It wasn't so much a miracle as it was a light turning on. There *is* a way to end food-related obsession, maintain a healthy weight, and feel completely normal around food again. It requires learning something new about what I call 'deceptive foods.'

To understand what we are trying to achieve, consider the case of a man who knows that cigarettes are killing him. This man may hate the effects of the cigarette, despise himself for continuing to smoke, and know very well that his health and life depend upon a behavioral change. Yet, the problem is he doesn't know how to make himself *do* it. You see, although he hates the *effects* of the cigarette, he simultaneously *likes smoking*. Thus, whenever he attempts to stop, he feels deprived – as though he is missing out on something good. Even if he desperately yearns to be free of the negative health consequences of smoking and the shame his continued behavior brings, as long as he *still wants the cigarette,* he remains ensnared in an internal battle of wills.

The issue is not that the smoker doesn't know what to do (stop smoking) or even that he doubts this is the best course of action. The problem is that part of him *doesn't want to do it.*

What the smoker needs is not so much a practical method of stopping, but a new way of looking at the situation – a more accurate way – so that he *no longer desires the cigarette.*

The moment he achieves this mindset, the jaws of the trap open, and walking away from the cigarette becomes not only possible, but *easy.* This is because, as the great stop-smoking guru Allen Carr discovered, leaving behind something that you no longer want is no hardship at all.

Of course, in the case of overeating, the situation is not nearly so clear. Unlike smoking, it isn't widely accepted that anything in the food supply is addictive at all – nor is it obvious what this addictive element might be. For example, if sugar is the culprit, why do so many studies tout the benefits of eating fruit? If refined carbohydrates are to blame, why do many populations consuming large amounts of white rice remain lean?

Furthermore, unlike smoking, it isn't at all clear whether abstinence is the best approach. Attempting to abstain from every 'problematic' food can seem impractical, unworkable, or downright impossible. In short, when it comes to overeating, neither the culprit nor the cure is clear.

We will get to these questions soon. For now, just imagine that someone *could* wave a wand and take away every speck of desire within you for certain foods. Can you see that this would immediately solve the problem?

The moment you no longer want the thing that is harming you, you're free.

Changing Your Mind Requires New Information

Desire is not a fixed, constant state. Your desire for any particular item fluctuates as your knowledge of a situation changes. The human brain is responsive and adaptive, calculating and recalculating needs so that you are primed to take the best course of action at any given moment.

To understand how new information can alter the way you respond to the same circumstance, consider the following thought experiments:

- You are walking alone through a park at sunset. Upon hearing a rustling in the bushes, your heart starts to race, as you imagine a predator lurking. When a rabbit bounds out of the undergrowth, fear instantly transforms into relief.
- You are at an office party, seated opposite an attractive colleague whom you have been dreaming of for

months. When they begin to play footsies under the table, you feel a rush of euphoria. This emotion ceases immediately when you discover it is not your crush but the office sleaze.

- You have a dull ache in your side after pulling a muscle. The ache is annoying but not severe, and you mention this in passing when seeing your doctor about something unrelated. After examining you, the doctor says there is a small chance the discomfort is caused by a tumor rather than a strain. Immediately, the dull ache throbs and swells into a panic-filled pain.

These examples illustrate that it is more than possible to respond to the *exact same stimuli* in a different way when new information comes to hand. There is nothing you can do to *will* yourself to think about food differently unless this is accompanied by new information that reorganizes your existing interpretation of the world. Behavioral change occurs when *what we know* changes – when new information shifts or dismantles prior beliefs and understandings.

This book offers a new way of looking at eating behavior – a more accurate way. It explains how sensory deception within the food supply provokes measurable changes within taste and smell receptors and how this undetected bodily manipulation leads us to *misinterpret what is happening*.

It can seem impossible to contemplate at the outset, but there *is* a way to escape the endlessly demoralizing cycle of losing and regaining weight. It involves changing how you define and view the substances that are to blame.

This approach works because all addictions have at their root the same fundamental error in perception. And when this error is corrected, you are free.

Who am I?

I am a mother from New Zealand. I have no relevant work experience or nutritional qualifications (I have two degrees in a field completely unrelated to nutrition). What I do have, however, is almost two decades entangled in what can only be described as a dietary nightmare...and the complete and utter joy of being free of it.

This is not my autobiography, but by way of introduction, I will offer a brief summation of my dietary history and the events leading up to the moment when the final pieces of the puzzle fell into place.

I began dieting at age seventeen, abstaining from breakfast and lunch on school days without my parents noticing. Such strategies are now known as 'intermittent fasting' or 'time-restricted feeding,' but back then, I knew it simply as *not eating.* My parents did not own a bathroom scale, so I could not easily measure my weight loss progress, and I soon gave up on this endeavor and returned to eating as I had always done.

My next serious dieting attempt began at age nineteen while at university. I had little nutritional knowledge (there was no internet in those days to conduct research, and I was too embarrassed to borrow weight loss books from the library). From popular magazines, I learned that fat has more calories per gram than carbohydrates or protein and was informed that restriction in both calories and fat was the answer (it is not). For breakfast, I poured a drizzle of fat-free milk upon manufactured cereal and stirred it around so the bowlful became mildly damp. I purchased scales, drew a graph, and tracked my weight loss weekly. I lost 37 pounds (17 kilograms) in three months. This left me at the very bottom of the normal BMI range. I was not thin enough to qualify as anorexic, but I no longer menstruated, needed a heater even in summer to keep warm, and was once so fatigued that I passed out in the shower.

At age 20, I embraced vegetarianism, combining this with strict calorie counting. I had read that 1,200 calories was a good daily target for a dieting female (it is not – to put this ridiculous total in perspective, this is fewer calories than is needed to sustain many active 2-3 year old children).[1] Wanting to ensure that I did not exceed this intake, I decided to eat 1,200 *kilojoules* instead (this is approximately 290 calories). I rationalized that this would help me lose weight faster. During this period, I became intimately familiar with the calorie value of virtually every food.

For obvious reasons, consuming a daily target of 290 calories was doomed to fail, and this is where my appetite really seemed to get 'out of control.' During dietary lapses, I would consume anything I could get my hands on, eating vast quantities of food in horrifying combinations.

I played out versions of the above over and over again until age 23, when I introduced exercise. At one point, I ran every single day for 409 days in a row, often for more than an hour at a time. Sometimes, my eating would feel 'under control,' at other times, it would not.

During this period, I began reading frantically, devouring every diet-related book I could find. I also read about those with eating disorders and discovered the rather terrifying notion that *something might be wrong with me.*

In the years to come, I broadened my reading to cover topics about depression, behavior, decision-making, and addiction. With the advent of the internet, I began scouring websites, blogs, forums, and scientific papers for anything that might offer a clue as to how I could get my eating and my weight 'under control.' At various points, I tried diet pills (the kind that purportedly fill your stomach with fiber), hypnosis, extended fasting, and low-carbohydrate diets.

Eventually, at age 28, I thought I had stumbled upon the holy grail. I finally understood the value of nutrition and had worked out that feeding my body wholesome, natural foods from all food groups allowed me to eat until I was satisfied while losing weight. I devised a home exercise plan, coupled with a running schedule, and at last became fit and lean in a way that felt manageable. I consumed a meat and fat-rich diet, along with lavish quantities of fruits, vegetables, full-fat milk, eggs, nuts, and whole grains.

Much of the knowledge I had acquired by this stage was invaluable, but I still had the enemy squarely in the wrong corner. I considered the problem to be an addiction to refined carbohydrates, and I believed that addiction meant a *lack of control over these things.* I feared that if I consumed just a little white sugar, white rice, or white flour, I would tumble spectacularly from the wagon and eat much, much more. I believed this because, on the rare occasions that I consumed these things, this is exactly what I did.

About a year after the birth of my first child, by which time I had fallen from the wagon and gained weight once more, I began eating a 'normal' diet combined with reasonable quantities of whole foods and fresh smoothies.

Suspecting that something in my eating behavior had gone horribly wrong and not wanting to introduce disordered eating patterns to my children, I vowed, with increasing fervor, to eat *normally*, aiming to consume the generally wholesome (but imperfect) diet that I had eaten as a young child.

Unfortunately, this strategy did not reliably result in weight loss, and there seemed to be no clear definition of what 'normal' *was.* As such, I eventually resorted to restricting my intake. And, as with every attempt prior, I soon put all the weight back on and more.

Finally, I abandoned the idea of *any form of dietary restriction*. By this stage, I felt as though I hated dieting with every cell in my body. Yet, despite attempts to repeatedly nourish myself for years on end, it seemed as though I had acquired a persistent overeating problem – a behavior that gripped me in a way that only felt like an addiction.

After the birth of my second child, by which time I was at my highest weight ever, I had a permanent tug-of-war in my brain.

As the years passed, attempts to reform my eating became fewer and farther between. It seemed increasingly difficult to summon the strength to start again. And, as my weight climbed, despondence, shame, and self-hatred grew.

At last, after years of desperate research and personal trial and error, the final pieces of the puzzle began to fall into place. A key insight came in the aftermath of a personal health scare brought on by my poor diet. As the health scare unfolded, I promised myself that this was *it*. I made a vow like I had never made before and prayed to God, despite not being religious, vowing with every speck of my being that, *this time*, I would change.

What horrified me was that I did *not* change. Although this event appeared directly attributable to my diet, I was soon continuing on as if it had made not an ounce of difference.

The utter horror that I would pass through such a situation and then *keep on going* with the same damaging behavior, with barely a blink of hesitation afterward, made it terrifyingly clear that nothing was going to stop me.

By that point, I felt as though I had exhausted all of the known nutritional strategies – had tried every viable weight loss approach known to man. It seemed, at some level, that I knew *what* to do (eat less junk food) but that I could not or would not do it.

For years, I had hoped that some external event might spur me into action because earlier dieting attempts were often made in response to a particular life change. But now it seemed evident that nothing was going to throw me from this awful rollercoaster that I had climbed upon.

About a month after this event, by which time my junk food intake had escalated above previous levels once more, I came to the indisputable conclusion that if I wanted to fix this thing, it was going to have to be up to me. The world would not rearrange itself into a circumstance that would propel me to change. *I would have to do it.*

This prospect left me blanketed with fresh despair and hopelessness. It seemed, by this stage, that I had lost all shred of food-related self-discipline and willpower. I broke dietary promises to myself so frequently that I don't think I even believed my own word anymore.

But despite fearing that the situation was hopeless, I sat down, pulled out a piece of paper, and began to bullet-point the things about the situation that I believed were true.

You see, the one thing I clung to was that something so *fundamental to life as eating* could not possibly be so complicated that it was beyond me. I had excelled academically, had a great childhood, and a rewarding career. It seemed infeasible that I could not do something so basic as feed myself appropriately. I desperately clung to the notion that *there must be something I wasn't understanding*.

And as I jotted down ideas on that piece of paper, one tiny fact poked its head out at me – something that, until that moment, I had not seen. Fleshing the idea out further, I drew a diagram with two overlapping circles. Inside one circle, I wrote, 'tastes great,' and inside the other, 'low nourishment.'

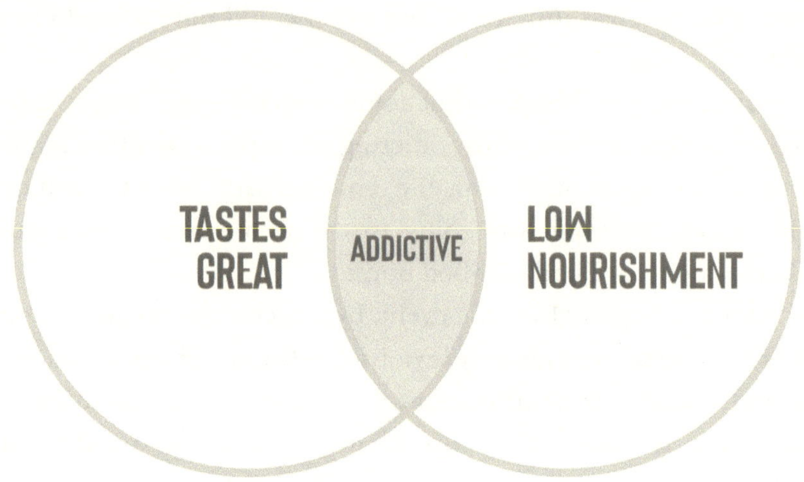

As I stared at that diagram, it occurred to me that all the foods that were killing me were in the central overlapping region.

Of course, during my extreme dieting phases, I had binged on anything and everything I could get my hands on. For example, I once ate an entire week's supply of fruit in one sitting, followed by a whole cooked chicken. On other occasions, I ate entire batches of fat-free, sugar-free muffins and whole loaves of freshly baked bread. This is just the tip of the embarrassing iceberg. However, since abandoning food restriction completely, my overeating focused predominantly upon items in the central region of the graph. I no longer overate fruit, salmon, or chicken. Nor did I binge upon bland, low-nourishment items, such as bowls of white rice or plain white bread. And despite experts telling me that sugar was the dietary equivalent of cocaine, I never once took a cupful of sugar from the cupboard and chowed it down. Instead, my overeating centered, almost exclusively, upon foods that were both low in nutrition *and* tasted great.

As I stared at that diagram, I realized that this implied the problem had *something to do with flavor.*

I thought about how almost all the experts were preoccupied with the balance of macronutrients (fats, proteins, and carbohydrates) or the effect of a single ingredient (such as refined sugar) on the body. Yet very few people appeared to consider the fact that whether or not we seek out or enjoy a particular food *depends upon how it tastes.*

As I contemplated this, a whisker of hope emerged.

I knew, at this point, that something about my behavior mimicked the patterns I saw in other addictions. I was familiar with the great work of Allen Carr, whose stop-smoking method allows people to instantly (and most importantly *happily*) end a lifetime's addiction to nicotine. I had also read extensively about alcoholism, drug addiction, and emerging research about pornography and gaming addiction. Yet, at this point, two things remained very unclear.

Firstly, I didn't know what the addictive element in food *was,* and none of the popular theories seemed to make sense. Secondly, I didn't know what addiction even *meant.*

Of course, I could recognize the familiar pattern – the growing obsession, the escalating usage, the withdrawal period, the endless broken promises – but nowhere had I read of a universal theory or convincing explanation as to *why* this pattern of behavior played out in certain circumstances.

As I studied those two overlapping circles, I sensed that flavor and nutrition were not *all* that mattered. For example, I suspected it would not suffice to take a plateful of chocolate, sprinkle vitamin pills over the top, and call this a 'tasty, high-nourishment meal.'

I suddenly wondered whether the flavor and nutrition *had to be in the right place.* In other words, I suddenly questioned whether flavor had a *purpose*. Perhaps, in some way, flavor was acting as a *signal*, telling my body what kind of nutrition a food contained. For instance, BBQ-flavored crisps, chips, or crackers seem to promise the appearance of protein with their savory aroma, yet the protein never comes.

I thought back to how I had initiated diets, escalating hunger, and then tried to satisfy this elevated hunger using foods spiked with manufactured flavors. Perhaps this had muddled the stream of flavor signals that my body was using to regulate food intake, such that my body could *no longer reliably predict what type of nutrition was coming in.*

This new possibility soon led to a dramatically different way of viewing and perceiving food. The most miraculous part is not just that weight began to fall off me, but that the near-constant food-related obsession that had haunted me for decades lifted. And in its absence, a glorious peace returned – a blissful space for *life* to move back in.

As my health and weight normalized, I began documenting these ideas on a website, www.eatlikeanormalperson.com, in an effort to establish exactly why this change had been so dramatic and different from all dietary approaches I had tried before.

As I documented these ideas, I continued to research the role of flavor. Important insights came from Mark Schatzer's book, *The Dorito Effect* (2016), which introduced me to the research of Fred Provenza and Clara Davis, whose findings further support the critical importance of the relationships between flavor and nutrition.

It was when I finally understood the impact of intermittent reinforcement (the mechanism at the heart of gambling machines, whereby a single action *sometimes* leads to a reward and sometimes does not) that I realized I had stumbled across a hypothesis that explained not only the obesity epidemic but *every single addiction*.

Some Warnings

This is not a typical 'diet' book. Nor is it a typical 'stop dieting' book. It is a logic-based explanation of what causes overeating and how to stop.

The premise is that deceptive flavor signals and other forms of molecular mimicry within the food supply create intermittent reinforcement, provoking a cascade of short-term bodily adaptations that increase appetite and drive overeating – including the overeating of genuine, nourishing foods. As such, this book presents a solution for overeating of all kinds.

It is important to note that 'deceptive food' is not necessarily synonymous with 'junk food.' Many individuals who believe they consume quite nourishing fare unwittingly take in a large number of deceptive flavor molecules. On the other hand, many foods that are commonly thought to be 'fattening' are not deceptive at all.

This book explains how ongoing exposure to deceptive foods promotes 'disordered' eating behaviors – particularly when deceptive foods are encountered during a state of extreme hunger, such as in the wake of a conventional diet. It provides a simple blueprint for normalizing eating patterns, extinguishing dietary obsession, and achieving an optimal weight that can be maintained for the rest of your life.

From a practical perspective, the method involves prioritizing nourishing, 'flavor-honest' foods (those that do not deceive the sensory system) and eating until full at regular meals, providing the body with a reliable stream of flavor cues that rapidly resets appetite to normal levels.

The method does not require 'giving up' anything. Rather, it involves seeing deceptive foods in a different light, such that you *no longer want them* (improbable as this prospect may seem at the outset). With this new mindset, deceptive foods are no longer sought out and are avoided where possible – sidestepping the practical dilemmas that often accompany moderation and abstinence. Consequently, the intake of misleading molecules falls close to zero, leaving you feeling unbelievably *free*.

The cure is informational. That is, it works by communicating something new so that you view both food and yourself in a different way.

If you have ever tried to convince someone of a new idea – particularly when that viewpoint is novel or controversial – you will know that reciting a single fact rarely does the trick. What is needed is a careful sequence of arguments, each building upon the previous one, so that the person gradually comes around to seeing things in a new light, with all doubts and uncertainties laid to rest.

For this reason, chapters in this book are designed to be read in the order given. Furthermore, since behavior change requires reframing how you think about the situation, you cannot expect to turn to a single page and find the 'solution.' Skipping to the end will be about as useful as a smoker who reads that the solution is to *stop smoking*. Of course, understanding where the deception hides is slightly more complex than in the case of nicotine, but the real power of this book is found in the cumulative sequence of ideas that work together to change your mind.

Please be aware that this book includes material that some individuals may find offensive or controversial, such as descriptions of graphic animal experiments and passing references to pornography. It also includes discussion of many other addictions unrelated to food. This is because it is often easier to identify the error in another's behavior than it is our own.

This book is the culmination of over twenty years of my own

personal research into this topic. It synthesizes ideas from multiple scientific fields, presenting a new way of understanding eating behavior and addiction. While I have endeavored to ensure that ideas are well-referenced, scientific knowledge is constantly evolving and often subject to debate, with numerous conflicting arguments advanced by individuals on all sides. It is almost impossible to produce a treatise that remains 100% accurate in every tiny detail across every scientific discipline at all times. Furthermore, as the concepts in this book have been woven together over the course of two decades, there may be instances where I have inadvertently misattributed an idea or failed to give credit where it is due. If you discover an error, please get in touch via libby@eatlikeanormalperson.com, and I will endeavor to update subsequent editions as necessary.

However, as you read, please remember that many of the concepts presented here are not only novel but challenge the conventional assumptions about addiction, obesity, and eating disorders. If you encounter something that *seems* incorrect, do not automatically assume that it is. For example, while reviewing an earlier draft of this manuscript, some beta readers initially found the emotional eating material difficult to accept. Yet, by the end of the book, many of these same readers had tearfully changed their minds. In short, please allow me the opportunity to lay out the argument in full before you decide whether the ideas have merit. Importantly, *keep an open mind* and consider the possibility that if all other strategies have not worked, *a new way of looking at things might help.*

The book begins with a general discussion about behavior and decision-making. This material may initially seem rather abstract and unrelated to eating issues. Some readers may fear they have opened an obscure scientific textbook and find themselves impatient to get to the topic at hand. Rest assured that these brief introductory passages provide a vital foundation for the understanding of eating behavior that is to follow. As you continue to read, the pieces of the puzzle will gradually fall into place, and everything will become clear.

To fully grasp a problem, we must start at the beginning.

2

BEHAVIOR

> At some point, a particular arrangement of particles got so good at copying itself that it could do so almost indefinitely by extracting raw materials from its environment. We call such particle arrangement *life*.
>
> — MAX TEGMARK, *LIFE 3.0* (2017)

To grow, repair, and move, humans must obtain a supply of chemicals from the environment. Some of these chemicals are known as *nutrients*. We typically extract these nutrients from other lifeforms, such as plants, animals, and fungi.

Nutrients are required in particular quantities and combinations. People who attempt to survive on only lean protein, for example, with insufficient fat, eventually die from protein poisoning. Those who consume the wrong variety of plants (poisonous mushrooms, for instance) or prepare an item incorrectly (such as failing to soak or cook kidney beans) may suffer adverse health effects. Complicating matters further, items that are beneficial in smaller amounts can be dangerous when consumed to excess. For example, overdosing on nutmeg leads to convulsions, hallucinations, pain, and delirium,[1] yet small amounts appear to offer anti-inflammatory,[2] antioxidant, and antimicrobial[3] benefits. Similarly, while vitamin C is essential for immune function and collagen synthesis, excessive vitamin C supplementation can lead to diarrhea, nausea, and acute kidney failure.[4 5]

Not only are particular quantities and combinations of these nutrients needed in order to thrive, but the optimal range varies with the individual and circumstance, fluctuating according to a myriad of factors, including age, nutritional status, the presence of injury or illness, circadian rhythm, parasite load, level of exertion, pregnancy/breastfeeding needs, and so on. Yet, despite this complexity, your ancestors somehow managed to carry out this task without the benefit of modern science.

To get an idea of just how skillful lifeforms are at optimizing their food supply, consider the case of a bonsai tree. Bonsai trees are ordinary trees grown in shallow plant pots. With only a small area of soil and limited room for growth, you might suspect the tree would wither and die. Instead, it becomes a perfectly formed miniature tree.

Something similar happens when certain breeds of baby mice are fed a nourishing yet low-calorie diet immediately after weaning. Instead of growing into thin, bony, full-sized adults, they become perfectly formed miniature mice.[6] These tiny mice live longer and in greater health than controls. Such studies are often cited as evidence that low-calorie diets lead to an increased lifespan; however, it is worth noting that these miniature mice now consume, on average, 30% more per gram of body weight than the controls. In other words, these brilliant mice adapt so well to the reduced food supply that *they are no longer deprived.*

Even newly weaned human babies, with limited vocabulary and zero formal nutritional knowledge, self-select appropriate foods when given the chance. In the 1920s, a Chicago pediatrician called Clara Davis set out to see if children possessed the capability to choose appropriate foods.[7] Davis cared for fifteen children in an orphanage (aged 6-11 months at the outset), recording every item they ate for up to four and a half years while tracking their height, weight, and other health parameters. At each meal, the children were presented with an array of food, including fresh fruit, vegetables, oats, wheat, meat, fish, liver, brains, bone jelly, bone marrow, cod liver oil, sea salt, water, orange juice, and milk. The adults did not comment on food intake nor direct the children toward particular items. At every meal, the children were free to consume as much or as little as they desired.

To begin with, the babies gnawed or chewed on virtually every item within reach (including the plates, spoons, trays, and so forth). However, they soon began to exhibit distinct preferences. Although the food combinations were sometimes unusual – for example, one baby chose liver and orange juice for breakfast – all the children thrived. They recovered from illnesses quickly and spontaneously increased their intake of beef, beets, and carrots while recovering from glandular fever. One child entered the experiment with rickets – a bone disease caused by insufficient vitamin D – and voluntarily swigged down cod liver oil (a known cure for rickets) until his body healed. The participants were evaluated as being "uniformly well-nourished, healthy children."[8]

Just as these children somehow knew how to seek out the nutrition they needed, animals, too, hunt out specific substances to medicate, nourish, or heal themselves. Sheep, who seem, to our ill-informed human eyes, to eat only 'grass,' carefully select from hundreds of different plant species, each of which interact and combine in potentially harmful or beneficial ways.[9] When cats, dogs, geese, bears, bonobos, chimpanzees, and gorillas are infested with worms, they consume extra-fibrous plant matter to flush out the digestive tract and expel the worms.[10] Even primarily herbivorous animals turn to animal food sources when a particular nutrient is lacking.

Although human knowledge is expanding at an unprecedented rate, we remain novices in the field of nutrition.[11] Some doctors are adamant that a vegan diet is optimal; others advocate 100% carnivorism. The entire spectrum in between is filled with various competing strategies, all marketed by seemingly intelligent, well-educated folk who are convinced they are right.

To put our novice status in perspective, humans only realized that vitamins existed in 1911.[12] There are likely many aspects of our food supply that we have not even identified, let alone researched or understood, such as the function or impact of the hundreds of 'secondary compounds' present in the plants we eat.

Luckily, our novice status in this area does not have to prohibit health. The fundamental processes for regulating food intake must operate perfectly without the direction of modern man.

In case it is not obvious, wandering around aimlessly and hoping that whatever enters the mouth will do the job is not a viable survival strategy. The business of knowing what and how much to eat is far too important to be left to the mercy of chance. You, like all lifeforms, carry within you an inbuilt system for finding and consuming the raw materials you need.

This book presents the argument that human food intake is

regulated by *relationships between flavor and nutrition* – that eating behavior, like all behavior, is driven by pattern and prediction.

The Survival Game

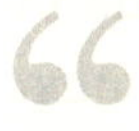

> The goal of behavior is to make the right choices; to choose the course of action that maximizes the survival of the organism's genetic code.
>
> — PAUL GLIMCHER, *DECISIONS, UNCERTAINTY, AND THE BRAIN* (2004)

Eating is a type of behavior. To alter an eating behavior, it helps to first understand the principles that govern *all* behavior.

It can often appear that human actions are mysterious, carried out according to some deep and unknown personal whim. But, as you will soon see, behavior follows rules. This is very good news because it means that eating behavior, no matter how excessive, disordered, or 'out of control' it may seem, can be understood, predicted, and changed.

In a very real sense, life is a survival game. Whether you consider yourself to be the result of billions of years of trial and error or the creation of a wise and all-knowing God (or some combination of the two), one thing is certain: your genes are good at this game.

Across the vast, dangerous expanse of history, every single one of your ancestors survived at least until childbearing age. Every single ancestor conceived viable offspring. Every maternal ancestor gave birth to at least one live child: a squalling, defenseless infant who somehow managed to grow up and do the same thing all over again. This long, unbroken chain of survivors managed to achieve this miraculous feat without any scientific studies, formal nutritional guidelines, or books.

Whether your ancestors made it through each round of this brutal and rather unforgiving game depended, in very large part, upon their behavior.[13] Although luck, fate, and circumstance play a role, *the way you act* enormously impacts your odds of survival. Once the cards are dealt, so to speak, what matters next is *how you play*. In fact, as any good card player knows, when several rounds of a game are played, *skill at playing the game becomes the most important variable of all.*

This means that *behavior* cannot be a trivial aspect of this survival game. If your genes are optimized to survive across time (which they must be), your behavior cannot be a random, happenstance affair. It must follow rules.

To understand eating behavior, therefore, we must first understand the rules of the game. And there are only three:

1. **Seek survival rewards:** things that improve the odds of your genes surviving and replicating across time – sought in order of priority. (This includes seeking nutritious food that provides energy and building blocks for growth, reproduction, and health.)
2. **Avoid survival threats:** things that reduce the odds of your genes surviving and replicating across time – avoided in order of priority. (This includes avoiding unnecessary, harmful, or contaminated foods that lead to sickness or death.)
3. **Ignore everything else.**

The third rule sounds unimportant, but it is vital because misdirected attention compromises performance in the first two areas and quickly becomes a survival threat itself. In a world where resources are limited and competition is fierce, time and energy spent on the wrong thing can be the difference between surviving or not.

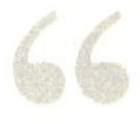

> In the game of life, life must win every moment of every day, while death has to win only once.
>
> — MARTIN SELIGMAN, PETER RAILTON, ROY BAUMEISTER, CHANDRA SRIPADA, *HOMO PROSPECTUS* (2016)

Even if an individual does not die outright from a tendency to pursue the wrong thing at the wrong time, subpar performance is not a mild survival issue. Unhealthy lifeforms are less able to escape predators or produce viable offspring. They are less desirable mates and less able to select optimal partners. In short, those who do not wish to play this game, or who play it badly, are outcompeted by better players over time.

Suppose there were two otherwise identical species, but one behaved so that *every* action was predicted to improve their odds of survival, whereas the other only did so 80% of the time. Which species would be more likely to outperform the other?

Unsurprisingly, lifeforms who spend a greater percentage of their time behaving in such a way that improves their odds of survival are *more likely to survive.*

It can be hard to fathom, but *all* of your actions – from choosing what food to put on your plate to the microscopic cellular responses in the body – aim to improve your genetic odds in this survival game. Of course, not every action achieves this outcome or is the right thing to do. But it is implemented – whether you know it or not – with this as the goal. This is very important to understand because it means that no matter how bizarre or irrational your feeding behavior may appear, there is *logic at the heart of it.* And when you understand this logic, you can see how to change.

Even single-celled organisms follow the rules of this game. Their outer cellular membranes detect changes in the nearby environment, such as adjustments in temperature, light, or chemical concentrations, allowing them to rotate their tail-like appendages, tumbling toward things that are likely to benefit their survival and away from things that are not.[14]

> "A bacterium does not bounce around in its world like a ball in a pinball machine. [...] They can sense where there is food and propel themselves to that spot. Similarly, they can recognize toxins and predators and purposely employ escape maneuvers to save their lives.
>
> — BRUCE LIPTON, *THE BIOLOGY OF BELIEF* (2016)

Humans are complex creatures, it is true. But our goal is the same: move toward survival rewards; move away from survival threats; ignore everything else.

To make *good* decisions, the brain has an inbuilt system for identifying and prioritizing survival rewards and threats, predicting what to pursue or flee at any one moment. This system also determines which foods are *desired* or *avoided.*

Emotions

What we call an *emotion* is the feeling of a carefully calibrated chemical signal that is crafted for a specific survival-related function. Emotions are the mechanism by which the brain prods the cellular teams that make up the body this way and that.

If the brain detects the presence of a survival reward in the nearby vicinity, such as a piece of ripe fruit on a tree, it issues a chemical signal that we call *desire*. Desire depends upon one's interpretation of the situation (see chapter 1: *Changing Your Mind Requires New Information*) as well as the need for that item. Hence, what is desirable to one person is not necessarily desirable to another.

If the acquisition of a survival reward is impeded, attention is refocused on the task with a chemical signal that we call *craving*.

As the reward draws closer and its acquisition appears more likely, a chemical signal that we call *anticipation* or *excitement* is issued, ensuring we maintain a state of high alertness and attention until the reward is captured.

When the reward is obtained or brought within the body, a chemical signal that we call *pleasure* is issued. It is essential to note that *pleasure is not the reward itself* but rather a *signal* that a predicted reward has arrived. The reward is the *genuine survival benefit obtained* (such as nutrients arriving in the gut), and it is this that shapes the behavior going forward. We 'like' pleasure because this sensation coincides with the prediction of a survival win.

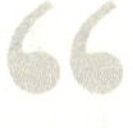

> Men have generalized the feelings of good things and called them pleasure and the feelings of bad things and called them pain, but we do not give a man pleasure or pain, we give him things he feels as pleasant or painful.
>
> — B.F. SKINNER, *BEYOND FREEDOM AND DIGNITY* (1971)

If subsequent examination of the situation deems that the reward really did arrive in the anticipated and necessary volume, a chemical signal that we call *satisfaction* arises.

Satisfaction is the instruction to disengage, to end the pursuit. *Enough.*

If the acquisition of survival rewards is reliable and successful across time, a chemical signal that we call *happiness* is issued. Happiness implies one's rules of operation are accurate; position in the game is tracking upward;[15] the world is understood.

Pattern and Prediction

Although the rules of the game are simple, following them is no easy matter. The business of navigating in and around survival rewards and threats is complicated due to the sheer volume of potential data. Each decision involves an enormous array of fluctuating variables. Consider the stream of information coming in via the senses (sight, sound, smell, taste, and touch) and the vast array of internal data the body must keep track of (temperature, glucose load, nutrition status, and so on). Numerous external factors must also be evaluated and monitored, such as the accessibility of tools, availability of resources, impending weather conditions, and so on. Complicating matters further, each survival reward is required in a particular quantity at a particular time, with both deficiencies and overdoses posing a threat. Too much oxygen, you die. Too little oxygen, you die. The same applies to water,[16] heat, nutrients,[17] and almost every other survival reward that exists.

To avoid carrying out immense and paralyzing calculations at every turn, lifeforms act according to *predictive behavioral rules* that summarize reliable relationships between action and outcome.

Without reliable links between behavior and its consequences, navigating the world would be impossible. If the world were not comprised of cause-and-effect relationships, we would have no idea what to do. In fact, life could not exist. But when something *reliably occurs* (that is, when a particular outcome can be predicted with a reasonable degree of certainty), lifeforms can estimate the impact of a particular action and *select behavior accordingly.*

Operating using predictive behavioral rules speeds up the decision-making process and frees the brain from the burden of continual analysis.[18] Behavioral rules condense experiential data into a useful, short-hand format, allowing energy and attention to be reserved for unfamiliar situations that may harbor a reward or threat or for deciphering challenging environmental circumstances that still need to be attended to and understood.

Behavioral rules that are inherited across generations are called *instincts* or *reflexes*. These are passed down from parent to offspring, giving each new organism the best chance of survival.[19] Long-lived lifeforms, like ourselves, however, are vulnerable unless these rules can be updated and adjusted via experience. If behaving in a certain way does not result in the anticipated outcome, and such variation is not within the expected margin of error, *adjustment of the behavioral rule is required.*

Recalibration of the Rules

If behavioral rules were not updated, a lifeform would be stuck with an inappropriate rule whenever the environment changed. To act appropriately in a rapidly changing world, therefore, we must possess a method for updating the rules.

To achieve this, the brain carefully monitors key survival consequences after particular actions occur, automatically adjusting the relevant behavioral rule upward, downward, or extinguishing the rule altogether, based on the new value of the survival rewards or threats received.[20] In this way, behavioral rules are constantly updated to reflect the current anticipated outcome.

Because survival is fraught with risk, and errors are costly, behavioral rules are maintained with mathematical precision. As complicated as this sounds, this process operates without conscious awareness and has been observed in a wide range of animal species.[21][22]

> "The surprise isn't so much that choices track consequences in some way. (Imagine how haywire things would be if they didn't.) What was eye-opening were the mathematically consistent and elegant ways in which they did so across so many species, consequences, and behaviors.
>
> — SUSAN SCHNEIDER, *THE SCIENCE OF CONSEQUENCES* (2012)

It turns out that lifeforms assign *precise statistical estimations* to behavior, reflecting the anticipated consequences upon survival (positive or negative). These behavioral rules translate relevant prior and inherited experiences[23] into a single numerical estimation (a kind of running average), predicting whether a particular action is likely to help or hinder survival, and to what degree.[24][25] These mathematically precise rules govern every decision you make, including *what to put into your mouth.*

When updating behavioral rules, recent outcomes are most important and are weighted more heavily in the calculation.[26] This is because things that occur *today* are more likely to accurately reflect the current environment than things that happened weeks, months, years, decades, or generations ago.

Selecting behavior according to mathematically precise predictions sounds like an excellent plan. In fact, it is the best plan there is. It would work well in all circumstances...if it weren't for the loophole in the system.

You see, certain species have discovered that there is a tremendous survival advantage to be had in *manipulating the behavioral rules of another lifeform.*

Deception

In her book *Supernormal Stimuli* (2010), Deirdre Barrett describes the work of Nobel Prize-winning biologist Niko Tinbergen, who showed that animal behavior is often elicited in response to a narrow range of stimuli.

Tinbergen and others found that animals can be fooled into responding to artificial objects that mimic key cues in the natural environment with more enthusiasm than they show for the real thing (often with dire consequences). Supernormal stimuli are exaggerated versions of natural stimuli that provoke a stronger response than the natural item. This response can occur even when the fake object is absurdly unrealistic in other ways.

For example, herring gull chicks will beg for food more vigorously from red knitting needles with white bands painted around them than they will from a realistic 3D model of an adult herring gull head (adult gulls have a red spot on the yellow bill, and the chicks normally peck the red spot to signal that the mother should regurgitate her food). Similarly, small songbirds will sit on fake eggs that are much larger and more intense in pattern and color than their own. They will sit on fake eggs that are so large they repeatedly slide off them, ignoring their own paler, dappled eggs. Likewise, a Greylag goose will roll any nearby round-shaped object into her nest, even a doorknob or football-sized fake egg.

The supernormal stimuli effect occurs because nature prioritizes efficiency. If a lifeform can get away with an uncomplicated rule for survival (i.e., round shape = egg) and arrive at the correct behavior faster than a competitor who uses a more complex rule, the faster, more efficient strategy will win.

Because simple behavioral rules are prioritized and because all creatures rely on such rules to navigate the world, deception is a constant threat.

Cuckoos exploit the supernormal stimuli effect by laying their eggs in other birds' nests. The appearance of the cuckoo egg is similar to that of the victim species but is typically a little larger and brighter, ensuring it is preferentially warmed in the nest.[27] Once hatched, the cuckoo chick often develops a larger and redder beak than the victim species, so it monopolizes the food supply and is more likely to be fed by the unwitting foster mother.

Deception occurs when one lifeform mimics a feature of the environment that another is using as a cue to implement a behavioral rule. By mimicking key environmental stimuli, lifeforms can manipulate the behavior of another for their own gain.

Manipulation of this kind can offer tremendous survival rewards for the perpetrator, often for minimal effort. For this reason, deception is widespread within nature, as explained by evolutionary biologist Robert Trivers.

> When I say that deception occurs at all levels of life, I mean that viruses practice it, as do bacteria, plants, insects, and a wide range of other animals. It is everywhere. Even within our genomes, deception

> flourishes as selfish genetic elements use deceptive molecular techniques to over-reproduce at the expense of other genes. Deception infects all the fundamental relationships in life: parasite and host, predator and prey, plant and animal, male and female, neighbor and neighbor, parent and offspring, and even the relationship of an organism to itself.
>
> — ROBERT TRIVERS, *THE FOLLY OF FOOLS: THE LOGIC OF DECEIT AND SELF-DECEPTION IN HUMAN LIFE* (2014)

Trivers describes the eternal dance between the deceived and the deceiver. As deception arises, those individuals who can detect the mimicry have improved survival odds, and their offspring proliferates. Over time, the population fills with those who are better at detecting and avoiding that precise deception. In retaliation, the deceiving species acquire more cunning manipulation tactics. The balance thus continually oscillates, swinging back and forth between deceiver and deceived.

When faced with a deceptive circumstance, abandoning pursuit of a survival reward is not a viable option (just as ignoring a looming survival threat is untenable). A cuckoo victim, for example, cannot refuse to sit on all eggs without eliminating her own offspring in the process. A victim of deception thus remains at the mercy of their enemy *until they can reliably discern between the genuine item and the imposter.*

Until this happens, the victim remains trapped, operating via a faulty behavioral rule that now leads to *unpredictable outcomes*. Sometimes, sitting on an egg leads to hatching one's own offspring; sometimes, it leads to raising the offspring of the enemy.

Although it can be hard to comprehend, deception often presents a far more serious threat to survival than natural disaster or attack. This is because, in the act of being deceived, the victim is fooled into *willingly returning for more.*

Deception applies the illusion of a reward where it does not belong and thus dupes a lifeform into *pursuing a threat.* In other words, deception coerces a lifeform into *violating the rules of the game.*

3

THE ROLE OF FLAVOR

> “When we eat, we attend to the concentration of chemical stimulus in our food (e.g., judging whether our food is too salty or contains a hint of onion).
>
> — DANIELLE RENEE REED AND ANTTI KNAAPILA, *GENETICS OF TASTE AND SMELL: POISONS AND PLEASURES* (2012)

THE PREVIOUS CHAPTER introduced the idea that behavior stems from predicted associations between action and outcome. Let's now explore how this concept relates to eating.

We tend to think of 'chemicals' as artificial manufactured substances, but chemicals are the building blocks of life. James Kennedy, an Australian chemistry teacher, publishes posters illustrating the wide array of naturally occurring chemicals found in fruits and vegetables. His poster of a banana, for example, lists approximately 50 substances (this excludes pesticides, fertilizer residue, contaminants, and "thousands of minority ingredients").[1] In other words, every time you eat *anything*, you take in a very large number of chemicals.

As food enters the mouth, some of these chemicals slot into taste bud receptors, aided by chewing and the release of saliva. Taste buds are found in many locations within the oral cavity, such as on the tongue and throat. Each taste bud has 80-100 receptors,[2] which are activated by precise chemicals only – those with a specific molecular shape – just as a key fits into a lock. When a particular chemical activates a taste bud receptor, a signal is sent to the brain.[3] If many receptors are activated, a stronger signal is sent,[4] indicating a higher concentration of that particular chemical in the mouth. In this way, the type and quantity of chemicals within food can be estimated while you are eating.

Scientists describe the taste bud as a "complex signal processing unit."[5] There are currently five known types of human taste bud receptors (sour, salty, bitter, sweet, and umami),[6] each of which detects the presence of broad categories of food.[7] Umami sensors, for example, detect the presence of glutamate and ribonucleotides, which are commonly found in cooked and aged meats and other easily digestible protein sources.[8] New research also indicates that taste bud receptors for other substances, such as fatty acids,[9] starch, calcium, and water,[10] may soon be identified.

In addition to those chemicals sensed by taste buds, another important subset (those that vaporize and float through the air) are perceived as *smell*. These volatile chemicals enter the nasal cavity through the top of the mouth while chewing, as well as via the nostrils, and activate odorant receptors. Humans have approximately 350 – 400 types of odorant receptors,[11] which can be activated in various combinations, purportedly allowing us to distinguish between more than a trillion odors.[12] *Specific smells are associated with specific nutrients* and hence provide "important information about the nutritional makeup of foods."[13]

Although humans are not renowned for having an incredible sense of smell, Gordon Shepherd, emeritus professor of neuroscience at the Yale School of Medicine, argues that our sense of smell is far better than we realize. In his book *Neurogastronomy* (2013), Shepherd explains that there are two types of smell – 'orthonasal,' which occurs when *breathing in* chemicals from the outside environment, and 'retronasal,' which occurs when *breathing out,* whereby volatile chemicals released while chewing food are swept into the nasal cavity.[14]

Dogs are great at detecting and tracking smells in the outside environment (aided by a long snout close to the ground) and hence have an advanced sense of orthonasal smell. Shepherd argues that humans, on the other hand, have a particularly advanced sense of retronasal smell, *specifically to detect and analyze food flavors.* He suggests this advanced sense of smell is largely hidden from our conscious awareness because we perceive it to be *part of taste* (he notes that holding one's nose while eating makes it clear how much flavor perception is derived from smell).

Humans typically consume a much wider range of foods than other species due to the many ways we grow, store, and prepare food (such as cooking, preserving, and fermenting), as well as our tendency to inhabit vastly different environments. Shepherd believes that navigating this complex food environment and selecting between such a wide array of foods demands a highly advanced sense of retronasal smell.

The information gleaned via taste and smell receptors, along with other sensory data (such as the color, texture, and temperature of food), together creates our perception of flavor. And our perception of flavor *strongly influences how we act around a particular food.*

For example, an intense, undesirable flavor may trigger immediate rejection, such as spitting out or retching. A *pleasant* flavor, on the other hand, may initiate a cascade of digestive responses, such as increased saliva and gastric juices,[15] helping to prepare the digestive tract for the incoming nutrition.

The *reason* we have taste buds and smell receptors strategically positioned within the mouth and nasal cavity is to ensure that helpful or harmful chemicals are detected *before* they enter the body. In a very literal manner, smelling, chewing, and tasting the food lets sensory receptors carry out a complex chemical analysis, the result of which *directly influences whether a substance is permitted entrance to the body*.

Finding and acquiring nutrients (while avoiding toxins and other harmful chemicals) is essential to life. The rules governing eating behavior are thus just as deliberate and mathematically precise as all other behavioral rules. In fact, distinguishing between flavors is so important that there appear to be *more human genes dedicated to coding smell than to almost any other activity* (genes specific to the olfactory system are second in number only to those dedicated to the immune system).[16]

If flavor were a trivial detail, our brains would not pay so much attention to it. There is zero survival benefit in detecting and transmitting useless information (remember the third rule of the game). Cats, for example, cannot taste sweet flavors because their traditionally meat-based diets contain little sugar.[17] Chickens, who predominantly eat starchy grains, also have no functioning sweet receptors.[18] Aquatic mammals, on the other hand, often have very few taste receptors at all, presumably because visual cues and other sensory stimuli are more important when distinguishing between swimming prey that is swallowed in one gulp.[19]

Initial flavor rules are passed down as instincts. As such, babies emerge from the womb liking their mother's milk and disliking bitter tastes.[20] Toddlers are also predisposed to enjoy flavors present in their mother's milk and flavors consumed by the mother during pregnancy.[21] Moreover, inherited flavor preferences can reflect the local conditions where your ancestors resided.

> You are predisposed to prefer your own culture's culinary customs because following them, at least in the distant past, favored survival in the local habitat, which had its own unique variety of edible plants and animals and traditions for safely preparing them...
>
> — KATHLEEN MCAULIFFE, *THIS IS YOUR BRAIN ON PARASITES* (2017)

Although we begin with inherited flavor rules, we do not depend on these alone. Lifeforms are sometimes flung from one habitat to another, such as following a natural disaster or the exhaustion of a prior food source – not to mention the constant adjustments due to changes in season, weather, and climate. To thrive, humans must be able to adapt to a new food environment quickly. Thus, flavor preferences can be shaped, molded, and extinguished via experience.

Flavor-Nutrition Relationships

Although foods contain hundreds or even thousands of naturally occurring chemicals, only *some* of these chemicals contribute toward our experience of flavor: those that slot into taste and smell receptors. This subset represents only a fraction of the food as a whole. Many chemicals (including those with nourishing properties) are not detected by the mouth or nose at all. To establish whether an edible substance is beneficial for survival, therefore, the brain makes a *prediction* about what is entering the body based on the flavor profile detected.[22] To do this, flavor at the mouth is linked with the subsequent nutrition (or harmful substances) that arrive in the gut.[23] In this way, flavor acts as a *nutritional marker* or *environmental cue*, alerting the body that a particular set of chemicals is coming in.

Flavor detection thus has a very specific survival-related function. A *delicious* flavor indicates that a *beneficial* set of chemicals appears to be arriving (i.e., nutrients that you need); a *revolting* flavor indicates an incoming survival threat (such as the ingestion of toxins or parasites).

Positive flavor responses can be learned, even if a flavor is initially disliked – as long as consuming that flavor reliably leads to needed nutrients. This is how people 'acquire' tastes for things and why parents are encouraged to feed their children a new food several times to ensure that adequate exposure to the flavor has occurred.

The ability to learn new flavor preferences is demonstrated in many species, including rats, chickens, sheep, goats, and humans. Fred Provenza, professor emeritus of Behavioral Ecology at Utah State University and author of *Nourishment: What Animals Can Teach Us about Rediscovering Our Nutritional Wisdom* (2018), discovered that sheep make "multiple flavor-feedback associations with minerals."[24] In one experiment, Provenza fed a group of sheep a diet deficient in phosphorus. He then gave these same sheep maple-flavored feed for six days while simultaneously dosing them with phosphorus. The aim was to see whether the sheep would learn to associate maple flavor with phosphorus. When he subsequently gave these phosphorus-deficient sheep a choice between maple-flavored feed or another flavor, they ate the maple flavor enthusiastically, even though it contained zero phosphorus.[25] To ensure that sheep do not naturally prefer maple flavor, Provenza fed another group of sheep a *different* flavor along with a dose of phosphorous. When given the choice, these sheep preferred the *other* flavor. If phosphorus was subsequently associated with a different flavor altogether, the sheep changed their preference, avoiding the previously preferred flavor.

It takes only a few days for new flavor-nutrition associations to be learned, but *liking* a particular flavor can be extinguished immediately if nausea or vomiting follows ingestion (indicating a serious survival threat – such as the presence of a high level of toxins). Flavor aversions can endure for a lifetime if the perceived threat to survival is severe. Furthermore, when an aversive flavor is added to another food, this item is avoided too.[26]

Flavor aversions can occur even when multiple foods are consumed simultaneously. Provenza describes sheep eating four familiar grains as well as a new type of grain (and a capsule that induces nausea). In this circumstance, the sheep quickly learn to avoid the new grain only – and associate this with the onset of nausea.[27] Even inherited flavor preferences (such as liking sweet flavors) can be extinguished in some circumstances. This is necessary because not all sweet flavors are harmless, and not all bitter ones are dangerous.[28]

> “...it is relatively easy to make the taste of sugar change from palatable to unpalatable. For example, experimental pairing of sugar taste with upper gastric malaise and nausea can render sugar unpalatable...
>
> — PAUL A.S. BRESLIN, *AN EVOLUTIONARY PERSPECTIVE ON FOOD AND HUMAN TASTE* (2013)

Over time, the learned relationships between each particular flavor and the chemicals that subsequently arrive in the gut are adjusted and refined, so we are more likely to act appropriately when the flavor is next encountered. In other words, through repeated exposure, flavors are linked with their nutritional and metabolic consequences, and these learned associations *influence future eating behavior*.

Is it really plausible that flavor is the driving force behind food choices? Do humans really determine where nutrients are located based on the memory of a flavor in the mouth? Does the brain really have the capacity to track and monitor so many complex variables?

To get an idea of how adept the human brain is at remembering patterns, think of how many songs people can distinguish between. Each song is an arrangement of musical notes, yet many people can remember and hum these complex patterns with ease. Avery Gilbert, author of *What the Nose Knows (2015),* mentions that our interpretation of smell has been likened to a fingerprint or musical chord. As another example, think of how many words you can recognize. Each word is imbued with meaning, and relationships between words are incredibly complex. Nonetheless, most young children learn to master these verbal patterns with ease. Alternatively, consider how many faces you can keep track of. People are mobile collections of visual stimuli – mouths, eyes, hands, heads, limbs – all in slightly different shapes, colors, and sizes. Yet, you can probably distinguish between a great number of people. What is more, you can probably detect slight changes in the expressions on these faces and attribute meaning. Humans are exceptionally proficient at reading facial expressions because doing so, *just like finding the raw materials necessary to build and maintain the body,* is crucial for survival.[29]

Each unique smell (remember, smell is the largest

component of flavor) creates a unique pattern of activity in the brain.[30] When we think of a food, we recall its flavor. This alone indicates the brain is capable of tracking and storing such information.

To successfully navigate through life, seeking nutritional rewards and avoiding dietary threats, we learn the patterns between flavor and nutrition.

People often view flavor as an inherent, fixed property of a particular food – a pleasant side-effect of eating. However, our flavor perception fluctuates according to the expected nutritional payload and *our need for that nutrition*.[31] [32]

Hunger and Satiety

The amount of food one consumes on any given occasion is influenced by both *hunger* (the signal to eat) and *satiation* (the signal to stop eating). As the supply of nutrients and energy is used up between meals, satiety decays until hunger is the predominant signal once more. Hunger for specific flavors rises and falls to ensure that, over time, the correct balance of nutrients is obtained.

Because hunger is often directed toward a specific flavor, it is possible to feel full of one food while hungry for another. *Sensory-specific satiety*, as this phenomenon is known, is observed in numerous species. For example, when people consume bananas until satiation, the smell of bananas is no longer perceived as pleasant; however, the aroma of other foods remains appealing.[33] Similarly, protein-depleted individuals prefer savory over sweet foods.[34] Studies of the brain show that feeding to satiety on one flavor results in a decreased neuronal response to that flavor but not others.[35]

Sensory-specific satiety explains why people can feel like they still have room for dessert despite having eaten a full meal and also why buffet-style dining opportunities often result in a greater ingestion of food. 'Overeating' in this context is the sensible attempt to source the wide array of nutrients predicted by the many different flavor profiles.

When the body needs a particular nutrient, the brain signals a desire for flavors associated with that nutrient (this is the method by which the body then *obtains* that nutrient). As the need for a particular nutrient grows, hunger for the associated flavors becomes more pronounced, prompting the individual to take action and seek out that item. Hunger rises at regular mealtimes to focus attention on the necessary task of gathering nutrition at a time when food is predicted to be readily available.

If a desired flavor is accessible in the nearby environment, cravings mount to ensure you proceed toward the item and acquire the necessary nutrition.

As you bite into the food, flavor molecules slot into taste and smell receptors. If the appropriate flavor is detected, pleasure is issued to signal the arrival of an incoming nutritional reward.

Although seeing delicious food on a shelf or discovering a piece of ripe fruit on a tree may elicit a burst of excitement, the most reliable predictor of incoming nutrition is the *immediately preceding stimuli:*[36] flavor in the mouth. The initial mouthful is thus accompanied by an *increase in desire*, ensuring you are not distracted at this crucial moment and keep on eating until the optimal volume of nutrition is obtained.

> If we were to define hunger in terms of strength of behavior regardless of the presence or absence of discriminative stimuli, we should have to agree that a small amount of food increases it.
>
> — B.F. SKINNER, *SCIENCE AND HUMAN BEHAVIOR* (1965)

In addition to the burgeoning signals of desire and pleasure, flavor in the mouth stimulates the release of "an extensive array of enzymes, hormones, and transporters,"[37] which help to prepare the body for digestion[38] and metabolic responses.[39]

Just as the mouth and nasal cavities are filled with sensory receptors, so too are the stomach, small intestine, and large intestine.[40] As food is digested and broken down into its molecular parts, the gut and the organisms that reside within (the microbiome) carry out a far more comprehensive and accurate assessment of the chemicals consumed.

If harmful toxins or bacteria are detected, the entire volume may be ejected via vomiting or hastened through the digestive tract as diarrhea.

Whereas pleasurable flavors act as a cue to initiate eating, signals from the stomach and intestine indicate when it is time to *stop*.

Despite the popular belief that it takes twenty minutes before fullness signals 'register,' alterations in fullness occur on an almost real-time basis. The combined influence of flavor at the mouth and chemicals in the gut "act concurrently shortly after a meal begins."[41] Consequently, nourishing, genuine foods taste progressively less appealing the more you eat of them. (If you wish to test how rapidly satiation can kick in, take a block of 100% butter from grass-fed cows and begin to eat. You will quickly discover that 'stop eating' signals can register in a very short space of time.)

When the gut detects that the optimal volume of nutrition has arrived (or when the presence of harmful substances indicates that continued consumption is unwise), hunger is terminated, satiation occurs, and the eating episode ends.

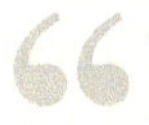

...the gut continuously sends information to the brain regarding the quality and quantity of ingested

> nutrients... [...] By acting not only on brainstem and hypothalamus, this stream of sensory information from the gut to the brain is in a position to generate a feeling of satisfaction and happiness as observed after a satiating meal...
>
> — H. BERTHOUD, *VAGAL AND HORMONAL GUT-BRAIN COMMUNICATION* (2008)

However, if the predicted nutrition does *not* arrive, the feeling of *wanting more* remains. It is, as you are probably quite aware, possible to have a full stomach and *still feel hungry*.[42]

Sham Eating

Note: The following sub-chapter discusses animal experiments that some readers may find unsettling. These are helpful for understanding the concepts within this book, but reader discretion is advised.

To understand the importance of the learned relationships between flavor and nutrition and the critical role of gut signals, it helps to examine a set of animal experiments that explore a concept known as *sham eating*. Sham eating refers to a kind of 'fake' eating experience in which an animal chews and swallows food, but the food does not reach the digestive system. This is accomplished by a surgical modification that allows the food to exit the body via the esophagus or stomach immediately after being swallowed. As you can imagine, these experiments result in much longer eating episodes than usual.

When rats undergo sham feeding after three hours of food deprivation (a standard length of time for a rat to go without eating), they consume about twice as much food as usual before giving up on the fruitless activity. The rats soon attempt to eat again, halving the typical gap between meals.[43]

If another sham eating episode follows, the rats eat even more and wait an even shorter time before attempting to feed again.

The most shocking outcomes occur, however, when *very hungry* animals are sham fed. When rats are subjected to 17 hours of food deprivation, they sham feed for *7.5 hours straight*. After not eating overnight, monkeys will also sham eat *continuously*.[44]

Hungry animals sham feed for extreme durations because starvation is a serious threat to survival. If the presence of flavor at the mouth indicates that nutrition has been found, it makes sense to grab the opportunity and persevere in the hope that the expected survival reward may eventually arrive. Severe hunger thus predisposes a lifeform to sham eat for an extraordinary length of time.

It might not sound particularly surprising that satiation does not occur when nutrition fails to arrive in the gut. After all, how can you feel full when the stomach is empty? But a lack of satiety occurs even when the procedure drains food out of the small intestine,[45] rather than the esophagus or stomach. In other words, even with a full stomach, satiation does not occur if the small intestine does not detect the required nutrients.

Human patients report similar findings. The following description was given of a woman who, in 1858, had an opening in her small intestine, through which most of her food drained out:

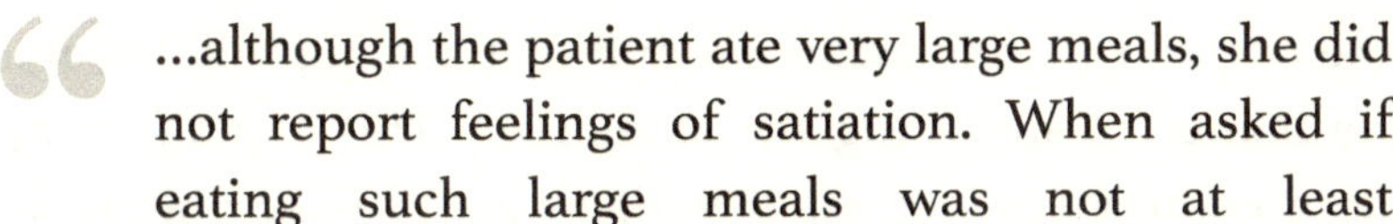

> ...although the patient ate very large meals, she did not report feelings of satiation. When asked if eating such large meals was not at least

> momentarily satiating, this patient answered that her stomach was full but she still felt hungry.
>
> — DANIELLE GREENBERG, *SATIATION: FROM GUT TO BRAIN* (1998)

Other sham eating experiments illustrate how accurately the digestive tract monitors nutritional reward. If only a *portion* of the food is removed from the stomach, the animal keeps eating until the withdrawn volume is replaced.[46] In such cases, nutrition arrives in the gut at a slower rate than is predicted by the input at the mouth, yet the animal keeps eating until sufficient nourishment is obtained.

Similar outcomes occur when nutrients are directly introduced to the first part of the small intestine during sham feeding. Nutrient infusion will bring sham feeding to a rapid halt in rats, rabbits, pigs, dogs, and humans, with the speed of satiation relating to the concentration of nutrients introduced.[47] In fact, termination of sham feeding with nutrient infusion occurs even after 17 hours of food deprivation.[48] In other words, *as soon as the required volume of nutrition arrives in the body, the eating behavior stops.*

Further sham eating experiments investigate what happens when the food is replaced with different substances, such as saline solution (salty water), so there is a *mismatch* between the flavor at the mouth and the chemicals arriving in the stomach. In these experiments, the stomach grows fuller while the animal eats, but satiation *still doesn't occur* (unless these solutions have an aversive quality – i.e., unless the digestive tract detects the presence of something harmful). This means that *volume alone* is not the crucial satiating factor[49] – and that 'feeling full' is not a simple matter of stretching the stomach.[50] This explains why drinking endless cups of water with meals to reduce appetite makes not an ounce of difference. (This is no surprise. If the digestive system were so primitive that it could not distinguish between water and nourishment, we would not last very long.)

Other sham eating experiments explore what happens if the nutrients arrive in the stomach or intestine *at the wrong time* – for example, if the chewing and digestion are disconnected by more than a few minutes. In this scenario, the nutrition *no longer appears plausibly connected to the flavor consumed at the mouth*, and satiation *still does not occur,* even if the nutrition arrives.[51] This has important implications for vitamin pills (which typically deliver nutrition without any preceding flavor profile) and is discussed in more detail in chapter 4: *Supplements and Fortification.*

Similar studies involve the insertion of valves or 'inflatable cuffs' between the stomach and small intestine. These control how long food remains in the stomach and allow signals from the small intestine to be isolated and analyzed separately from those of the stomach. It appears that both the stomach and intestine are responsible for sending separate, synergistic signals to the brain.[52] This is likely one reason why gastric bypass patients report a reduction in hunger in the weeks and months following surgery, as these procedures severely disrupt the complex and critical signaling from this region.[53] (It is worth noting that this reduction in hunger is often temporary and gastric bypass is not recommended for many reasons, as will be discussed in chapter 10: *Bariatric Surgery.*) Furthermore, when the brain cannot receive signals from the stomach or small intestine at all (such as following a vagotomy procedure removing the vagus nerve, which connects the digestive tract to the brain), nutrient infusions do *not* halt sham eating.[54]

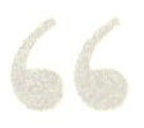

It is as if the gut, with its myriad chemoreceptors, conducts an ongoing analysis and keeps a record of

> what is being consumed and secretes a specific cocktail of hormones into the blood in response. These hormones then customize the digestive process (the secretion of the proper digestive hormones and juices, and in the right concentrations and points in the process, and so on) to the meal being eaten, as well as inform the brain as to the total nutrient load consumed. At some point, the cumulative impact of these various factors stops the eating process.
>
> — STEPHEN C. WOODS, *THE EATING PARADOX: HOW WE TOLERATE FOOD* (1991)

Sham eating experiments closely parallel those in which the *food itself* is manipulated – such as when a single food is altered to contain fewer calories than before while the flavor profile stays the same. In such circumstances, animals quickly learn to increase their intake to account for the reduction in expected energy.[55] [56]

To maintain accurate flavor-nutrition rules, the body tracks two kinds of sensory information: the flavor coming in at the mouth and the chemicals that subsequently arrive in the gut. Together, these two inputs create a predictive loop that guides future eating behavior.

Sham eating experiments offer insight into what has gone wrong with the modern food supply. Manufacturing processes have *disrupted the relationships between flavor and nutrition* so that the flavor at the mouth does not accurately reflect the nutrition coming in.

4

DECEPTIVE FLAVOR

BECAUSE ONLY *SOME* chemicals create the sensation of flavor, it is possible to dramatically change what a food tastes like without substantially altering the nutrition. Sometimes, only the aroma of a food needs to change for flavor perception to alter. Textural or thickening additives can also modify flavor perception, as can changes to visual stimuli. Some drinks, for example, have clouding agents added to mimic the natural juices after which they are named.[1] Many otherwise identical products are multicolored to simulate variety, even though the core ingredients remain the same.

Refined sugar was one of the first chemical compounds to be isolated and used in food production. Extracted from cane or beets, refined sugar strengthens the flavor of any naturally sweet item. However, this flavor manipulation is child's play compared to the complex flavoring strategies now used in modern food manufacturing.

In *The Dorito Effect* (2016), Mark Schatzker describes how the invention of gas chromatography dramatically advanced our capability to mimic flavor. Along with tools such as mass spectrometers, gas chromatography allows manufacturers to identify the precise chemical compounds that contribute to a particular aroma, identifying the exact ingredient list down to the molecular level. By the mid-1970s, this technology was becoming automated and spreading throughout the world.[2] Consequently, flavor technologists can now imitate flavors in exceptionally convincing ways. As Morley Safer from *CBS News* explains, flavor chemists can travel to exotic fruit orchards, acquire flavor samples, and bring these back to the laboratory for simulation.[3]

Many of the flavor molecules used in this process are extracted from food sources. This is convenient, as it allows these additives to be described innocuously with 'clean label' wordings, such as *so-and-so extract* on the ingredient list. Non-food sources are also commonly used as these can be cost-effective, stable, and easier to produce in larger quantities. However, in terms of flavor, it makes little difference whether the additives are 'natural' or 'synthetic' in origin, because, at the molecular level, these are the same. The issue is not the origin of the molecule but the *misleading flavor signal* this sends to the brain.

Concealing Flavor

A common tactic used in modern food production is the concealment of unpleasant flavors that naturally exist in some ingredients. Such strategies include masking bitter or metallic aftertastes, hiding saltiness, down-playing sourness, or concealing a wide variety of 'off-notes.' This concealment process is known in the industry as "neutralizing the base."[4]

Neutralizing flavors is useful if ingredients have unpleasant tastes that are disliked by consumers. For example, pea protein – a popular ingredient used by manufacturers hoping to boost the protein content of plant-based foods – has an off-putting flavor that is often described as "grassy, beany, earthy, bitter and chalky."[5] Similarly, fruit juices may contain 'bitter notes' due to the pith, seeds, and peels being crushed during large-scale pressing.[6] Ingredients derived from aged fruits and vegetables consumed out of season may also have bitter flavors or off-notes. Unsurprisingly, these unpleasant flavors "deter consumers from craving"[7] these products. Some ingredients require "multiple masking solutions"[8] before they are accepted by customers.

Flavor-masking of this type benefits food manufacturers a great deal. It is much more cost-effective to mute an unpleasant flavor than to revamp a manufacturing plant or pay for higher-quality ingredients.[9]

Catering to these needs, many flavor-solution companies offer handy products, such as *astringent taste blockers* (which eliminate the mouth-puckering sensation derived from sour ingredients), individual *flavor maskers* (which conceal specific flavors, such as *stevia masker*), and a huge range of *bitter blockers.*[10] Bitter blockers work by overpowering an existing flavor or directly inhibiting the function of taste receptors so consumers cannot detect the presence of a bitter ingredient in the mouth.[11]

Another method of concealing bitterness involves hiding 'troublesome' ingredients within encapsulating technologies. Microencapsulation is the process of enclosing tiny particles or droplets of a substance within a coating or shell. These textural elements act like minuscule pills within the food and are often so small they can be consumed without being fully crushed by the teeth while chewing. This tactic is especially useful for concealing bitter substances such as caffeine within ice cream or for adding fish oil to orange juice. Microencapsulation technologies are widely used by modern food manufacturers[12] and allow "ingredients with unwelcome tastes to pass through the mouth without eliciting negative feelings."[13]

Strategies of altering, minimizing, hiding, or eliminating flavors are integral to the modern food industry – facilitating the use of cheaper, inferior, and less desirable ingredients. Unfortunately, identifying this kind of manipulation within products can be challenging, with additives often appearing on labels merely as a natural or artificial flavor, flavor 'enhancer,' 'taste modifier,' e-number, or chemical name.

Remember, an unpleasant flavor is not a trivial inconvenience to be muted at leisure. It is a vital survival signal, predicting the presence of something harmful that the body does not want or need.

By masking unpleasant flavors, food manufacturers disarm the natural taste alarm system, fooling consumers into eating substances their bodies would otherwise reject.

When unpleasant flavor signals are muted, taste and smell receptors cannot do their job properly nor warn you about what is coming in.

Transporting Flavor

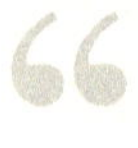

> Spraying unfamiliar foods with a known and liked substance, such as molasses or high-fructose corn syrup, encourages livestock – and humans – to eat unfamiliar foods. For livestock, this trick works well to ease the animals into eating weeds such as thistles.
>
> — FRED PROVENZA, *NOURISHMENT: WHAT ANIMALS CAN TEACH US ABOUT REDISCOVERING OUR NUTRITIONAL WISDOM* (2018)

Another common strategy used by food manufacturers is to uplift a flavor from one place and transport it to another. This usually involves taking cheap, bland ingredients (or a pre-neutralized base, as described previously) and making these things taste like something much better.

Mark Schatzker explains how original versions of the corn chip were considered a flop until flavors were added, at which point the market exploded.[14] Rather than eating a plain concoction of corn and oil, each mouthful now tastes as though it delivers numerous nutritious ingredients.

Similar deceptions occur with flavored drinks, sweets, savory crisps, crackers, and so on. These foods are a kind of chemical hoax.

> Would a seven-year-old girl be interested in drinking a bottle of water mixed with sugar? The answer is no. [...] But add some flavorings to sugar water and the child thinks it tastes like juice and will finish a whole bottle.
>
> — MARK SCHATZKER, *THE DORITO EFFECT: THE SURPRISING NEW TRUTH ABOUT FOOD AND FLAVOR* (2016)

This kind of flavor manipulation fools consumers into believing they are eating a wide range of foods without it ever being obvious that the same few core ingredients are consumed over and over again. Flavor manipulation of this type creates a kind of sham eating experience, whereby the flavor at the mouth does not match the nutrition that arrives in the gut.

Wholesale transport of flavors is obvious trickery, but the real terror lies in much more subtle deception.

Strengthening Flavor

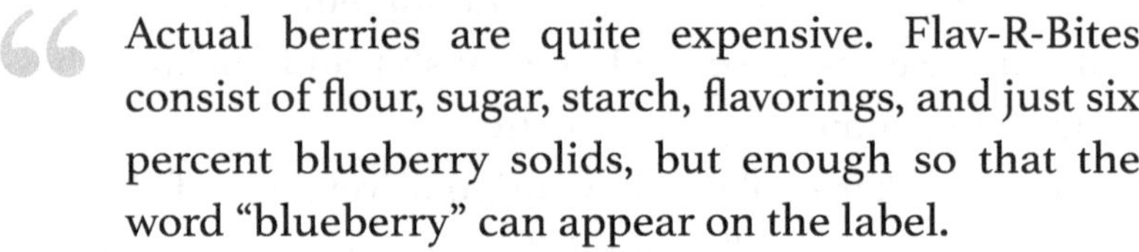

> "Actual berries are quite expensive. Flav-R-Bites consist of flour, sugar, starch, flavorings, and just six percent blueberry solids, but enough so that the word "blueberry" can appear on the label.
>
> — MELANIE WARNER, *PANDORA'S LUNCHBOX: HOW PROCESSED FOOD TOOK OVER THE AMERICAN MEAL* (2014)

The most convincing way that food manufacturers manipulate flavor is by taking an existing flavor and making it stronger. Butter, for instance, can be made even more intense and 'buttery' in flavor through the addition of diacetyl,[15] a compound known for its buttery aroma.

Flavor strengthening is widespread and found in almost all types of manufactured food. Crumbed chicken, orange juice, and pasta sauce, for example, often have 'natural flavors' or 'extracts' on the ingredient list. These flavoring agents contain a mixture of undisclosed chemicals that, in many countries, need not be declared or specified. Even fresh meats can be pre-soaked, injected, or marinated in flavoring solutions.[16]

It is worth noting that flavor concentration of this sort is a far cry from traditional methods. When a rich soup boils on the stove, water is evaporated, causing the flavor to intensify. In this case, the strengthened flavor *correctly signals the increased nourishment of the soup*. As each spoonful now contains less water, the concentration of nutrients is higher; thus, the strengthened flavor accurately 'labels' the meal. When manufacturers add a few drops of flavoring solution to a soup, however, the soup does not change in nutrient density at all.

Just as sugar strengthens the flavor of naturally sweet items, glutamates, responsible for the umami taste, amplify the flavor of savory foods. Synthetic monosodium glutamate (MSG) has received negative press in recent times; hence, these added glutamates often hide under a variety of guises, such as hydrolyzed vegetable proteins (which can contain 10-30% MSG), and extracts from yeast, tomatoes, and mushrooms.[17] Marketers of these products reassure consumers that the glutamates in these extracts are 'naturally occurring' and in far lower concentrations than pure MSG. Nonetheless, these additives artificially concentrate glutamates and are used predominantly for flavor manipulation.

Just as sugar water is unappealing, so too is plain rice with added MSG. Yet, if MSG is added to *fried* rice, the fried rice is perceived as tasting better than it did before.[18] In the latter case, the presence of the few genuine savory ingredients helps to cement the deception. As author Robert Greene explains, the best way to seduce a victim is to merge illusion and reality – to embellish and build fantasy upon the truth.[19]

Flavor-strengthened products have several advantages for the manufacturer. Firstly, the nourishing ingredients (which are typically the expensive ones) can be reduced, offering significant savings.

> ...why clog up your cold storage area with vats of real cream when you can use a 'powdery, homogeneous and free flowing cream to yellow powder with a cream taste and smell' that doesn't need to be chilled, and takes up a fraction of the factory space?
>
> — JOANNA BLYTHMAN, *SWALLOW THIS* (2015)

Secondly, due to the reduced nutrition, consumers must eat more to meet survival needs (a win for the manufacturers). Thirdly, unlike complete sham foods, such as flavored drinks or sweets, flavor-strengthened items deliver both taste *and* satisfaction if enough is eaten. In fact, the boosted flavor is perceived as superior – because it predicts a heightened survival reward. It is thus no surprise that many of the most commonly craved foods contain trace amounts of nourishing ingredients, supplemented with a heavy dose of added flavor (cookies, pizza, ice cream, and so on).[20]

To understand the lengths that manufacturers go to in creating flavor-enhanced products, consider the case of a typical mass-produced pizza. A nationwide pizza chain in New Zealand,[21] for example, adds "natural flavor" to the dough; "maple flavor," "smoke flavor," and "flavor" to the bacon; "flavor" and "autolyzed yeast extract" (which contains glutamate) to the beef topping; "natural flavor" to the cheese; "hydrolyzed yeast protein," "autolyzed yeast extract," "color," and "flavor" to the BBQ and tomato sauces; and so on. These additives take the few scraps of nourishing ingredients – the trace amounts of meat, vegetables, and cheese – and exaggerate the flavor so that the sub-par nutritional reward is marketed under the illusion of tremendous gain.

As these misleading concoctions are eaten, flavor molecules slot into the taste and smell receptors, sending the brain the message that a *huge load of nutrition* is coming in. Because *some* nutrition arrives in the stomach (but far less than is predicted based on the strength of the flavor), these items eventually lead to satiety if enough is eaten.

If something tastes great and eventually leads to satiety (albeit delayed), what is the problem?

The problem is not just that a larger volume must be consumed before fullness is achieved (delivering more calories than is optimal – not to mention the influx of harmful and unwanted chemicals) but that the *learned relationships between flavor and nutrition weaken.*

If flavor-enhanced foods are consumed on a regular basis, the strengthened flavor soon predicts the sub-par nutritional reward. Genuine flavors, by comparison, seem inadequate. To get ahead, food manufacturers must sell *even more* intensely flavored products.

Supplements and Fortification

Intensive farming techniques, modern agricultural practices, long shipping and storage times, unforgiving manufacturing processes, and a preference for cheap and durable ingredients can result in foods that are lower in nutrition than those our ancestors plucked fresh from the ocean, field, or tree. To compensate for this deficiency, modern humans are often advised to take vitamin and mineral supplements.

Some supplements are recommended to be taken on an empty stomach. In this case, the nutrition from the pill is *disconnected from any preceding flavor signal.* From the body's perspective, nutrients spontaneously arrive in the stomach without the ordinary forewarning, providing far less opportunity to release appropriate hormones and enzymes as required to digest and utilize the material. This may be one reason why some supplements cause gastrointestinal discomfort, nausea, or diarrhea when consumed on their own.[22]

Other nutritional supplements are recommended to be swallowed with meals, as this can improve absorption. For example, some nutrients are fat-soluble and are absorbed better when taken with a meal containing fat.

The problem with consuming supplements at meals, however, is that the nutrition from the pill is now *arbitrarily connected to the random assortment of flavors present in the accompanying meal.* As Provenza's sheep experiments might suggest (see chapter 3: *Flavor-Nutrition Relationships*), this adds infinite confusion to the learned relationships between flavor and nutrition.

Something similar happens when products are 'enriched' with vitamins or minerals without this being signaled by a corresponding change in flavor. In some countries, for example, certain brands of bread have folic acid added, while others do not – despite the loaves being indistinguishable in appearance and taste. Sporadic fortification between brands makes it very difficult for the body to predict when and where a nutrient will appear.

The muddling of flavor-nutrition relationships may help to explain why a number of vitamin and mineral studies report *worse health* in the cohort who supplement their diet.

> Betacarotene, when you get it in the form of a carrot, is undoubtedly good for you. When they took betacarotene out of the carrot and gave it as a supplement to patients with cancer, it actually seemed to make them worse.
>
> — MICHAEL MOSLEY, *THE FAST DIET* (2013)

Another reason why supplements may lead to detrimental outcomes is that the isolation of a particular compound can exclude other potentially beneficial elements found in the original food source, which are sometimes necessary for utilizing that particular vitamin.

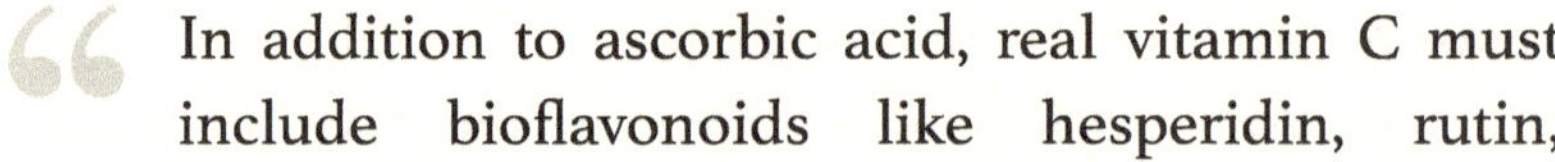

> In addition to ascorbic acid, real vitamin C must include bioflavonoids like hesperidin, rutin,

> quercetin, tannins, along with other naturally occurring compounds. Mineral cofactors must be available in proper amounts. If any of these parts are missing, there is no vitamin activity.
>
> — SCOTT TREADWAY, QUOTED BY RANDALL FITZGERALD, *THE HUNDRED-YEAR LIE* (2007)

Others express legitimate concerns about the safety of additives included in these formulations. However, the primary issue with supplementation is that both the nutrients and any additives within the pill now arrive in the body without a reliable preceding flavor signal.

Nutrients can be harmful in elevated doses, with the optimal amount varying due to circumstance. Even if a test indicates that an individual is deficient in a particular nutrient, there is no way to know whether the test is reliable, the target amount optimal, or whether the proposed pill contains the solution. This leaves consumers reliant on the wisdom of marketers from the supplement industry,[23] who have a tremendous incentive to convince people that they cannot perform optimally without these products.

This does *not* mean that vitamin pills cannot deliver a tangible improvement in health in some circumstances. There are certainly occasions where emergency usage of vitamins or minerals is warranted. However, to acquire optimal nutrition on an ongoing basis, the body must have *a reliable method* for locating, acquiring, and monitoring the intake of each nutrient. Although supplementation can solve an emergency problem, it does not protect the body from enduring that same deficiency again. In fact, as the hypothesis presented within this book might suggest, supplementation is almost certain to confuse flavor-nutrition relationships further, hindering the body's ability to source the nutrition it needs going forward.

Your body already has an incredible system for hunting out and locating chemicals in this vast, complicated world: it learns the patterns between flavor and nutrition. Attempting to artificially remedy a deficiency by delivering a nutritional win that is disconnected from a preceding flavor cue can alleviate a short-term crisis, but it does nothing to restore a reliable method of acquiring that nutrient in the future.

Flavor: The Most Important Dietary Stimulus

Flavor compounds may deliver very little in the way of calories and can be added in tiny quantities – sometimes the very last item on the ingredient list. As such, they often fly under the radar. But flavor is the *driving force behind our food choices.*

If foods had no flavor and everything tasted the same, nothing would seem any more appealing than anything else. Eating would be boring – a chore. You wouldn't be able to distinguish the edible from the non-edible, let alone be able to hunt out and isolate the nutrients you need.

When it comes to the human food supply, flavor is king. If something looks odd but has a delicious flavor, the pleasing flavor almost always overrules the appearance. Greengage plums, for instance, are ripe when they are green. Those new to this variety of plum may eye them with distrust, convinced the fruit is unripe. However, once bitten, the flavor overrides any uncertainty.

Flavor is the crucial, defining characteristic of human food. Size, shape, location, and cultural wisdom may *suggest* that an item is suitable to eat – but only once it is within the mouth and subjected to a detailed chemical analysis via the taste and smell receptors, do we know for sure.

In a very real sense, it is as if the body is protected by a series of gatekeepers or guards. Cultural wisdom prevents most things from getting near the mouth at all. Rather than risking your life sampling any old plant, fungi, insect, or animal, you improve your survival odds by selecting only from those items that other trusted individuals verify are good to eat. (Interestingly, this is one reason why livestock shifted from one part of a country to another are more likely to die from a toxic overdose, as they haven't yet built up a repertoire of appropriate cultural wisdom about which local plants are optimal to eat.)[24]

Visual cues provide further information about whether something should be brought toward the mouth. If a food looks foul or has a soiled or dirty appearance, you may discard it outright rather than risk contaminating the body with rotten food, dangerous bacteria, or toxins. To clarify the age or status of a particular food, you might bring it nearer to the nose and sniff cautiously. In this way, the appearance, location, and external aroma act as preceding cues, helping you navigate toward or away from the substance as appropriate.

But if something passes all these tests and makes it into the mouth, the taste and smell receptors act as the final gatekeeper. Sensory receptors carry out a detailed chemical analysis, sending this vital information to the brain. Only once the mouth and nose have directly sampled the flavor does the brain have solid chemical data upon which to make a final prediction and act. In response, you know whether to spit the item out, continue chewing dubiously, or swallow in delight and begin to eat.

As food manufacturers know well, flavor cues are the *single most important stimuli* when it comes to human food. And, as food manufacturers also know well, these flavor cues can be concealed, manipulated, and exaggerated. Just as a Greylag goose will roll a football-sized object into its nest, humans will gobble down almost anything *as long as it tastes good.*

When we crave food, the mind doesn't fill with information about vitamin C, magnesium, or any other nutrient. Instead, we fantasize about the *flavors predicted to deliver the nutrition we need.* It is the experience of *engaging with a particular flavor* that is craved.[25]

People come up with a million psychological theories to explain their bizarre eating habits, but if something doesn't taste good, we don't overeat it. It doesn't matter how bad someone's childhood was, how dysregulated their emotions are, how depressed or anxious they feel, how much they hate their body, how long their dieting history has been, or how hopeless their willpower seems to be... If something doesn't taste nice, we don't overeat it.

Masters of Deception

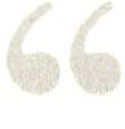

> For obvious reasons, every producer tries to step up the need of the consumer for the goods manufactured by him.
>
> — KONRAD LORENZ, *CIVILIZED MAN'S EIGHT DEADLY SINS* (1974)

Humans rest atop the food chain not as the result of brute force, sharp teeth, or slashing claws. We dominate and outwit other species by leveraging our intellect, communication skills, and our ability to deceive.

Ants line up to drink the poison we feed them. Fish and mice voluntarily take our bait. Cows are confined by flimsy fences that could be broken easily if the cows only realized.

Sometimes, humans develop mutually beneficial

relationships with other species; at other times, we trick and fool animals into doing our bidding.

The Machiavellian Intelligence hypothesis posits that human intellect was honed in response to the *threat of deception from within our own species.* If an unscrupulous individual can defraud and mislead another without being caught, he or she stands to profit. Those who can detect and evade such deception benefit enormously, as they cannot be taken advantage of.[26] Some scientists believe that our cognitive ability is the result of an escalating arms race between the deceiver and the deceived, playing out within the human species over time.

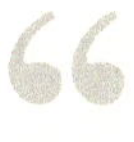

> ...many signs suggest that the keys to our intelligence lie in the harsh, unflattering light of social challenges, the arena of zero-sum games in which one person's gain is another's loss.
>
> — KEVIN SIMLER AND ROBIN HANSON, *THE ELEPHANT IN THE BRAIN* (2018)

Flavor-manipulated foods offer a tremendous survival advantage to those who sell them. If manipulating flavor causes products to fly off the shelves, companies that don't employ such tactics risk being outcompeted.[27] A shopkeeper may *wish* to sell only authentic, traditional foods, but if their products are more expensive and less flavorsome by comparison, they may be driven out of business.

The retailer, like the manufacturer, the flavor technologist, and every other individual in the production chain, each plays their own survival game. Sometimes, the combined effect of many individuals acting in their own interests results in beneficial outcomes; at other times, it results in horrors on a magnified scale.

> Economists and mathematicians have developed elegant game-theory explanations for how people can be incentivized to actions that ultimately cause a catastrophic outcome for everyone.
>
> — MAX TEGMARK, *LIFE 3.0* (2017)

It can be hard to believe that humans would deliberately taint the food supply. But it is worth remembering that almost every addictive substance is manufactured and promoted by *other humans* – those with an economic motive in the behavior continuing.

David Courtwright, professor emeritus at the University of North Florida and author of *The Age of Addiction* (2019), describes how the process of finding and monetizing addictive substances has become "increasingly calculated" due to advances in technology. He notes that nicotine addiction exploded when factories could finally mass-produce cigarettes. (Interestingly, cigarettes, like alcohol and caffeinated beverages, are now heavily flavored.)[28] Furthermore, when addictive substances are first discovered and their lucrative potential emerges, the threats of engagement are downplayed and denied for as long as possible. It takes time for harm to be proven beyond reasonable doubt and for products to be socially frowned upon. As recently as 1910, for example, shopkeepers were still selling candies laced with morphine.[29]

Nourishing food is expensive. It takes considerable resources to grow, store, and prepare. Those who can substitute cheaper ingredients without detection have an edge over their competitors. Jonathan Rees, history professor at Colorado State University and author of *Food Adulteration and Food Fraud* (2020), explains that humanity's first documented laws involved the prohibition of food adulteration. Gail Jarrow, author of *The*

Poison Eaters (2019), provides examples of the widespread food fraud that took place in the late 19th and early 20th centuries. She describes how sugar was used to disguise the taste of rotten corn, formaldehyde used to prevent aged milk from turning sour, lead used to make cheap wine clear, and coloring agents used to mask the appearance of rotting meat. Jarrow explains how inexpensive and sometimes inedible ingredients were used to bulk-out products, such as 'pepper' made from ground corn, charcoal, and cracker crumbs, with a sprinkling of real pepper thrown in to cement the deception – and 'bread' containing ground beans, peas, chalk, and sawdust. In a textbook from this period, Dr William Krohn details how bread could be lightened with ammonia and milk thinned with unsanitary water before being colored white to conceal the dilution.[30]

The influx of food adulteration at this time occurred because people were leaving rural lifestyles in droves, and many no longer grew the majority of their own food. As such, products were often prepared in factories away from public view and it became "particularly easy to fool customers."[31]

You may suspect that food adulteration of this type is now prohibited due to food safety regulations, but it is perhaps more accurate to say that modern manufacturers simply undertake more devious forms of manipulation. Larry Olmsted, author of *Real Food/Fake Food* (2017), describes modern food manufacturing as a "massive industry of bait and switch." He notes that 58% of the fish recently tested at New York City retail outlets were not the species of fish claimed by the seller. Expensive species were often substituted with fish from dubious sources,[32] and farmed salmon (full of antibiotics) was dyed pink to imitate premium, wild-caught salmon. According to Olmsted, most olive oil in America is diluted or substituted with inferior oils, including those that are rancid or heavily refined with chemicals. He describes colored and flavored soybean oil, marketed as organic, extra virgin olive oil from Italy.

Product substitution of this type is blatantly illegal, yet apparently occurs on a wide scale throughout the modern world – with certain countries faring worse than others.

> In the United States, as much as 10 per cent of the food on supermarket shelves might be adulterated. In Bangladesh, the problem of food adulteration is so bad that it has been likened to genocide.
>
> — JONATHAN REES, *FOOD ADULTERATION AND FOOD FRAUD* (2020)

If this kind of rampant illegal deception occurs, do you really think that manufacturers who can lawfully substitute cheaper ingredients and then add back flavorings so that your tongue doesn't know the difference will not do so? In fact, companies are almost compelled to use such tactics because those who offer cheaper, tastier products make more money than those who do not.

Modern technology has facilitated the creation of edible illusions. When we overeat these items, experts issue a diet prescription that exacerbates hunger for the same misleading substances. When we still overeat these things, they say we are disordered and broken.

We point in fear at different parts of the food, wondering if this or that ingredient is to blame, in a hopeless game of Whack-A-Mole. We blame fat, so the food manufacturers take out fat and put the flavor of fat back in. We blame sugar, so they remove naturally sweet ingredients and add artificial sweeteners back in. We demand low-calorie items, so they bulk up foods with filler ingredients and fiber while adding flavor to disguise the substitution. We seek cheap goods, so they use preservatives to extend shelf life while nutritional quality degrades, demanding yet more flavor manipulation.

This entire charade occurred gradually, involving thousands of different chemicals, each mapped onto naturally occurring stimuli, so that the sensory system finds it almost impossible to discern. Flavors are mixed and matched in unpredictable ways, exaggerating and transporting flavor signals from one location to another, leaving learned flavor-nutrition relationships in disarray.

To get an idea of how widespread this problem is, consider a single example: strawberry flavor. Historically, strawberry flavor was associated only with the plant compounds that naturally occur in fresh strawberries. Today, strawberry flavor is associated with sweetened strawberry jam, strawberry desserts, strawberry ice cream, strawberry yogurt – and an almost infinite array of foods that contain no genuine strawberries at all. The relationship between strawberry flavor and nutritional outcome has become wildly unpredictable. The odds of the body finding the nutrition it expects after consuming strawberry flavor are about the same as winning at a slot machine. A similar madness exists with almost every other known flavor.

Modern manufacturing processes scramble the relationships between flavor and nutrition. It is like taking the face of your lover and applying it to your enemy. It is like making a word mean one thing today, and the same word mean ten different things tomorrow.

Your body contains a sophisticated biological flavor-detection system. This inbuilt capability is how your ancestors (and all animals) survived across millennia without any formal nutritional guidance. But this sophisticated system can only do its job when there are *reliable relationships between flavor and nutrition.*

Rather than reliable flavor-nutrition relationships, we now have a situation where a single flavor leads to *multiple nutritional outcomes.* When outcomes vary in this way, we have something far worse than *weakened* flavor-nutrition relationships. We have something that we might call *the intermittent reinforcement of flavor.*

5

INTERMITTENT REINFORCEMENT

We have thus far discussed how lifeforms navigate the world according to learned or inherited relationships between action and outcome. We have discussed how this introduces the risk of deception, whereby lifeforms can manipulate environmental cues that influence another's behavior. In the case of food, we have examined how manufacturers conceal unpleasant flavors and strengthen positive flavors, manipulating sensory signals that influence human eating behavior. It is now vital to understand the effect of *intermittent reinforcement.*

The concept of intermittent reinforcement was popularized by a series of experiments conducted by American psychologist B.F. Skinner in the 1940s. In these experiments, pigeons were placed in small wooden chambers with a glass front for several hours each day. The pigeons were fed less food than usual, so they maintained 75–90% of their original body weight (the precise weight reduction varied depending on the experiment, as Skinner wanted to examine how different levels of deprivation affected the pigeons' behavior). Daily food rations were adjusted as necessary to keep the pigeons' weight stable. In other words, the pigeons in these experiments remained underweight and hungry.

Each testing chamber featured a lever mounted on the wall, connected to a food dispenser, allowing the birds to access additional food. The pigeons quickly learned that pecking this lever would dispense a pellet of food into the chamber.

To begin with, the birds received one pellet for every peck, a scenario known as *continuous reinforcement*, whereby a single action (pecking the lever) reliably leads to the same reward (a pellet of food).

After a certain period, Skinner removed the pellets from the dispenser so the pigeons no longer received a pellet when they pecked the lever. When this happened, Skinner observed that the birds learned to disassociate the behavior from the reward and stopped pecking the lever. This termination of a learned behavior is known as the *extinction* of that behavior.

If a pigeon has only a few reinforced pecks of the lever, extinction occurs rapidly. If a pigeon has had *many* reinforced pecks, extinction takes a little longer. However, in either case, the pigeon soon learns that pecking the lever no longer delivers a food pellet and stops pecking.

The most interesting of Skinner's findings involved what happened when the pellet *sometimes* appeared and sometimes did not – a situation known as *intermittent reinforcement*.

A particular type of intermittent reinforcement is known as a *variable ratio schedule*. In this situation, the pellet arrives in a random pattern, varied by frequency. For example, the pigeon might receive a food pellet every third peck on average – yet, sometimes, the pellet might arrive after the first peck, sometimes after the fifth peck, and so on (as long as it works out to be every third peck on average). In other words, although the pellets arrive in an unpredictable pattern, the average number of pecks can be held constant, allowing Skinner to test the effect of varying the average gap between rewards.

In this scenario, the pigeon has *no way to determine precisely which peck will deliver the reward.* However, it learns that if it keeps pecking, soon enough, another pellet will arrive. Here, we have a single environmental cue (the lever) which, when a particular action is taken (pecking the lever), *sometimes* leads to a survival win (the food pellet) and sometimes a survival loss (the lack of a pellet is a loss because pecking itself uses energy, attention, and time).

Although the appearance of the food pellet is unpredictable in this circumstance, the pigeon's *behavior* is highly predictable.

It pecks like crazy and does not want to stop.

Increased Engagement

When subjected to intermittent reinforcement, Skinner's pigeons pecked at an extreme rate, far faster and more frequently than is ever observed with continuous reinforcement. Although it may seem counterintuitive to *peck more when rewarded less*, this is a surprisingly logical response.

Firstly, if an action delivers a survival reward (i.e., something needed for survival) on an intermittent basis, and there are no other known options for acquiring this reward, you *must engage more frequently* to obtain the same volume of reward. For example, if a food pellet now arrives every third peck on average, the pigeon must peck three times as often to obtain the same number of pellets.

Secondly, pecking itself uses energy. Thus, the pigeon now has a *heightened need* for food and must consume more pellets than previously to cover this additional energy expenditure.

Thirdly, and most importantly, the pigeon is now forced to endure long periods without any reward, and it *cannot predict when these will occur or how long they will last*. Because the pellets arrive randomly, sometimes with very long gaps between them, the pigeon *cannot rely on a food pellet being there when it needs it*. To optimize survival, the pigeon must now build up a *buffer of pellets* – an emergency store of energy reserves – so it can survive any long gaps when pellets do not arrive.

These three factors (the reduction in reward-to-peck ratio, the increased energy expenditure, and the need for a buffer to endure long periods without reward) lead to a *dramatically increased peck rate*.

To understand why responding at an extreme rate is not only predictable but essential in this circumstance, imagine a scenario in which you are the sole income earner for your family. In this fictional scenario, you are paid $600 every Monday – the exact amount needed to support your family. To earn this income, you work 20 hours per week, with the remaining time spent on essential survival pursuits, such as caring for young children, growing vegetables, and doing chores. One day, your boss – a previously reliable employer – announces that the business is in a precarious position and that your pay rate must drop by half. Your boss can no longer guarantee payment every Monday but promises to pay you as soon as money comes to hand. Due to the reduced pay rate, your boss is happy for you to work as many extra hours as you need.

Ordinarily, in such circumstances, you would seek another job, but let's assume that no other employment options are available and no government subsidies compensate for the reduction in income. In this scenario, you suddenly change from continuous reinforcement to intermittent reinforcement, whereby you are paid half as much as before, on average. The question is, how many hours should you now work?

If you double the hours worked, you would earn $600 a week again, which you previously needed to survive. However, simply doubling your work hours is no longer sufficient because working more requires *spending more* (for example, you now have increased childcare costs and added fuel costs) because the extra time spent working can no longer be spent on other activities.

Finally, and most importantly, *you can no longer rely on the money being there when you need it.* Due to the irregular payment schedule, you quickly discover that sometimes three or four weeks might pass without any payments coming in. To survive these weeks, you must *stockpile savings.* Even with enough cash on hand to pay rent and bills a few weeks in advance, you can never feel secure about it because the gaps between payments are unpredictable and sometimes extreme, and you can never be sure when long gaps will occur or how long they will last. The sensible and predictable response in this situation is to *work as many hours as you can.*

In a very real sense and for very logical reasons, intermittent reinforcement *drives engagement up.*

How frequently do pigeons peck when exposed to intermittent reinforcement? Skinner describes pigeons pecking *2-3 times per second for fifteen hours,* with breaks of no longer than fifteen or twenty seconds throughout the entire period.[1]

In fact, they peck so rapidly that someone who didn't understand what was happening might believe the bird had a pecking disorder.

Resistance to Stopping

The second predictable response to intermittent reinforcement is a *resistance to extinction.* In other words, even when the reward is withdrawn completely (so food pellets no longer arrive at all), the pigeon takes a very long time to give up pecking the lever. Skinner described one pigeon that pecked *10,000 times* before it gave up, while another took *six years* to stop pecking the lever (this is half the normal lifespan of a pigeon).

Resistance to stopping the behavior seems a bizarre and ridiculous response. Why continue pecking the lever when no reward is forthcoming – especially as pecking itself quickly becomes a survival threat, consuming energy, attention, and time? Why doesn't the pigeon give up on this 'bad habit'? Why doesn't it realize that even doing *nothing* is better than this?

As we shall soon see, resistance to extinction is also a surprisingly logical response.

Firstly, intermittent reinforcement *trains the bird to expect long gaps between rewards*. Because this is part of the training, it is never immediately clear when a reward has disappeared for good.

Compare this to what happens when pellets disappear following *continuous reinforcement*. When the pellets are withdrawn following continuous reinforcement, the pattern changes from 'reward always here' to 'reward never here' – an obvious and noticeable change. Extinction following continuous reinforcement thus occurs relatively quickly. However, this is *not* the case when a reward disappears following intermittent reinforcement because *it is never clear when the pattern changes*. It can seem that the lack of reward is simply the beginning of an ordinary gap between rewards.

Secondly, despite the lack of rewards, pecking the lever is *the only known behavior* that the pigeon has associated with increasing its food supply. All other trialed actions deliver *zero additional food pellets*. Even though the odds of a pellet arriving become infinitely small as time goes by, *these odds remain better than zero*. Continuing to peck the lever becomes an increasingly poor option, but it remains *the best option the bird has.*

To understand this more clearly, imagine you are trapped in a room, imprisoned by an enemy whom you cannot see or communicate with. Although the food supply is adequate, no water is provided. As your thirst escalates, you investigate every item in the room in a desperate attempt to solve your water crisis. Eventually, through a process of trial and error, you discover that pressing a small button on the wall emits a stream of water below. To your great relief, you take one of the many empty bottles lying around, fill it, and drink until your thirst subsides.

Unfortunately, after a few weeks of imprisonment, the button begins to malfunction and only *sometimes* delivers water. To ensure that you have enough water to survive, you press the button more frequently, filling as many spare bottles as possible so that you always have an emergency supply of water on hand.

But what should you do if your captors one day disable the water button completely? How long should you keep fruitlessly pressing the button?

Initially, of course, you won't notice the difference. It will just seem as if the button has temporarily stopped working again. Yet, as the days pass and your store of water dwindles, a sense of panic may set in. Despite this, pressing the button remains the only viable option you have. You cannot give up attempting to acquire water unless you are prepared to die.

In fact, your captors could make your button-pressing 'habit' much worse by turning the water back on one day after a very long gap. Skinner discovered that by gradually increasing the gaps between rewards and stringing together different reinforcement schedules so the pattern becomes exceptionally unreliable and hard to predict, he could train a pigeon to be *extremely resistant to extinction.*

In short, intermittent reinforcement leads to both increased engagement and a resistance to stopping the behavior. We can summarize both of these things as *the urge to keep pecking.*

Obsession

Robert Sapolsky, Professor of Biology and Neurology at Stanford University, describes how the release of dopamine – a neurotransmitter associated with motivation and learning – increases when an individual is exposed to intermittent reinforcement.[2] According to Sapolsky, the greatest dopamine release occurs when a reward appears 50% of the time (such as the result of a coin toss). Sapolsky argues that this is because, in such circumstances, *uncertainty about what will happen is the greatest.*

Compare this to a situation where a reward appears only 1% of the time versus a situation where the reward appears 99% of the time. Although these two scenarios are vastly different (one almost always delivers the reward, while the other hardly ever does), we have an *equal level of certainty* about the outcome in both cases and can make a reliable prediction about whether engaging with these odds is worthwhile.

In a 50/50 scenario, however, the outcome can go exactly either way. It is impossible to predict what will happen and very difficult to know what to do because the probability of winning or losing is identical.[3] In this situation, any additional information we can glean that helps refine the probability one way or the other is *highly valuable*[4] because it allows us to make a far more accurate decision about how to act.

Dopamine plays a fundamental role in *monitoring prediction errors* (the violation of expectation that occurs when a reward arrives in a larger or smaller quantity than expected). To help identify the cause of this error, dopamine facilitates an *increase in attention* – which we might describe as a heightened obsession toward the relevant stimuli.

This increase in obsession is vital because situations that are not well understood and only *sometimes* deliver a reward, cannibalize time and resources, and risk exposing a lifeform to unexpected threats. To establish exactly how to act in this circumstance, we must *pay close attention* to what is going on in the hope of identifying precisely where the reward or threat is found.

If the need for a particular survival reward is high, and the probability of receiving that reward is uncertain, attention is maximized. Attention rises and falls in response to both the *urgency of a perceived need* and our ability to *reliably meet this need* as required.

For this reason, the third and final predictable response to intermittent reinforcement is an *increase in obsession*. Obsession is the tuning of sensory organs toward a narrow set of stimuli – those environmental cues predicted to reveal information that solves the problem. If this increase in obsession does not yield adequate results, the pool of focus is widened, and the individual begins to scan the environment, searching for relevant patterns, attempting to discover where a reliable relationship between action and outcome is found.

When a pigeon is constrained within an experimental box interacting with a rigged lever, no amount of extra focus helps. But in real-world situations, this is almost always not the case.

In *The Science of Consequences* (2012), Susan Schneider gives the example of butterflies released into a field where only some of the flowers contain nectar. In this scenario, butterflies quickly learn to distinguish between the rewarding and unrewarding flower colors.[5] Similarly, Skinner ran experiments in which pigeons were rewarded for pecking a certain spot on the wall but not others – requiring the pigeon to discriminate between spots of different shapes, colors, sizes, and locations. Initially, the pigeons pecked many different spots, hoping these would deliver a food pellet.[6] With repeated engagement and focused attention, however, the pigeons learned to distinguish between the rewarding and unrewarding spots.[7] For example, the pigeons might learn that the shape of the spot is relevant but not the color, or vice versa. With each engagement, the pigeon has more information and can refine the learned relationship between action and outcome until, at last, it has a reliable rule to operate by.

To understand the value of heightened attention, consider a hunter whose tribe depends upon the acquisition of meat. The hunter who learns from experienced elders, studies animal behavior, and practices various trapping techniques is far more likely to improve hunting prowess. Perhaps particular terrain, weather conditions, weapons, or hunting companions lead to improved results.

There is always uncertainty with hunting, but *any reduction in uncertainty* pays off enormous dividends. By getting better at finding the reward, the hunter is no longer obligated to hunt non-stop out of frantic necessity, and can instead fit hunting in at optimal times, reducing risk exposure and attending to other pressing survival needs.

Heightened attention helps an individual *discriminate between the important properties or characteristics* of a situation, allowing the identification of a more accurate set of behavioral rules.[8]

Minimizing uncertainty – bringing intermittent reinforcement closer toward a reliable continuous relationship – provides *enormous survival benefits*. Obsession is the lifesaving attention necessary to solve a problem. It facilitates the discovery of a better behavioral rule and helps a lifeform escape the costs of engaging with intermittent reinforcement.

The moment it becomes evident that two situations that previously seemed identical are, in fact, subtly different from each other and that one variation *always* delivers the reward, whereas the other *never does*, it is finally clear how to act. The moment the correct operational rule is found, attention can be turned toward other matters, and you can get on with living the rest of your life.

Species that acquire defenses against deception do so by inheriting *heightened sensitivity to relevant stimuli*. For instance, birds who are able to discern an imposter egg from their own are more likely to raise their own offspring. As the genes of these discerning birds proliferate, surviving descendants are also more likely to carry the same traits. Over time, a victim species thus develops increased sensitivity to relevant environmental cues, inheriting the ability to identify and reject the imposter egg.[9]

Those who escape intermittent reinforcement during their own lifetimes also do so by learning to distinguish between relevant stimuli, detecting important differences between the genuine and imposter item.

Obsession is vital. It illuminates the pathway out.

The Normal Response

Increased engagement, resistance to extinction, and heightened obsession are highly predictable responses to intermittent reinforcement across a wide range of species.[10] This pattern of behavior occurs in goldfish, mice, rats, cats, dogs, monkeys, and humans.[11]

This means that this response is not a sign of malfunction or disorder. Rather, it is the *normal and optimal response* of any lifeform attempting to decipher a set of unreliable data that threatens survival.

Such behavior may seem absurd from the outside, but when understood in this context, it makes perfect sense.

Intermittent reinforcement is the mechanism behind gambling addiction, constant email checking, and refreshing of the Facebook feed. What is less well known is that this phenomenon lies at the heart of every single addiction.

6

ADDICTION

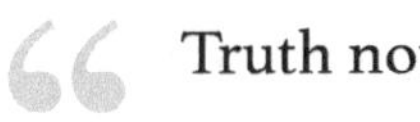

Truth nourishes; illusions kill.

— ALLAN COHEN, *A COURSE IN MIRACLES MADE EASY* (2015)

WHAT WE CALL addiction is the logical pattern of behavior that emerges over time when a lifeform engages with intermittent reinforcement. It is obvious that the pull of a slot machine creates variable outcomes. Just as with Skinner's pigeon experiments, we have an environmental cue (the lever) that an individual responds to by implementing a particular action (pulling the lever). This action then leads to variable and unpredictable outcomes – sometimes a financial win; sometimes a financial loss (as well as the loss of time, energy, and attention).

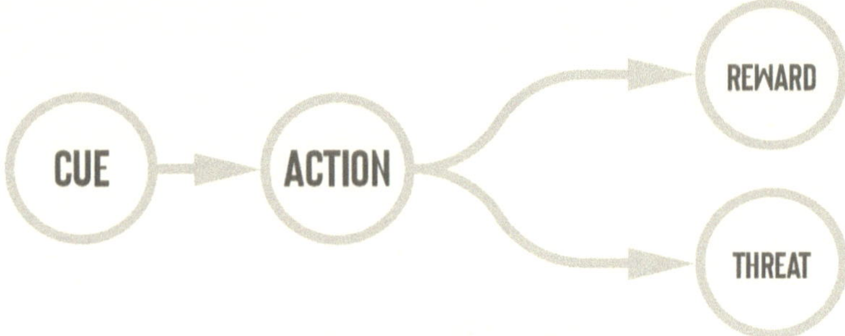

A situation in which a single behavior leads to an unpredictable outcome is easily recognized as intermittent reinforcement. However, it is critical to see that intermittent reinforcement also arises when *two or more subtly different environmental cues* (each leading to different outcomes) *are perceived by the sensors as the same thing*. This might occur, for example, if a butterfly cannot distinguish between two types of flower, yet only one delivers nectar. In this case, the two similar flowers *act as a single cue* and are treated in the same way, initiating a single action that now leads to variable outcomes.

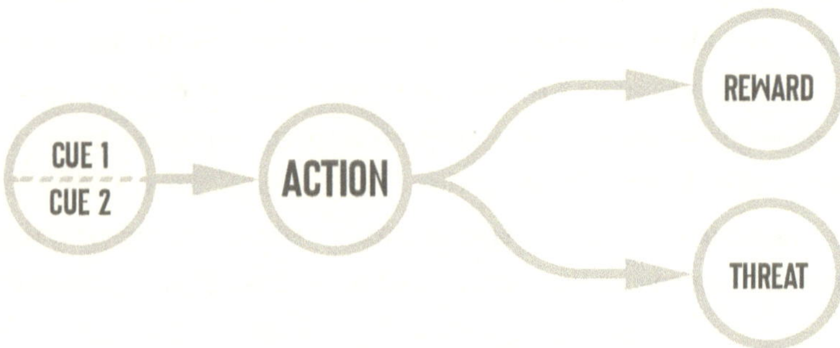

This is what happens with all drugs. Nicotine, alcohol, and all other drugs mimic chemicals that are naturally found within the human body. In order to impact a particular bodily response, a drug must imitate an aspect of natural chemical behavior. If this mimicry did not occur, the drug would have no pharmacological effect.

When the molecular shape of a drug is similar enough to a naturally occurring chemical within the body, it slots into the same receptors. In a very literal sense, it is as if the body mistakes the drug for the genuine item and *treats them the same.*

OxyContin, heroin, and Fentanyl,[1] for example, are chemically similar to natural endorphins. Human bodies create endorphins in precise quantities, at precise times, for specific survival-related functions. For instance, immediately after childbirth, natural endorphins ensure that the shock of having propelled an infant from the uterus is superseded by appropriate feelings of warmth and love for the child. As with all bodily chemicals, these natural endorphins communicate *an essential signal that is intrinsically connected to the specific circumstance and its predicted impact on survival.*

Just as with external behaviors, internal bodily responses follow predictive rules. For instance, the release of hormones, neurotransmitters, and so on directly inhibits or increases the release of other bodily chemicals in a reliable and organized fashion. Without these carefully controlled rules of operation, life could not exist.

When a drug is introduced to the body, two versions of a chemical are suddenly experienced: the genuine item (produced by the body for a specific survival function) and the artificial version (appearing spontaneously whenever injected or ingested). If the artificial version closely mimics the genuine item, it slots into the same receptors.

To understand why this creates intermittent reinforcement, let's consider a common drug, caffeine. Caffeine is a bitter chemical used by plants as a pesticide to discourage other insects and animals from eating the leaves, seeds, or nuts. It just so happens that caffeine mimics a chemical found in the human body called *adenosine* and binds to the very same receptors.[2]

In the human brain, adenosine contributes to a sense of drowsiness, encouraging sleep. Levels of adenosine increase every hour someone is awake, communicating their present state of fatigue. When there is a sufficient volume of adenosine, the body knows it is time to rest and sleep.

However, when caffeine slots into adenosine receptors, it doesn't activate these in the same way. You see, although caffeine and adenosine are very similar, they are not quite the same. Rather than *activating* the receptor, caffeine occupies and *blocks* it, preventing adenosine from binding to the receptor. When some adenosine receptors are blocked by caffeine, only a portion of the body's vital sleep signal gets through.

Caffeine, which imparts several adverse health effects, such as an increase in the stress hormone cortisol, reduced iron absorption, and increased calcium loss, hence creates the illusion of a well-rested body.

From the body's perspective, ingesting caffeine introduces *variability in adenosine signaling*. Sometimes, adenosine levels appear to correctly communicate how tired you are; at other times (when receptors are blocked by caffeine), an incorrect sleep signal is received. In other words, the body's production of adenosine now appears to deliver intermittent results.

Because good sleep is vital for decision-making and health (and is hence critical for survival), the body cannot sit back and accept this situation. With ongoing caffeine use, the body thus begins to produce *more adenosine receptors*[3] [4] [5] in the hope that, on average, the correct tiredness signal once again gets through. The more caffeine one consumes, the more adenosine receptors are generated. Hence, whenever someone attempts to cut back on their caffeine intake, they feel far more tired than before, making it seem as if they cannot cope without their regular caffeine dose.

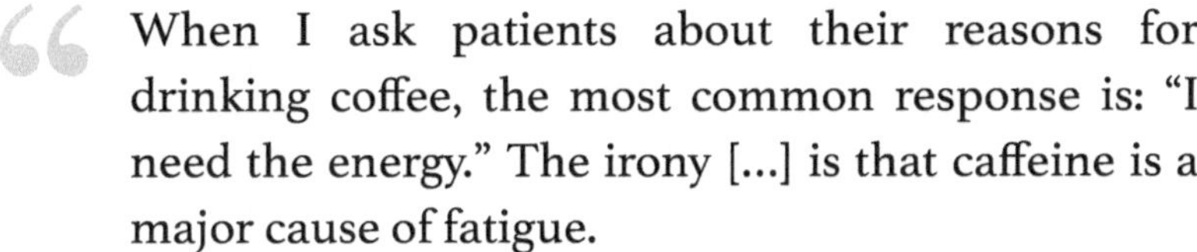

> When I ask patients about their reasons for drinking coffee, the most common response is: "I need the energy." The irony [...] is that caffeine is a major cause of fatigue.
>
> — STEPHEN CHERNISKE, *CAFFEINE BLUES* (1998)

Consider another common drug: nicotine. Found within tobacco, cigarettes, and vaping solutions, nicotine mimics a neurotransmitter called acetylcholine, which has diverse roles in the human body. For instance, in the peripheral nervous system, acetylcholine helps regulate muscle contraction, heart rate, blood vessel dilation, and so on.[6] As with other bodily chemicals, acetylcholine is released in carefully controlled quantities at specific times, ensuring (among other things) that an individual is focused, energetic, and primed to take action at precisely the right moment.[7] If nicotine is inhaled, however, an unpredictable acetylcholine signal is now experienced. Sometimes, activation of acetylcholine receptors indicates that a particular survival action is warranted; at other times, it indicates only that a wad of smoldering tobacco has been raised to the mouth – bringing with it a slew of associated negative health effects. Activation of the acetylcholine receptor is now associated with intermittent outcomes: sometimes a reward, sometimes a threat.

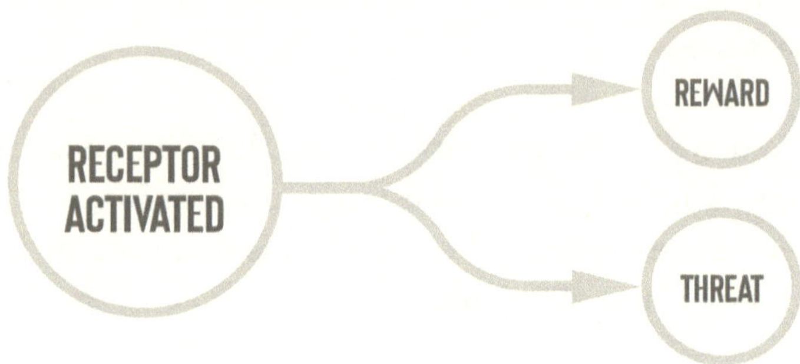

Every addiction has intermittent reinforcement at its core. This is true even in the case of so-called 'behavioral' addictions. For example, social media content arrives via informational feeds that are themselves unpredictable and intermittent. Pornography mimics the shapes and sounds of attractive, sexually available human forms – yet fails to deliver the genuine connection, intimacy, cooperation, pooling of resources, and offspring that may result from genuine, real-life engagements. Similarly, video games imitate battles, quests, and other goal-orientated activities, simulating a sense of accomplishment and progress – without the tangible rewards that accompany such achievement in real life.

Some individuals might suspect that the visual and audio mimicry that occurs with video games or pornography is not at all the same as the molecular mimicry seen with drugs. However, this visual and audio data is transmitted and communicated to the brain by *activating sensory receptors* in the eyes and ears, just as drugs activate internal bodily receptors. A pornographic scene, for example, might activate a similar pattern of photoreceptors in the retina and trigger similar sound vibrations in the cochlea as experienced with a real-life romantic encounter.

Every addictive situation involves a genuinely rewarding

scenario and a *misleading counterfeit*. The 'fun' in early phase addiction is a temporary miscalculation – a *prediction error* that arises as the result of a deceptive circumstance that appears to signal a survival reward *but does not*.

When misleading data interacts with bodily receptors, a false signal is transmitted. Because the human body is an amazing survival machine, it cannot tolerate error signals. With mathematical precision, it begins recalibrating internal systems to account for the error.

Tolerance and Escalation

Abandoning a survival reward when intermittent reinforcement is detected is not a viable long-term solution because, by definition, these rewards are necessary for survival. The only feasible option in this circumstance is thus to *alter the behavioral rule to account for the variability*.

This sub-chapter uses basic calculations to illustrate how intermittent reinforcement prompts *increased engagement, resistance to extinction,* and *obsession,* as described in the previous chapter.

Readers with an aversion to mathematics should not fear. This material includes only very basic addition, multiplication, and division. When beta readers evaluated this part of the book, a significant percentage commented that although they "hated math," the calculations were invaluable.

I have included quotes from some of these readers below as reassurance:

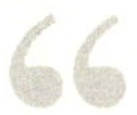

> I found this VERY HELPFUL to support your whole theory despite me being rubbish at maths.

> The equations require a slow down of reading, but they definitely set the scene to drive the above point home. Mind blowing stuff!

> I love this way of presenting the facts. Seeing it all expressed in equations and numbers makes everything extremely clear.

> Wow! What a fantastic illustration of how and why I seek out junk food obsessively! At first I worried when you mentioned equations but it really struck a chord with me! [...] This chapter was an 'a ha' moment for me. Fantastic!

> This chapter is not simple but it is The key! Congratulations on the investigation. It has made me see everything different.

This sub-chapter is perhaps one of the most important parts of the book. The equations are not nearly as complicated as they may first appear. Seeing the ideas laid out in black and white, summarized in numerical form, is incredibly helpful.

With that out of the way, let's begin.

We will start by assuming that engaging with a genuine environmental cue (let's call this $\mathbf{C_g}$ for short) reliably leads to a survival reward, **R**. In other words, let's imagine that engaging with a particular environmental cue (such as eating a specific flavor) reliably leads to a survival reward (such as the arrival of a particular nutrient in the stomach).

We can summarize this as follows:

$$\mathbf{C_g \rightarrow R}$$

For the sake of simplicity, let's now assume that the *value* of **R** is **10 'survival units'** of some hypothetical reward, with only minor variation. In other words, we will assume the brain has a way of assigning a numerical value to survival outcomes in order to prioritize one action above another (this is a reasonable assumption and appears to be exactly what the brain does).[8 9 10] In other words, we can think of this as a certain volume of nutrition arriving.

We can hence say that engaging with the genuine cue, $\mathbf{C_g}$, reliably leads to **10 survival units.**

$$\mathbf{C_g \rightarrow 10\ survival\ units}$$

Now, let's imagine that a counterfeit cue (let's call this $\mathbf{C_c}$) enters the environment, which the lifeform *cannot readily differentiate from the genuine item*. In this case, rather than a benefit, a threat, T, arises:

$$\mathbf{C_c \rightarrow T}$$

In other words, engaging with the counterfeit results in a survival *loss*, as might be expected, due to the wastage of time and resources, as well as the inadvertent ingestion of unnecessary or harmful substances.

Although many addictive behaviors deliver a low and almost negligible threat, let's keep the calculation simple and assume that the counterfeit delivers a loss of **minus 5 survival units.**

$$\mathbf{C_c \rightarrow -5\ survival\ units}$$

Let's now imagine that **120 survival units per day** are needed of this particular reward in order to optimize survival. This means that on an average day, we can assume a lifeform seeks out the genuine cue, C_g, twelve times, resulting in a string of rewards as follows:

R, R, R, R, R, R, R, R, R, R, R, R

The sum of these twelve rewards meets the daily target:

12 x 10 = 120 survival units

If the lifeform cannot differentiate between the genuine cue and the imposter, however, a string of different rewards and threats may inadvertently appear as the counterfeit infiltrates the environment. For example:

R, R, R, T, R, R, T, R, T, R, R, T

In this case, the lifeform set out to engage with the cue twelve times, as usual. But on some of these occasions, the imposter was encountered, and a threat was received instead. In this example, the lifeform engaged with the genuine item eight times and the counterfeit four times.

The sum of these twelve engagements is:

(8 x 10) + (4 x -5) = 60 survival units

In other words, the lifeform expected that engaging with the cue twelve times would deliver **120 survival units**. However, due to the undetected emergence of the counterfeit cue, only **60 survival units** were received. If this pattern continues for a few days (and is thus not a one-off occurrence), the lifeform is forced to *adjust the learned relationship* between the environmental cue and the expected outcome to *better account for the new data.*

Because 60 survival units are now received from twelve daily engagements, the average reward per engagement drops to **5 survival units** (because **60 ÷ 12 = 5**).

The lifeform applies this new prediction to *both versions of the cue* (**C_g** and **C_c**) because the lifeform *cannot yet distinguish between the genuine item and the counterfeit* and hence treats them both as the same thing. The lifeform thus now predicts that engaging with the cue leads to **5 survival units.**

Because two days have passed, at a shortfall of **60 survival units per day** (recall that 120 survival units are needed to optimize survival, yet only 60 were received), the lifeform now has a *heightened need* for this particular reward. On the third day, the following is thus required:

120 + 60 + 60 = 240 survival units

If **240 survival units** are now needed, and each engagement with the cue is predicted to deliver only **5 survival units on average**, the daily target must rise from 12 engagements to **48** (because **240 ÷ 5 = 48**).

This *increased daily target* is experienced as an *increase in desire for the cue*. The greater the desire, the more urgent the action, reflecting a more serious survival need.

If the lifeform attempts to maintain only 12 engagements as previously, cravings are issued to ensure that the new target of 48 is met. Prior levels of engagement no longer result in the same level of satisfaction because the lifeform does not predict that this will provide the necessary volume of survival rewards.

As a result of this new prediction, receptors in the lifeform adjust, just as the pupil in an eye expands or contracts to let in the correct amount of light after experiencing a change in lighting conditions. This adaptive phenomenon is known as *tolerance*. Tolerance is reflected throughout the organism via adjustments in specific sensory receptors, which increase or decrease in number so that subsequent encounters with the cue *accurately reflect the predicted change in survival value.* If detrimental substances are anticipated as part of this exchange (such as the inhalation of tar within tobacco smoke), other bodily systems adjust to cope with the incoming poison.

Addiction experts typically describe tolerance as a natural 'habituation' that results from repeated or prolonged exposure. However, it is worth noting that sensory recalibration of this sort does not occur with daily exposure to other substances like water or oxygen. Tolerance is better understood as the *purposeful adjustment of sensory receptors to account for the new value of a predicted survival reward.*

As the relationship between an action and outcome moves away from a stable continuous relationship toward intermittent reinforcement, *desire for the cue grows*, reflecting the increased daily target. Because the lifeform cannot yet distinguish between the counterfeit and the genuine item, this increase in desire *applies to both versions of the cue*, which are perceived by the sensors as the same thing.

This increase in desire prompts the lifeform to be more efficient in seeking the cue, prioritizing sources that promise to deliver the reward in higher volumes for less effort, as is necessary to meet the rising daily target.

Unfortunately, high concentrations of the cue are *almost always found in the counterfeit.* Cuckoo eggs are slightly bigger and brighter than eggs of the victim species. Pornography presents heightened and distorted sexual stimuli in endless supply at the click of a button. Recreational drugs deliver molecules in higher concentrations than naturally occur. Flavor-manipulated foods are typically more intense in flavor than their genuine counterparts. After all, if the imposter contained lower concentrations of the cue than were readily available elsewhere, the genuine item would always be perceived as superior, rendering the counterfeit 'ineffective.'

Because it is the counterfeit that typically contains higher concentrations of the cue, as the urgency of the survival need climbs, an *increasing preference for the counterfeit* emerges.

The following string of 48 engagements is thus much more likely to contain a *higher ratio of threats*, as per the following example:

R, T, R, T, R, T, T, R, R, T, R, T, T, T, R, T, T, R, R, T, R, T, T, T, R, T, R, T, R, T, T, T, R, T, R, T, T, T, R, T, T, T, R, T, R, T, T, T

The sum of these 48 engagements is as follows:

(18 x 10) + (30 x -5) = 30 survival units

In other words, despite the lifeform having now spent all day frantically engaging with the cue, the net effect is a mere **30 survival units** – far less than was received via the original 12 genuine engagements. The expected outcome of engaging with the cue now plummets to ***less than one survival unit per engagement*** on average.

> Like the character in "Alice in Wonderland," the addict must run as fast as he can just to stay in the same place.
>
> — FLOYD P. GARRETT, *WHY IS RECOVERY SO HARD* (2012)

These basic calculations provide conceptual illustration only. They do not take into account the spread between rewards (which exacerbates things further due to the necessity of acquiring a buffer to sustain survival through long periods when no reward is forthcoming), nor do they account for historical data (which impacts the value of present-day engagement to a lesser degree), nor is any consideration given to the complex interplay between competing rewards. Finally, it goes without saying that addiction does not usually advance in a dramatic three-step fashion.

Despite the simplicity of these calculations, the general principle illustrated here plays out in every form of addiction. The speed of escalation depends upon many variables, such as the severity of any pre-existing survival need, the gravity of losses incurred by the counterfeit, the prevalence of the imposter, and many other environmental factors that influence access, concentration, and availability of both the genuine and counterfeit cues.

With potent drugs, escalation typically occurs quickly. Lower-impact counterfeits, such as nicotine, incur a slower death slide. Consequently, these 'milder' addictions are often trivialized despite the consequences spanning decades and the death toll being far greater.

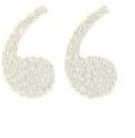

> ...the further they take you down, the greater your perceived need becomes. With alcohol it can be so gradual you barely notice you are falling.
>
> — ANNIE GRACE, *THIS NAKED MIND* (2018)

In short, engagement increases with the prevalence of the counterfeit cue. At each step along the curve, the propensity to take one more step grows because prior levels of engagement are no longer enough. Addictive substances steal the very thing they pretend to deliver. The more you seek the reward, the more the counterfeit takes it away.

Tolerance – sensory recalibration – is not an error by the brain, nor is it damage or malfunction. It is the correct and purposeful response – the only thing a sensible lifeform can do when faced with a misleading circumstance that it does not yet understand.

Note: Those who are interested in the mathematical aspects of this topic might wish to see the elegant formulas proposed to track reward predictions across time, such as a formula published in 1955 by Robert Bush and Frederick Mosteller, which provides a way to mathematically predict whether an action is likely to occur in a given circumstance (for example, the probability that Pavlov's dogs might salivate when a bell is rung). This formula considers not only the current value of an anticipated reward but also the value of past engagements. As such, it more accurately simulates the way a brain might track survival value across time. See more here: www.eatlikeanormalperson.com/foods-that-lie/flavor-formulas/

The Downfall

As a lifeform pursues higher and higher doses of the counterfeit, the threats mount, and the downward trajectory becomes evident. As the lifeform scrambles to meet the growing demand, other survival needs begin to fall like dominoes. As psychologist Abraham Maslow described in 1943, survival needs are organized in a hierarchy.[11] Some actions *must* be prioritized above others. If access to oxygen is compromised, for example, it is ridiculous to worry about mating opportunities, social status, or future achievements. As intermittent reinforcement tightens the noose on a particular survival need, other less urgent needs are placed on hold.

As the severity of the situation unfolds, each competing need is put on standby in order to dedicate more time and resources to meeting the obscene daily targets and solving the problem. The brain strategically withdraws resources from less essential survival pursuits, such as work, relationships, and community ties. This is experienced as a *lack of motivation* across the board.

One by one, less-essential facets of life are offloaded. If the deceptive circumstance remains unresolved, eventually, every spare moment is dedicated to thinking about the cue, engaging with it, and desperately trying to be free of it. In this situation, the individual knows that something is wrong. Sometimes, a cue delivers a survival win, sometimes a loss. This situation captivates attention because solving this dilemma is critical for survival.

If no solution appears forthcoming, *anxiety* is the instruction to cast the net wider, to scan haphazardly over the horizon: the relevant stimuli are undetected, unfound, unknown. Anxiety is the result of an unaddressed survival threat. It arises when an individual does not yet have a plausible course of action but *knows* that something must be done.

The unfolding drama is a kind of trauma – the unpredictable emergence of a survival threat that one's own actions do not appear to mitigate.

The summation of this nightmare is known as *withdrawal.*

Withdrawal is the aftermath of engaging with a counterfeit cue. It is the misery of downregulated sensory systems, combined with the physical damage as the body weakens and atrophies due to the harmful effects of engaging with the counterfeit and compromised progress in other areas of life. It is the shame of being the apparent architect of your own demise and the sheer horror of not knowing how to escape the trap that you are in.

> The feeling must have been closely akin to that experienced by one who suddenly steps into quicksand and realizes that every effort to extricate himself carries him just so much deeper.
>
> — NAPOLEON HILL, *OUTWITTING THE DEVIL* (1938)

Misfortune, calamity, and environmental disasters are devastating enough, but manipulation at the hands of deception has an added layer of horror: the feeling of voluntarily walking to one's death and not understanding why.

Withdrawal is the restless malaise that infests the addict's life like a slow-blossoming poison. It is the pale background misery that is almost ever-present, *except* when encountering high volumes of the counterfeit cue.

For a blessed, fleeting moment, stockpiles of the counterfeit appear to meet the heightened demand. Of course, they do not. Each engagement delivers only another threat, driving the learned relationship between cue and reward lower. Afterward, anxiety roars back to life, louder than before.

In this state, downregulated sensory systems make normal levels of engagement feel inadequate, insufficient, not enough. Large volumes of the counterfeit appear to be the only thing that can alleviate the accumulated survival need.

Addiction is a death spiral.

Like lobsters, chickens, and chimpanzees, humans monitor their position in the social hierarchy. Addiction causes one's status to free fall. In response to this free fall, the brain issues another signal: *depression*.

By this stage, the individual may believe they have two problems – a bizarre behavioral pattern called *addiction* and a mysterious chemical imbalance called *anxiety* or *depression*. It may seem that if mental health issues could just be brought under control – or home and work environments modified so that life was *a little more pleasant* – it might be possible to get a handle on the excessive usage.

But the anxiety and depression that engulf an addict are not a sign of abnormal brain regulation. They are the *correct and accurate evaluation of the circumstance.* They are a desperate call to focus single-mindedly on the stimuli most likely to contain the solution. They are the instruction to throw every speck of brainpower at deciphering the problem.

> “When you're ill, you spike a fever, lose your appetite, and become depressed and listless. Contrary to popular belief, these symptoms don't mean that the disease agent is weakening you but just the opposite—they demonstrate that the brain, in conjunction with the immune system, is mounting a multipronged campaign against the invader.
>
> — KATHLEEN MCAULIFFE, *THIS IS YOUR BRAIN ON PARASITES* (2017)

Rumination is a gift. You have your attention exactly where it needs to be. Lifeforms with a tendency to respond to dire threat with a relaxed, lackadaisical manner do not make it through this survival game. You are the offspring of a long line of winners. And winners don't smile while a con artist takes them out of the race.[12]

Anxiety and depression are the impetus – the unbearable instruction – to escape the trap that you are in.

Hypothesis Testing

Addictions have only one escape hatch: you must *expose the deception* and separate the genuine item from the counterfeit.

Ordinarily, the more one engages with a particular circumstance, the more precise and accurate the relevant set of behavioral rules becomes (recall the example of a hunter who gets better with practice, as discussed in chapter 5: *Obsession*). However, when deception muddles the data, it is much harder to initially understand what is going on.

Although repeated engagement with a deceptive circumstance may not immediately deliver a workable behavioral rule, it does achieve something. It alerts the brain that *something is wrong with its definition of the cue.* It informs the brain that *what is being treated as one thing must be treated as two.*

You see, deception is not only common wherever lifeforms compete for finite resources as they do on planet Earth – it is *expected.* As such, the human brain comes equipped with protective mechanisms preinstalled.

In order to troubleshoot the error, the brain strategically collates evidence from all sensory teams. It begins to meticulously examine the cue-set (the pool of fake and genuine cues), hunting for where the deception hides. The brain systematically redraws boundaries around relevant stimuli, focusing on each discreet aspect of the circumstance, approaching the situation in subtly different ways, rapidly testing behavioral hypotheses one after the other. This is why all addicts seem to hop from strategy to strategy, trialing different ways of behaving in and around the cue.

Some hypotheses are time-based, such as a plan to limit alcohol to the weekends, or to only smoke cigarettes at certain times of the day. These approaches test whether the misleading element is related to *timing.*

Other hypotheses are situation-based, such as a rule to gamble at the casino, but not online; to drink with friends, but not alone. These approaches examine whether the issue is linked to *place*.

Further hypotheses split the cue-set according to defining characteristics or methods of engagement – a rule to avoid spirits, but not wine; to snort heroin, but not inject; to vape, but not smoke cigarettes.

Eventually, hypothesis testing extends to all manner of surrounding circumstances, ascertaining whether modifications in social interactions, careers, spouses, living arrangements, sunshine exposure, or sleeping routines might help to isolate the threat.

Endless permutations are tested and discarded in the desperate hunt for the rule that corrects the problem. This rapid-fire hypothesis testing can feel like a kind of insanity. But it is the essential and life-saving process of defining and redefining the cue-set, as necessary to *identify the counterfeit.*

When deception interferes with access to a survival reward, you must proceed by trial and error until a viable operational rule is found. Establishing cause and effect when deception interferes with the data is hard – particularly when the deception is at a molecular scale and cannot be seen with the naked eye. It is especially challenging when the downsides of engagement accumulate gradually and the warning bells toll slow. It is even more difficult when the deception is novel and new, and protective strategies have not yet spread throughout society.

Eventually, pursuit of the counterfeit may drive the cue-reward relationship below zero – such that every engagement is predicted to deliver a survival loss. Exhausted by the intense trial and error process and burdened by the damage of excessive consumption, the counterfeit is at last thrown down.

But without a clear understanding of where the deception hides, it is never clear where to draw the line. As long as the counterfeit appears integrally connected to a genuine survival reward, abandoning the counterfeit can feel like giving up on the very thing that is needed.

In response, the individual may knuckle down, grit their teeth, enduring cravings and resentment one day at a time, yearning for the reward that appears forsaken.

If the quit attempt is sustained, the negative consequences of prior engagement fade away, yet the misleading allure of the counterfeit may remain.

While the true nature of the deceptive item is concealed, the quit attempt is vulnerable – precarious. And, one day, the counterfeit reappears, full of charm, and the whole miserable cycle starts again.

Vulnerability to Deception

It is well known that chronic stress predisposes an organism to the pattern of behavior that we call addiction[13] [14] [15] [16] [17] – yet, it is not well-understood *why*.

Chronic stress is caused by the presence of any ongoing survival threat, such as violence, abuse, bullying, ostracization, social isolation, solitary confinement, lack of money or resources, sleep deprivation, continual illumination, daylight deprivation, constant vibration, electrical shocks, excessive heat or cold, environmental toxins, parasites, viruses, injuries, sensory deprivation, loud noise, and so on.

Many of those who experience 'disordered' eating patterns find it difficult to identify any potential stressor that may have preceded this behavior. Although some individuals can point to a stressful circumstance, a significant percentage are high-achieving individuals with strong family backgrounds and no obvious abnormal stressors. It can seem a bizarre puzzle until it becomes evident that one of the most potent stressors is *hunger.* In fact, hunger is a very common tactic used in animal studies investigating stress, precisely because food deprivation is a fast and inexpensive way to recreate a state of chronic stress.

Hunger is stressful because insufficient food leads to death. Chronic hunger thus takes precedence over almost all other survival needs, with the chronically hungry individual dominated by the desire to alleviate this state.

> “All capacities are put into the service of hunger-satisfaction, and the organization of these capacities is almost entirely determined by the one purpose of satisfying hunger. [...] For the man who is extremely and dangerously hungry, no other interests exist but food.
>
> — ABRAHAM MASLOW, *A THEORY OF HUMAN MOTIVATION* (1943)

The combination of food deprivation and extreme exercise[18] (two strategies often used in tandem by those with weight loss goals) creates a double whammy of stress: a world where energy usage is up while food supply is down.

Chronic stress creates a vulnerability to addiction not because stressed individuals are damaged or malfunctioning in some way, but because *those who actively seek a solution have greater odds of stumbling across a deceptive item that pretends to solve the problem.*

Evolutionary biologist Kevin Laland notes that approximately half of the innovative behaviors witnessed in primates occur in response to a stressful situation, such as a “food shortage, a dry season, or habitat degradation.”[19] Laland explains that fish, who are ordinarily cautious about swimming into dark holes where predators might lurk, take greater risks while hungry, navigating experimental mazes more quickly in search of food.[20]

> A wolf cannot afford to go hunting in the coldest stormiest night of the polar winter and perhaps pay for a meal with a frozen toe. However, under circumstances, it may be advisable to take such a risk, for example, if the animal is on the verge of starvation and has to stake it all on the last card in order to survive.
>
> — KONRAD LORENZ, *CIVILIZED MAN'S EIGHT DEADLY SINS* (1974)

An individual who is proactively hunting for a solution is far more likely to encounter a deceptive item than someone who does not seek a solution at all. Furthermore, an individual with a heightened pre-existing need for whatever the counterfeit pretends to deliver is more likely to *engage with gusto* – because doing so appears to solve the problem.

Urgent needs dictate urgent action. If you are drowning in the ocean, and a man rows nearby and stretches out his hand, there is no time for careful character evaluation. There is no time to establish whether this is a kind, honest, trustworthy savior. You must grab the outstretched hand and haul yourself into the boat because your life depends upon it. When survival is at stake, detailed assessment is a luxury you cannot afford.

It is no mystery why those with battered childhoods are more susceptible to chemicals that mimic the feelings of love, or why exhausted people are more susceptible to caffeine, or why lonely young men are more susceptible to pornography, or why *hungry individuals are more susceptible to foods that pretend to deliver the nutrition they need.*

Just as a hungry animal will sham feed for extreme durations, hungry dieters are far more likely to consume large volumes of deceptive food. Unfortunately, binge eating deceptive flavor molecules dramatically disrupts learned flavor-nutrition relationships, impacting appetite in a noticeable manner, prompting further consumption of the same deceptive items (see chapter 6: *Tolerance and Escalation*).

But stress does not compel addiction, nor lack of it offer protection. *Anyone* runs the risk of stumbling into the influence of a con artist that they don't know is there, particularly if this behavior is condoned by others. When a counterfeit is widely accepted by society (as is the case with deceptive food), social verification appears to encourage engagement – bolstered by slick marketing campaigns.

The worst tricks of all occur when the mass population succumbs. When the majority are fooled, a deceptive item may swell to maximum capacity, achieving widespread adoption before protective or retaliatory methods are discovered and employed.

When the use of a deceptive item is commonplace, and welcomed as part of ordinary life, even individuals without a heightened need are vulnerable. Whereas those with a heightened need for whatever the counterfeit pretends to deliver are more likely to consume large amounts with a bang, others may find their intake gradually inches up over decades. This is why it can seem that there are two classes of people: 'addicts' and everyone else.

The difference between those who present with 'disordered' eating patterns early in life and those who slowly drift into obesity over decades is one of degree only. The former have primed the trap with hunger.

As the intake of a deceptive item climbs, the threats delivered by the counterfeit soon become the primary stressor. Once one addiction gains a foothold, a vulnerability to the next arises because the stress of the first addiction increases the odds that another counterfeit will be encountered. As each counterfeit is identified and discarded, another rears its ugly head and pretends to repair the damage left by the predecessor. This colossal downward nightmare is known as the 'addictive personality.'

Addiction is not a bizarre, mystical condition that strikes a subset of the population without warning. It is the predictable pattern of behavior that emerges whenever a lifeform is misled by a deceiving entity that *pretends to deliver what is needed.*

While a heightened pre-existing need may set the whole drama in motion and accelerate the descent, the good news is that the presence of stress does not ever prevent nor hinder escape.

Recognition

Addiction is over the moment a counterfeit is recognized for what it truly is. When a deceptive situation is fully understood, the door to the prison opens. When a counterfeit is seen to not only cause harm but to deliver *zero benefits* – its status as a lying thief is exposed. This is the realization that occurs within Allen Carr's stop-smoking seminars and books. It is the sudden, shocking knowledge that *this thing is not what you thought it was.*

The correct insight can arrive after a long process of trial and error. After testing numerous hypotheses, oscillating back and forth between strategies, the truth is finally seen.

Reaching this viewpoint via trial and error can take a long time – and the costs of failure are high. However, learning from the experience of others accelerates this process. Cooperative human teams solve problems far faster than the same individuals working alone.[21] [22] Even rats extinguish unrewarding behaviors more quickly when watching other rats fruitlessly carry out the same activity.[23] If animals are asked to differentiate between two similar cues (one of which is rewarding and one of which is not), they arrive at the correct response far faster when seeing other animals make the right choice.[24] Lifeforms often mimic others as a way of acquiring optimal behavior patterns without the danger and wastage of resources that comes with personal trial and error. For this reason, the correct viewpoint may arrive in a burst of clarity after watching a video by someone else who has already escaped, or reading a book. But however it comes, the correct insight is always the same. It involves finally seeing that the deceptive item delivers *nothing beneficial at all.*

The moment a counterfeit's true nature is revealed, it can be discarded not with white knuckles but with relief. Rather than feeling as though it *must* be set down, you instead feel unbelievably excited to be free of it. Rather than fighting desire, everything suddenly feels easy. This is because when a counterfeit is seen to deliver only a loss, *you just don't want it anymore.*

In the wake of this transformation, behavioral change emerges not as a painful theoretical possibility but as the glorious act of taking back your life.

Once a counterfeit is set down, the genuine cue provides continuous reinforcement once more. The relationship between the genuine cue and the survival reward rapidly resets, engagement abates, satiation emerges, and obsession lifts. Other survival needs are picked up again, and you get on with the business of living.

The majority of this recalibration process occurs within a matter of days, with the system becoming indistinguishable from normal over the following few weeks. Although the return of a healthy physique takes time, happiness may arise *from the very first moment the deception is fully understood.*

Of course, some readers might fear that such a transformation is remote or implausible. Luckily, it doesn't matter how 'addicted' someone perceives themselves to be, or how entrenched a problem feels, or how doubtful this outcome may seem. This is because all addictions have at their root the same fundamental error of misperception, and all such errors collapse when the truth is seen.

> "Imagine that in a dream you are being chased by a bear. In another dream you are being chased by a hundred bears. In which situation are you in greater danger? Before you answer, consider the first principle of miracles: There is no order of difficulty in miracles.
>
> — HELEN SCHUCMAN AND WILLIAM T. THETFORD, *A COURSE IN MIRACLES* (1972)

We can interpret this quote to mean that it is no more difficult to escape one hundred dream-bears than it is to escape one. Both are illusions, and all dream-bears disappear the moment you wake up.

Just as immune dysfunction arises when the body cannot reliably distinguish between the *self* and *non-self*, the pattern of behavior that we call addiction occurs when a misleading entity is *mistaken as an ally*, and the enemy is embraced and willingly taken on board.

As with the immune system, the brain is involved in a pattern recognition game. Viruses evade the immune system using decoys, camouflage, and other forms of molecular trickery.[25] [26] These tactics increase the odds that a virus will *not be recognized*, allowing an invading agent to gain unimpeded access to the cell. Once access to the cell is breached, the virus goes on to manipulate the existing signaling pathways and rules of operation within the organism for its own gain.

Addiction is the exact same phenomenon at a different scale. It is the result of a categorization error – an identification error – in which a deceiving entity is *mistaken as something good.*

Addiction is cured by exposure of the deceit. Seeing under the hood breaks the spell. The moment truth is thrown into the light, the whole charade falls apart, and the addiction is over.

This is the moment the cue-set irrevocably splits into two.

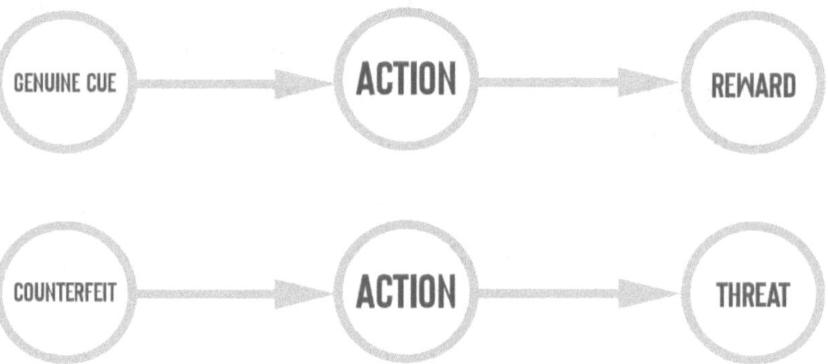

7

BODILY RECALIBRATION

LET'S now apply this new understanding of addiction to overeating.

As with other addictive substances, deceptive flavors are chemicals isolated from their source. Alcohol is a chemical extracted from decomposing plant matter. Nicotine is a chemical extracted from tobacco leaves. Heroin is a chemical extracted from poppy pods. Flavoring additives are chemicals extracted from a wide array of plants, animals, and fungi.

Flavor compounds are utilized because they mimic the flavor of a genuine nutritional reward (or, in some cases, conceal an unpleasant flavor). Remember, flavor acts as a label, providing the body with sensory data that indicates what type of nutrition a food contains. In the right quantities, these seemingly innocuous ingredients can fool people into eating bland or harmful substances that they would never ordinarily over-consume.

When deceptive flavors are eaten regularly, flavor-nutrition relationships weaken and become intermittent. Consequently, hunger rises to ensure that each flavor is engaged with more frequently to obtain the optimal volume of nutrition. Any attempt to reduce consumption to ordinary levels is met with resistance because this level of intake is no longer predicted to deliver the amount of nutrition required.

Chewing each mouthful of food provides a partial chemical analysis carried out by taste and smell receptors. The mouth and nose cannot reliably discern between fake and genuine flavors (this is the whole problem). The imposter molecules include thousands of different chemicals that are mapped so closely onto the genuine flavors that they activate the same taste and smell receptors.

Although certain 'junk foods' can be readily identified as problematic, the boundaries of this junk food category vary according to the expert followed. Hence, whenever people try to modify their diets, the boundaries are typically not quite drawn in the right place, and genuine nutritional rewards are often discarded or limited at the same time, while some deceptive elements remain.

When a diet arbitrarily limits access to *genuine* foods (or provides insufficient calories overall), the individual's need for nutrition increases, often to extreme and emergency levels, encouraging the consumption of larger volumes of food when the restriction abates. If subsequent binge eating includes deceptive food (which it often does, due to the improved perception of flavor), the resulting sham eating experience dramatically disrupts learned flavor-nutrition relationships.

You have been doing what any superb lifeform would do in this situation: test dietary approach after dietary approach until the correct operational rule is found.

Every time a potential culprit is identified, manufacturers leap in and fill the gap with more deceptive flavors: fake meat for vegans, sugar-free sweeteners for low-carbers, and so on. With every new potential culprit, the deceptive infiltration grows. As the added flavor molecules become more prevalent and the range of genuine food dwindles, the flavor selection appears ever more grand.

The more deceptive flavors are consumed, the more nourishment is needed, yet progressively less is received. Because the body no longer has a reliable method for predicting when or where nutrition will appear, an emergency buffer is required to sustain life during periods when insufficient nourishment is consumed. And, through it all, hunger climbs.

Conventional diets predispose the individual to consume high volumes of deceptive food, disrupting appetite and setting in motion a cycle that accelerates with time. Intermittent reinforcement is more devious than a loan shark. It is like someone who ratchets up the interest rate every time money is withdrawn. It provokes a runaway cycle facilitated by misled bodily systems that are doing their absolute best to save you.

Downregulation of Taste and Smell

> "Beware of false prophets, who come to you in sheep's clothing but inwardly are ravenous wolves.
>
> — MATTHEW 7:15, *THE HOLY BIBLE* (ESV)

When someone consumes flavor-manipulated foods, the average nutrition per unit of flavor drops. Let's consider the relationship between **banana flavor → potassium** (bananas are naturally a rich source of potassium).

Ordinarily, banana flavor in the mouth indicates that potassium is entering the body. Of course, not every human likes bananas (there are many sources of potassium, and for various reasons, you may prefer another one – flavors are liked and disliked on an individual basis, depending on your nutritional needs, inherited cultural preferences, prior experiences with a particular flavor, and so on).

When banana flavor is added to a wide variety of foods (such as banana milk, banana cereal, banana yogurt, and banana-flavored muesli bars), the relationship between banana flavor and potassium becomes intermittent and unreliable, with less potassium delivered per unit of banana flavor on average (not to mention the disruption to all other nutrients commonly found in bananas).

In this circumstance, the brain *cannot ignore this change.* Potassium is vital for survival – and helps with muscle contraction, relaxation of blood vessels, fluid balance, and so on.[1] Without potassium, the body cannot perform critical functions. While some dietary potassium is essential, *too much* can lead to heart problems and cardiac arrest. Although the body can filter out a certain amount of potassium through the kidneys and excrete the remainder in the urine, this creates an additional workload for the kidneys. Hence, as with all survival rewards, the body endeavors to maintain an optimal range.

The best thing the brain can do when it detects that banana flavor leads to *less potassium than before* is to recalibrate the sensory system to account for this change. It achieves this by *physically modifying taste and smell receptors*, such as by decreasing the "number of receptors on the membrane, thus altering sensitivity to a compound."[2] In other words, changes in learned flavor-nutrition relationships are reflected *directly within the sensory apparatus itself.*

This is an unbelievably efficient way for the body to store sensory data. If the brain had to maintain a complex database tracking every single prior engagement with a particular flavor across one's lifetime, this would be very labor-intensive compared to the wonderfully elegant solution of *updating sensory receptors.* Real-time recalibration of taste and smell receptors allows flavor sensitivity to be tuned to the current food environment, with sensitivity scaled up or down as required, based upon the results of each new engagement.

When deceptive foods are consumed, the brain receives a flood of misleading messages about the incoming nutrition. When the gut subsequently detects that this nutrition did not arrive in the volume promised, an error signal is detected. You can imagine the brain saying, "Look, taste and smell receptors, you're getting something wrong. You're giving me too many alerts about this flavor! You told me 10 units of potassium were coming in, but only 5 have arrived! You're too sensitive! Dial the volume down and notify me less often!"

Alterations to sensory receptors are initiated with the single goal of *altering an individual's response to the same stimuli going forward.*[3]

Most people have experienced a version of this adaptation process in real-time when switching between eating fruit and sugar-sweetened items. For example, if you bite into an apple, the flavor is usually delicious and sweet. However, if a piece of candy is eaten before biting the apple again, the flavor of the apple will seem remarkably less pleasant. Scientists often describe this as a 'fatiguing' of the receptors. However, it is better thought of as a rapid recalibration process seeking to redirect an individual toward the sweetest (and presumably most nourishing) item available.

Adjustments in flavor sensitivity are part of the ordinary "food intake control mechanism"[4] and occur on a flavor-by-flavor basis[5] (with specific receptors upregulating or downregulating as required).

These adjustments in sensitivity happen for a range of reasons. For example, flavor sensitivity often reduces when someone is injured or sick. At such times, it makes sense for resources to be prioritized toward healing rather than gathering and digesting food. Perhaps nasal congestion (a runny nose) is also a strategic effort, in part, to reduce smell sensitivity and minimize food intake while fighting off infection. Researchers have found that "upper respiratory infections are often accompanied by localized taste losses on the tongue."[6] When facing a serious health situation, such as chemotherapy treatment for cancer, flavor sensitivity may disappear entirely.[7]

In addition to short-term adjustments, changes to taste and smell receptors can persist for longer durations. When people suddenly lose their sense of smell (a condition called anosmia), they typically experience a loss of interest in food, perceiving eating as boring and tedious, which can lead to weight loss, illness, and malnutrition.[8] [9] Anosmia also appears to affect memory and has other hazardous side effects, such as an inability to detect spoiled food, smoke, or noxious fumes.[10]

Some might suspect that overeaters have *increased* flavor sensitivity and find flavors more pleasurable than usual. This is not the case. Overweight people typically have a weaker flavor response than normal-weight controls.[11] 'Dysfunctional' smell receptors are associated with a higher BMI.[12] (Of course, in light of the hypothesis presented within this book, these receptors are not dysfunctional at all, but are accurately dialed down to reflect the weakened flavor-nutrition relationships.)

Reductions in taste sensitivity of overweight individuals have been found for a host of different flavors, including umami. One study found that obese women could not detect normal levels of MSG and prefer higher concentrations in soups.[13] Obese children also have "significantly lower ability to identify the correct taste qualities."[14]

Why does reduced flavor sensitivity prompt overeating in some people but a loss of appetite in those who are injured or sick? The difference becomes clear when you see that in the case of illness or injury, both flavor perception *and* hunger dial down in unison. In contrast, the logical consequence of engaging with flavor-manipulated foods is that *flavor sensitivity declines while hunger rises.* Gradual reductions in flavor sensitivity are matched, lockstep, with an *increased need for nutrition*.

In other words, as with all other addictive circumstances, *desire goes up, while reward per engagement goes down.*

This two-pronged nightmare explains the obesity epidemic in one fell swoop. It also explains why overeating can occur with genuine foods as well as deceptive items – because *all versions of a flavor* (both genuine and counterfeit) are perceived as less rewarding. Ordinary concentrations of flavor no longer deliver an adequate sense of pleasure because the tongue and nasal cavity do not detect the strength of flavor as usual. Consequently, those with reduced flavor sensitivity are more likely to liberally apply flavor-enhanced seasonings and dressings[15] while prioritizing deceptive food whenever the opportunity arises.

Decreased flavor sensitivity is not just associated with obesity but Type 2 diabetes.[16] [17] In fact, some people with diabetes have *severe smell impairment*, and some have complete anosmia,[18] perhaps because, in such cases, flavor-nutrition relationships are deemed so unreliable that the brain shuts off smell sensitivity completely.

Just as smell 'dysfunction' is worse in morbidly obese people than it is in moderately obese people,[19] it worsens as diabetes progresses.[20]

Nutrients are not some quaint weight-loss variable; they are the building blocks of life. Anything that compromises your ability to reliably find these raw materials *is a direct survival threat.*

Those who navigate a food environment using unpredictable flavor-nutrition relationships (and who hence *cannot reliably source the raw materials needed to grow and heal their bodies*) are far more likely to incur breakdowns of function. It is perhaps no surprise at all that a diminished sense of smell *strongly predicts increased mortality risk*, with an effect that is "dose-dependent."[21]

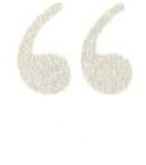

> It is now well established [...] that the olfactory system provides a unique probe into the general health of the brain. Thus, smell loss is among the first signs of neurodegenerative diseases such as Alzheimer's or Parkinson's disease and provides insight into elements of brain development. Importantly, smell loss is one of the best predictors of future mortality in older populations, being a stronger predictor than cognitive deficits, cancer, stroke, lung disease, or hypertension even after controlling for the effects of age, sex, race, education, socioeconomic status, smoking behavior, alcohol use, cardiovascular disease, diabetes, and liver damage.
>
> — CHRISTOPHER H HAWKES, *SMELL AND TASTE DISORDERS* (2018)

Could taste and smell loss in overweight populations be caused by some other factor unrelated to flavor? After all, smell loss can occur for numerous reasons, such as congenital conditions, illness, injury, and so on. Some suggest that diabetic populations might lose their sense of smell as a consequence of central or peripheral neuropathy (although evidence for this is "limited and inconsistent").[22] As yet, no studies directly examine whether intermittent reinforcement of flavor is to blame, because this is a new hypothesis, first documented within this book. It is worth noting, however, that in animal models, the taste and smell reduction that occurs with an obesogenic diet *reverts back as the diet returns to normal.*[23]

It is also interesting that taste and smell sensitivity often *restores* following obesity surgery,[24] suggesting that something about the **flavor → nutrition** feedback loop drives this change.

The crucial point is this: although people seek deceptive food for its strengthened flavor, it *systematically destroys the ability to experience flavor*. The more deceptive food is consumed, the less enjoyable each mouthful becomes, and the more mouthfuls are needed. Like every addictive substance, it steals the very thing it pretends to deliver.

This reduction in taste and smell sensitivity affects both deceptive and genuine flavor molecules alike; hence, *all foods taste worse*. This is why children raised predominantly upon junk food may refuse genuine, nourishing foods outright, because their sense of taste and smell has been driven so low that many ordinary foods no longer trigger a pleasure response. Consequently, genuine foods can appear boring, bland, and not good enough.

With a downregulated sensory apparatus and an upregulated appetite, ordinary quantities of food no longer satisfy. This is why it can feel impossible to return to 'normal eating' and why some find it challenging to summon energy and enthusiasm for preparing a simple, ordinary meal.

Attempting to resume 'normal eating' without understanding the role of flavor hence typically leads to weight gain, followed by another panic-stricken diet, causing the individual to ricochet back and forth between restriction and intermittent reinforcement.

From the outside, it appears as if hunger and satiety systems are well and truly broken – as if one cannot diet *or* stop dieting – the stomach has become a bottomless pit.

But the body is functioning *exactly as it should* in this

circumstance. Look around. *Two-thirds of the American population are overweight or obese.*[25] Of those who are a normal weight, many endure a private daily battle with food. These behaviors are the *normal and expected response.*

Misleading flavors elevate hunger, leaving the individual fatter and sicker while enjoying each mouthful less. In this state, returning to deceptive food can feel essential – the only way to achieve a fleeting sense of normality. But consuming these substances ensures that the state of normalcy creeps further from reach.

Deceptive flavors erode the ability to taste and smell food, presenting a dire survival emergency that captivates attention. Because this sensory recalibration occurs gradually at a microscopic scale, it is very hard to initially see what is going wrong.

If bodily senses are corrupted without one's knowledge, decisions are made using faulty data. But the capacity to *make* good decisions is *never compromised.* The error is only within the *data informing the decisions.*

The moment a deceptive situation is viewed correctly and the deception is understood, everything changes...because, at long last, you have *new* data to act upon.

Insulin Resistance

In addition to reducing sensitivity of taste and smell receptors, counterfeit flavors influence a number of other bodily systems. Let's speculate about the potential impact upon insulin.

When carbohydrates are digested, glucose travels from the small intestine into the bloodstream. At the same time, insulin is released from the pancreas into the bloodstream.

Insulin has several metabolic roles, one of which is to stimulate muscle, liver, and fat cells to take up excess glucose from the blood. Insulin does this by binding to receptors on a cell's surface[26] ('unlocking the door,' so to speak) so that glucose can enter the cell.[27]

When insulin levels are high, fat loss is inhibited. Proponents of low-carbohydrate diets often view this as concerning, but it is logical: there is no point in using energy from fat stores if a liberal supply of glucose already exists in the bloodstream.

Insulin has a very important role because both high *and* low blood sugar levels threaten survival. Low blood sugar (hypoglycemia) is particularly dangerous and can lead to fainting, seizures, and death. Sustained high blood sugar (hyperglycemia), on the other hand, can eventually lead to the diagnosis of Type 2 diabetes and associated complications,[28] including blindness, cardiovascular disease, and limb amputation. Because both high and low blood sugar levels present a severe health risk, insulin is released in a carefully controlled manner.

In some individuals, however, cells develop what is known as *insulin resistance* – a symptom of Type 2 diabetes – whereby changes in the number or sensitivity of insulin receptors (or alterations in downstream signaling molecules) make cells less responsive to insulin. As a result, higher levels of insulin are required to achieve the same effect.

In his book, *The Obesity Code* (2016), Jason Fung describes studies in which healthy individuals develop insulin resistance in a matter of days after having their insulin levels artificially raised. Fung also notes that insulin shots given to people with diabetes increase insulin resistance long-term. This implies that the body can deliberately implement insulin resistance in certain scenarios.

In fact, there is considerable evidence that the human body increases or decreases insulin resistance as part of ordinary life.

For example, during pregnancy, a mother's body increases insulin resistance so that glucose is spared for the baby's brain.[29] In this way, insulin resistance is sometimes described as the mechanism by which energy is 'rationed' within the body. By tuning insulin resistance across various tissues, the body can precisely control where and when energy is used,[30] responding to insulin production in an 'adjustable' manner,[31] according to the circumstances.[32]

Could it be possible, therefore, that the insulin resistance associated with Type 2 diabetes is not a 'dysfunction' as it is usually assumed but a deliberate bodily response?

Fung and others suggest that eating too many carbohydrate-rich foods spikes blood sugar levels and prompts high levels of insulin. These sustained high insulin levels are argued to eventually 'overwhelm' the system, so it is unable to return to baseline, resulting in higher-than-normal insulin levels even during fasting periods. These chronically elevated insulin levels are then argued to lead to insulin resistance.

However, Fung himself notes inconsistencies with this idea, describing Asian populations who have traditionally consumed large amounts of white rice; residents of Kitava who consume a diet rich in root vegetables like potatoes and yams; and people living in Okinawa who consume nearly 85% of their diet as carbohydrates. These populations traditionally report little obesity and type 2 diabetes. Fung also notes that low-carbohydrate diets have the same dismal long-term adherence as low-fat diets.[33]

In fact, the high-carbohydrate/insulin resistance hypothesis has many holes. For example, why do those who consume large amounts of potatoes anecdotally report *reduced* fasting insulin levels (such as Chris Voight, who ate only potatoes and oil for 60 days)?[34] Why do followers of *The Potato Hack* (a book that encourages 'potato fasts' – short periods during which you eat *only* potatoes) report such positive results?[35] Similarly, *Dr. Neal Barnard's Program for Reversing Diabetes* (2008) provides a method for curing Type 2 diabetes using a whole-food vegan diet with no limits upon carbohydrate intake.

There are also fascinating studies in which people who consume sucrose (refined table sugar) *plus* whole berries have better blood sugar levels in the following hours than those who consume sucrose alone, *despite the former consuming more sugar in total.*[36] (A similar effect was found when using berry nectar plus sucrose.) Studies also find that those who consume fructose (a type of sugar found in honey and fruit) in natural forms lose *more* weight than those who avoid fructose completely.[37] All of this makes it clear that the issue is not as simple as the amount of carbohydrates or sugar in the diet.

Let's consider another possibility. Perhaps insulin resistance is not caused by a high intake of carbohydrate-rich foods per se but by *the body's inability to reliably predict the amount of glucose coming in.* In other words, perhaps Type 2 diabetes is caused by an *intermittent relationship between flavor and glucose.*

Fung makes an interesting observation:

> In 1986, Dr. Michael Nauck noticed something very unusual. A subject's blood sugar response is identical whether a dose of glucose is given by mouth or intravenously. But, despite the same level of blood sugar, the subject's insulin levels differ greatly. Remarkably, the insulin response to oral glucose was much more powerful.
>
> — JASON FUNG, *THE OBESITY CODE* (2016)

In other words, when glucose is injected directly into a vein, *much less insulin is released than when the same amount of glucose is consumed orally*. Hence, it takes the body much longer to clear injected glucose from the bloodstream than when glucose is eaten, and blood sugar levels remain elevated for a longer period.

This is no surprise. After all, how can the body release the right amount of insulin if it doesn't know how much glucose is coming in? When glucose is injected into a vein, glucose spontaneously appears in the bloodstream, and the pancreas must scramble frantically to meet demand. When glucose is consumed orally, however, *gut hormones send an advance warning signal about the incoming glucose, aiding the insulin response.*[38] When glucose is injected, these gut signals are not received. Similarly, if glucose is eaten but signals from the gut are experimentally blunted, dysregulation of blood sugar ensues.[39] [40] In fact, a deficient insulin response even occurs if food is placed directly into the stomach (bypassing the mouth).[41] This is because *gut signals are modulated by signals from the taste buds.*[42]

It turns out that even just *tasting* a food (before anything is swallowed) triggers insulin release. This was shown in studies where various solutions were swirled around the mouth and then spat out.[43]

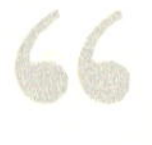

> Insulin increases prior to and during eating, as a response to unconditioned and conditioned food cues such as taste, odor, texture, appearance and peripheral environmental stimuli. The stimulus-response relationship between food cues and insulin secretion is much less recognized, and mentioned barely if at all by the advocates of diet and exercise.
>
> — TODD BECKER, GETTING STRONGER, *DIET* (2015)

Seeing, smelling, and even *imagining* eating can trigger insulin release. In other words, *any preceding environmental cue that suggests glucose intake is imminent* prompts an insulin response.[44]

Interestingly, patients with Type 2 diabetes often exhibit a deficient insulin response *regardless of whether glucose arrives orally or intravenously*.[45] In other words, it is as if the gut signaling in these patients (modulated by flavor signals) is not working as normal. When glucose is eaten, their body behaves as though the glucose has been dumped in the bloodstream without warning.

Although a range of environmental cues can indicate that glucose is forthcoming, the most potent and reliable signal is *flavor in the mouth*. For this reason, flavor plays a critically important role in signaling insulin release.

What are the consequences of mixing and matching flavor signals that are ordinarily associated with glucose (such as sweet or fruit flavors) in a random and haphazard manner? If relationships between flavor and glucose are unreliable and intermittent, isn't it reasonable to speculate that the body *no longer has a reliable system for predicting precisely how much glucose is coming in?*

When you consider insulin release from the perspective of flavor, it also becomes clear why insulin might be released in response to protein to a greater degree than is expected. In the modern food environment, protein is sometimes paired with glucose-associated flavoring agents (such as fruit-flavored protein shakes), which interfere with learned **protein → glucose** associations.

The notion that flavor manipulation might interfere with insulin signaling is supported by population studies (which find correlations between the use of artificial sweeteners and increased BMI, as well as between artificial sweetener use and insulin resistance).[46] Research also supports this line of argument, suggesting that using noncaloric sweeteners may disrupt learned flavor associations[47] and affect carbohydrate metabolism.

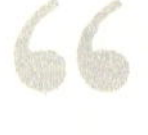

> Taste normally prepares the gut for the onset of certain nutritional components allowing effective processing to occur. Artificial sweeteners disrupt this and lead to a decoupling of taste from physiological consequences so that actual carbohydrate intake is not dealt with efficiently.
>
> — JAMES MCCUTCHEON, *THE ROLE OF DOPAMINE IN THE PURSUIT OF NUTRITIONAL VALUE* (2015)

Remember, the body cannot determine which glucose signals are misleading. Genuine and counterfeit flavors slot into the same receptors. The best the body can do in this scenario is to predict how much glucose, on average, is expected for each particular flavor (see chapter 6: *Tolerance and Escalation*).

The problem with using a type of average, however, is that sometimes this glucose prediction will be too high and sometimes too low (this is what an average means – it is a representation of the middle). As a consequence, on some occasions, *too much insulin* will be released and, on other occasions, *too little*.

If insufficient insulin is released, it takes the body longer than usual to clear the excess glucose from the blood (just as occurs when glucose is spontaneously dumped in a vein). This leaves blood sugar levels uncomfortably high for an extended period. This is not ideal, but it is not nearly as dangerous as what happens when *too much* insulin is released. In the latter case, a life-threatening emergency may unfold because very low blood sugar levels are fatal.

For this reason, the body must quickly ascertain that operating according to some form of average has a terrible flaw when it comes to insulin release. Because the human body is an amazing survival machine, it must take corrective action to ensure that this life-threatening emergency *does not happen again.*

Implementing a measure of insulin resistance is a simple and effective way to protect the body against unexpected low blood sugar drops that are otherwise unavoidable when glucose predictions are unreliable. Insulin resistance essentially adds a margin of error to the predicted glucose load (a safety zone), protecting the individual from the dangerous consequences of unpredictable low blood sugar drops.

Although this results in *vastly more instances of high blood sugar* (and thus the long-term complications of Type 2 diabetes), it is certainly preferable to immediate death.

In other words, it appears plausible that intermittent reinforcement of flavor (and the muddling of **flavor → glucose** signaling that results) might offer a logical explanation for insulin resistance and the development of Type 2 diabetes.

The more unpredictable a flavor environment becomes, the greater the mismatch between the predicted and actual glucose load, and the greater the buffer of insulin resistance required.

If we look at Type 2 diabetes from this perspective, we might speculate that insulin resistance is not a dysfunction, but the deliberate and life-saving response to variability in **flavor → glucose** relationships. In this context, insulin resistance can be viewed as a necessary and desperate bid to save an individual's life – a way to cope with nonsensical flavor signals in the best way the body can.

Despite the enormous differences between dietary

approaches, it is very interesting that *all of the eating plans that purport to help with insulin and blood sugar levels* (paleo, keto, carnivorism, vegan, whole foods, GAPS, etc.) *eliminate or significantly reduce flavor-enhanced foods*. Even fasting involves the complete removal of all misleading flavor signals. Mono-diets, such as the potato diet, have a similar effect: they remove *all misleading flavor signals* and deliver a single isolated flavor-nutrition relationship that can be quickly learned and relied upon.

Of course, restrictive dieting approaches are not viable long-term strategies – and, at some point, a wider range of nutrition must be consumed. If these approaches are undertaken without understanding the role of flavor, the issue is simply delayed, and the problem of *what to eat* remains.

Disruption of Circadian Rhythm

Just as a flower opens and shuts its petals at a certain time of day, humans operate according to daily circadian rhythms. Staying alive is complicated, and the multitude of protective, healing, and restorative functions that occur within the human body are synchronized in a carefully organized sequence over 24 hours. Different organs and bodily functions switch off and on as needed, adjusting in sensitivity at different times of the day.

What coordinates this great dance of activity? Two critical factors are the timing of light exposure and the timing of meals.

When flavor-manipulated foods are consumed regularly, the tendency is to move from ordinary mealtimes to sporadic binge eating or ongoing snacking and grazing. This is because when deceptive flavors recalibrate taste and smell receptors and exacerbate hunger, it is difficult to maintain a regular eating pattern unless consuming increasingly large volumes at each meal.

Satchin Panda, professor at the Salk Institute and author of *The Circadian Code* (2018), found that it is now common for modern humans to eat 4.2 – 10.5 times per day,[48] with only 10% of the adult population consistently eating within a 12-hour window or less. Many individuals also eat late into the evening, when the body would ordinarily rest.

Digesting and processing food is a resource-intensive task and involves many separate bodily systems. Panda suggests that eating at unexpected times causes the body to "drop everything it is supposed to do"[49] and divert resources towards digestion and food processing.

If digestive systems operate for an extended period or are forced to continue long into the night (when these systems would ordinarily be recouping and repairing), the balance between digesting and healing time is upset, placing undue pressure on various bodily systems. As a consequence, processes such as autophagy (whereby cells break down and recycle their parts for future use) have less time to occur.[50]

Both animal and human studies indicate that even modest reductions in eating windows lead to health improvements. For example, when mice consume an otherwise 'fattening' diet, shortening the eating window by a few hours per day improves health and longevity (despite the mice eating as much as they like when food is available).[51] A recent human study found that overweight individuals who adopt a 10-11 hour eating window (after previously eating across 14 or more hours per day) lose weight, increase energy, and improve sleep.[52]

Panda notes that the genes in the organs of mice become synchronized with their eating window and argues that genes throughout the body are regulated by our first bite of the day.[53] He recommends having breakfast early in the morning so that both signals from sunlight and diet are aligned. Interestingly, both insulin response and flavor-sensitivity are strongest in the morning. Nutrient absorption is also lower at night because the systems involved in processing and storing nutrients are circadian.[54] In other words, eating more frequently and for a longer part of the day has numerous detrimental effects upon health and weight regulation.

Compounding matters, as obesity climbs, people tend to become more self-conscious and may prioritize less-revealing attire, concealing as much skin as possible. With a heavier body that is harder to move around, people may spend less time partaking in outdoor activities, further reducing sunshine exposure and creating an additional blow for the body's circadian rhythm.

When retreating indoors, the eyes and skin receive less sunlight exposure, reducing vitamin D production. Just as many plants die without direct sunlight, sunshine is essential for the health of humans and many animals.[55] Disruption of natural lighting also impacts breeding cycles in some mammals.[56]

Not only does a lack of sunlight disturb the body's circadian rhythm, but it appears to compromise the ability to burn fat. Jeff T. Bowles presents the intriguing hypothesis that weight gain may be promoted by low vitamin D status and might be a form of hibernation response.[57] Bowles argues that a lack of direct sunlight upon the eyes and skin tells the body that it is winter and advantageous to stockpile fat reserves (partly as a buffer of energy to last until spring and partly as protection against colder winter climates).[58] Those with higher vitamin D levels do indeed appear to lose more fat when subjected to a low-calorie diet.[59]

In addition to receiving less sunlight, overweight individuals may turn to digital modes of communication to stay in contact with others, hiding weight gain behind a screen. This inadvertently increases exposure to other forms of intermittent reinforcement (social media, gaming, pornography, and so on), and may result in evenings spent eating deceptive food while staring at a brightly lit screen.

In *Why We Sleep* (2017), Matthew Walker explains that reading on an iPad before bed results in 50% less melatonin being released in comparison to reading a printed book, with the onset of sleepiness delayed by up to three hours.[60] This occurs because the artificial light from the screen confuses the body about what time of day it is, dysregulating circadian rhythm further and delaying sleepiness, so the individual goes to bed exhausted before waking up and repeating the cycle tomorrow.

As a final nail in the coffin, when attempting to lose weight in a sleep-deprived state, people are likely to lose more lean body mass than fat[61] and lose less weight overall.[62] Sleep deprivation also makes people hungrier and more susceptible to illness. In fact, total sleep deprivation can kill faster than total food deprivation.

> “Inadequate sleep—even moderate reductions for just one week—disrupts blood sugar levels so profoundly that you would be classified as pre-diabetic. Short sleeping increases the likelihood of your coronary arteries becoming blocked and brittle, setting you on a path toward cardiovascular disease, stroke, and congestive heart failure.
>
> — MATTHEW WALKER, *WHY WE SLEEP* (2017)

In other words, the consumption of misleading flavor molecules leads to several other behaviors that disrupt circadian rhythm and introduce further health consequences. With all of these confounding factors, it seems evident that returning to ordinary meal patterns, increasing sunshine exposure, and avoiding digital media after sunset might be a wise idea (at least in latitudes where natural sunshine hours make this feasible). However, attempting to implement these changes without first understanding the role of deceptive flavor can make it very difficult to resolve the problem.

Disruption of the Microbiome

In many respects, the human body is like planet Earth: a discrete world teeming with microscopic creatures that inhabit the environment the body provides. The skin, hair, mouth, nose, and all orifices are populated by millions of tiny organisms. The gut is filled with the largest community of all – more than one hundred trillion microorganisms.[63] This collection of lifeforms is known as the *microbiota* or *microbiome.*

The human body is very much a team effort. The relationship between the individual and the microbiota is bidirectional; each is adapted to the functions and needs of the other. The human host provides these microbes with nutrition and a home. In turn, they help the individual to digest food, extract nutrients, and manufacture mood-regulating hormones and neurotransmitters – GABA, dopamine, serotonin, and so on.[64]

The microbiota consists of thousands of different microscopic species, each adapted to certain food sources and microclimates. Some of these microbes are active during mealtimes; others are active while the human host is fasting, with active periods linked to the individual's daily circadian rhythm.[65] Unpredictable sleep patterns and a dysregulated circadian rhythm can wreak havoc with the microbiota.[66]

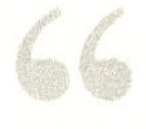

A recent study even linked jet lag to weight gain because disrupting your schedule through long-distance travel confuses the microbes in your gut.

— SUHAS KSHIRSAGAR AND MICHELLE D. SEATON, *CHANGE YOUR SCHEDULE, CHANGE YOUR LIFE* (2018)

Just as human behavior is modified by the world we live in – retreating indoors when it rains, wrapping up warm when the temperature plummets – the behavior of the species within the microbiota fluctuates according to the signals the body sends (and vice versa).

If deceptive flavor indicates that a load of nutrition is incoming, it seems plausible that certain bacteria might leap into action, ready to aid digestion. This might cause problems when the predicted nutrition is not forthcoming. For example, some species are known to resort to dining on the intestinal lining when starved of fiber.[67]

As an individual's diet changes, the balance of species within the microbiota adapts. Bacteria that are ordinarily helpful can become harmful when in plentiful supply.[68] Antibiotics also dramatically cull hundreds of beneficial bacteria, which can allow for an overgrowth of harmful species.

Many of the chemicals added to modern foods directly impact the function and health of the microbiome. Some additives, for example, can damage the intestinal wall.[69]

When much of the day is spent eating, the body has less time to heal and restore the gut lining. In this damaged state (a condition known as leaky gut syndrome), the porous lining can allow "undigested food particles, disease-causing bacteria, or allergy-causing chemicals to enter the body and activate the immune system."[70]

Emulsifiers – which are often added to foods to prevent fat and water from separating in mixtures such as ice cream – also cause changes in gut bacteria and gut inflammation in mice, leading to obesity.[71]

> When preservative-laden store-bought bread lasts weeks before spoiling, that means the microbes aren't eating it. 90 percent of the cells in the human body are microbial cells and these microbes do the heavy lifting for all our digestive processes including breaking down gluten. If the microbes won't eat the bread that's been in your cupboard for weeks, we can't expect the same microbes to digest that bread inside your belly.
>
> — JOHN DOUILLARD, *EAT WHEAT* (2017)

When a food supply disappears, lifeforms that rely on that food often die. You can imagine that if all of the plants on Earth died except for wheat and corn, most animals would also die. The planet would soon become overrun with the few species that thrive on wheat and corn, which would have numerous unpredictable consequences.[72]

The same thing happens within the gut when food intake narrows – such as when an individual takes up a restrictive diet. If the person later introduces new foods, it can seem as though they are suddenly intolerant to things they could previously consume without difficulty. This is because the microbes required to digest that item have not had time to repopulate the gut. This can lead people to believe they are allergic or intolerant to a growing number of items. Eating a narrow range of foods can also make it harder to deal with toxins (often present in small amounts in many natural foods) because the nutritional elements needed to counter and eliminate these compounds are missing from the diet.[73] The absence of these essential nutrients can further contribute to the perception that the individual has developed a sudden sensitivity to certain foods.

Obese people often have dramatically different microbiomes, with far fewer species on average. This makes sense when you consider that each bacterium is adapted to eating a different food source – just as each animal on Earth has its own preferred diet. Deceptive flavors can make it *seem* as though a wide array of foods are consumed, even though the core ingredients are often the same – fostering a narrow band of microbes within the microbiota.

Once someone *has* a limited microbiota, it can feel harder to alter the diet away from these foods. For example, if an individual has cultivated trillions of microbes who prefer the narrow ingredients within deceptive food, these may cry out in hunger whenever the individual attempts to stop feeding them – in a very literal sense by regulating or even directly producing hunger and satiety hormones.[74]

> ...from the start, gut bacteria have been in very close communication with the brain upstairs and maybe even quite dictatorial in their demands. After all, they greatly outnumber the rest of the cells in the body and clearly have a stake in the safety and welfare of their vessel.
>
> — KATHLEEN MCAULIFFE, *THIS IS YOUR BRAIN ON PARASITES* (2017)

In effect, when flavor-enhanced foods lie to the sensors, the gut becomes populated with a host of liar-supporters, crowding out those who survive on other foods. Interestingly, when helping people to break free from cigarettes, Allen Carr suggested that it can be helpful to imagine nicotine addiction as a "little monster" residing in the stomach that feeds on nicotine, which will rapidly wither away and die when nicotine is withheld. It is disconcerting to realize this may be the literal truth in the case of deceptive food consumption.

> Just as we have inadvertently domesticated rats to eat food out of the garbage, bacterial vermin have been domesticated to live in our bodies.
>
> — ROB KNIGHT AND BRENDAN BUHLER, *FOLLOW YOUR GUT* (2015)

The influence of these microbes is clear. When the microbiota from an overweight mouse (or from overweight people – including those who are sleep-deprived or jetlagged) is transferred to a healthy mouse, the healthy mouse becomes fat. Some thus suspect that fecal transplants might enable an overweight person to acquire the microbiome of a thin person.

Luckily, this dubious proposition is unnecessary. When deceptive food is avoided, the microbiome adapts. One study found that detectable changes in human gut microbiota occurred within *24 hours of changing diets.*[75] Another study found that when mice stopped consuming emulsifiers, gut bacteria gradually normalized.[76] In other words, when genuine, nourishing foods are consumed, a healthy microbiome repopulates over time.[77]

If someone regularly consumes deceptive foods, the systems in the body – including those lifeforms that reside within – are led astray. Taste and smell receptors desensitize, hunger rises, insulin resistance emerges, sleep and circadian rhythms fall out of whack, and the microbiota rages and tantrums for more.

One by one, the dominoes fall.

Degradation, Sickness, and Death

Let's not mince words. This is not just about aesthetics or social ostracism (which should not be minimized because these severely threaten a survival need, too). If genuine food is sacrificed for deceptive food on an ongoing basis, your life is in danger. Thirty-seven million Americans have diabetes,[78] making it the 8th leading cause of death in 2021. Another ninety-six million have prediabetes (this is more than *one-third* of US adults).[79] The leading cause of death – heart disease[80] – is also correlated with obesity,[81] as are cancer and stroke (which take out the 2nd and 5th positions, respectively). One hundred and thirty thousand people in America had lower limb amputations due to diabetes in 2016 alone.[82] According to a 2017–2018 survey, 42% of the American adult population is obese.[83]

Addiction doesn't just affect the individual. It spills from the victim and tars those nearby in ever-widening circles – not just via the transfer of faulty beliefs but also through the consequences of lack of achievement, depression, and never feeling good enough. These things rub off on loved ones, influencing others in countless ways. You don't know how much *good* you could do in the world if you broke free.

Deceptive food steals money, health, and life. Initially, it can seem only a cosmetic problem – a superficial struggle with weight. But deceptive food doesn't just make people fat; it cripples physical and athletic strength. It saps productivity and infests the consumer with a bone-deep lethargy that chases them from dawn until dusk. It erodes self-confidence, sacrifices career opportunities, compromises social engagements, and thieves *so much time.*

If someone doesn't have a reliable supply of the very building blocks needed to grow and heal the body, the body begins to break down. Eventually, organs and tissues buckle under the strain. The worst thing is the consequences pile up so gradually that it seems the individual is to blame.

Deceptive foods sicken the consumer in tiny increments, sabotaging every aspect of life. These items are slow-motion slaughtering the human race, and slow-motion is a terrible way to die. The only saving grace is that it offers a *window of opportunity to escape.*

8

GENUINE FOOD

THE DECEPTIVE STRATEGIES used within the modern food supply are varied and widespread, involving mimicry of thousands of different flavor molecules. As such, it is challenging to see precisely where the culprit hides. Popular diets often get some parts right, but because they don't understand the core mechanism, people are inadvertently encouraged to avoid different aspects of *genuine food.* Consequently, many nourishing, flavor-honest foods are discarded along with the counterfeit, restricting access to genuine nutritional rewards, ensuring these diets become increasingly difficult to maintain with time.

In the aftermath, the individual is left not only hungry and confused but fearful of many genuine foods. Some fear animal products for the saturated fat. Others fear carbohydrates for the insulin response. Some fear eggs for the cholesterol or dairy for the lactose and casein. Others fear fruit for the sugar or grains for the gluten. Some fear nuts and seeds for the antinutrients and oxalates, vegetables for the lectins, nightshades for the alkaloids, and so on. If you followed all of these recommendations, there would soon be nothing left to eat.

The aim of this chapter is not to insist that anyone must eat this or that, but to offer reassurance that (except in the case of allergy or intolerance) *all food groups offer valuable sources of nutrition.*

There is no consensus about what constitutes an optimal human diet. Around the world, indigenous diets vary widely. For example, the Inuit traditionally consume a diet rich in fatty fish and marine mammals; traditional Japanese diets focus on fish, seaweed, fermented foods, rice, and vegetables; the Maasai in East Africa consume predominantly meat, milk, and blood from cattle; and traditional Andean diets are rich in grains like quinoa, tubers, meat, and vegetables. Despite these vast differences, it is worth pointing out that no known traditional diet is exclusively vegan or exclusively carnivore: *all involve a broad mix of plant and animal foods.* The human species is evidently adaptable and flexible, capable of inhabiting all corners of the globe and thriving in a wide range of food environments.

As long as a variety of proteins, fats, carbohydrates, vitamins, and minerals are consumed within foods that *do not mislead the sensory apparatus*, the human body can competently direct food intake. This automated process of learning flavor-nutrition relationships has worked for every traditional human society and all animals across time – as it will work for you.

The danger is not with genuine foods but with their deceptive counterparts – the misleading substances that fool humans into consuming things their body does not need.

Traditional Processing

Most people suspect that *something* about modern food processing is to blame for the obesity epidemic. Yet, when pushed to explain why, there is very little clarity.

> What part of processing makes food bad? How does mere contact with a machine turn food from healthy to unhealthy? What food counts as "processed" or "not processed"? Is ground beef processed, since you grind it? Are scrambled eggs processed, since you scramble them? [...] Everybody I ask acts like the answers to these questions are obvious, but everyone has different answers, and nobody can tell me their decision procedure.
>
> — SCOTT ALEXANDER, SLATE STAR CODEX, *FOR, THEN AGAINST, HIGH-SATURATED-FAT DIETS* (2020)

It is critical to understand that although flavor manipulation is a *type* of processing, processing *per se* is not the problem. In fact, many traditional food processing methods are not just tolerable but beneficial. Humans have peeled, scraped, ground, chopped, pounded, soaked, dried, cooked, smoked, fermented, and preserved foods for thousands of years. Processing has many advantages. Heat can kill dangerous pathogens and make certain nutrients more bioavailable; grinding or pounding can tenderize food and make it easier to chew and digest. Even in circumstances where processing methods reduce nutrient density and increase calorie availability, survival benefits can result.

In his book *Catching Fire* (2010), Richard Wrangham, professor of biological anthropology at Harvard University, notes that humans now spend far less time gathering and consuming food than other primates. Our lips, teeth, mouths, jaws, stomach, and colon are smaller than they should be, given our size.[1] Wrangham argues that the human digestive tract shortened and our brain grew in response to our capacity to control fire and cook food. He suggests that the higher concentration of calories from cooked meals provided our ancestors with rapid and reliable fuel, encouraging brain growth while freeing up time for cultural and technological pursuits. In other words, once our ancestors were no longer required to spend all day foraging and chewing raw food, our most human qualities began to emerge.

Genuine foods (those that do not deceive the sensors) are not limited to raw, whole, unprocessed foods. In fact, attempting to survive exclusively upon such fodder is likely to result in a survival loss – something many raw-foodists quickly discover.

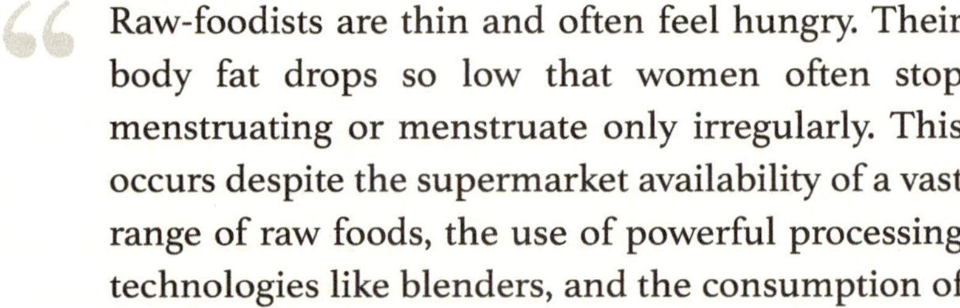

> Raw-foodists are thin and often feel hungry. Their body fat drops so low that women often stop menstruating or menstruate only irregularly. This occurs despite the supermarket availability of a vast range of raw foods, the use of powerful processing technologies like blenders, and the consumption of some preprocessed foods.
>
> — JOSEPH HENRICH, *THE SECRET OF OUR SUCCESS* (2015)

The reason that modern flavor manipulation tactics often lead to problematic outcomes, whereas traditional methods of food processing typically do not, is that historical processes almost always deliver *reliable flavor signals*. Cooked versions of a food reliably taste different from the same item consumed raw. Concentrated soups reliably taste more intense than watery soups. Milk with cream reliably tastes different from milk without cream. A peeled apple reliably tastes different than an apple eaten with skin. In each case, the change in flavor and nutritional outcome is predictable and reliable across time, resulting in flavor-nutrition patterns that can be learned and depended upon.

In contrast, the flavor manipulation tactics used by modern manufacturers involve refining substances into *isolated molecular building blocks* and then recombining these in an almost infinite variety of ways. Because every food manufacturer adds different molecules in different combinations, with some flavors manipulated while others are not, the resulting nutritional patterns are widely varied and unpredictable.

The best way to understand this in detail is to look at specific examples. Let's begin.

Sugar, Honey, and Fruit

To understand how modern flavor manipulation differs from traditional food processing, consider the lengths undertaken to isolate sucrose (table sugar) from sugarcane.[2] Though precise procedures vary depending on the manufacturer and scale of the operation, a common approach is as follows: After harvesting, sugarcane is washed, chopped, and shredded before being crushed through rollers to release the juice. The juice is then strained, mixed with calcium hydroxide and water, settled, and then spun like a washing machine to separate the juice from the solids. The extracted liquid is heated and concentrated, with chemicals added to separate more solids. It is then boiled until crystals form and spun to extract the syrup (known as molasses), leaving behind only the crystals, which are washed, spun, dried, cooled, washed, spun, melted, sieved, heated, crystallized, and spun once more. Chemicals are again added to extract more solids. The liquid is then decolored using activated carbon and a granular mixture of charred animal bones, which absorb further substances. At last, after the final heating and crystallizing, only sucrose remains, separated from all other chemicals that were naturally present in the plant. The tiny, translucent crystals are sorted via mesh screens and poured into bags.

Unlike traditional food processing methods, modern flavor manipulation involves *isolating chemicals at the molecular level*, with all other chemicals naturally present in the original source discarded (or used elsewhere).

If we liken the perception of flavor to reading a 'word' comprised of molecular 'letters,' modern processing methods strip away almost every other letter and then recombine the isolated letters into a completely new word with a different meaning.

In *Sugar: The Bitter Truth* (2009),[3] Robert Lustig notes that high consumption of fructose is linked to non-alcoholic fatty liver disease[4] (fructose is a sugar found commonly in honey and fruit – as well as within refined sugar and high-fructose corn syrup). Although Lustig directs his concern primarily toward *added refined sugars*, a growing number of people now avoid fructose altogether, minimizing the consumption of honey, fruit, and berries. It is critical to remember, however, that the *reason* humans desire sweet foods is because these are *associated with a survival gain*. If naturally sweet foods did *not* deliver a benefit, we would not like these flavors.

The natural sugars in fruit provide a critical marker of ripeness – appearing in the highest concentrations when harvesting is most beneficial to both the plant and the eater (a win-win relationship). Sweet-tasting fruit is thus perceived as more palatable than sour fruit and indicates that the item is ready to consume.

Fresh fruit offers a wealth of nutrition[5] and is associated with almost every health benefit imaginable. Fresh fruit is rich in vitamins, phytonutrients, and antioxidants and is well-known for its anti-inflammatory properties. Fresh fruit consumption is linked to improved cardiovascular health, better digestive function, enhanced immune response, and reduced risk of chronic diseases such as diabetes and cancer. Despite fears about high sugar content, those who regularly include natural forms of fructose within their diets appear to achieve greater weight loss than those who avoid fructose altogether (see chapter 7: *Insulin Resistance*).

Of course, many modern fruits offer less nutrition than historically. For example, fruit in grocery stores is often harvested while green (so produce doesn't bruise during shipping) and ripened artificially, compromising nutritional content. Modern cultivars may also contain fewer nutrients than heritage or heirloom varieties due to aggressive breeding for appearance, productivity, and hardiness rather than nutrition – an issue exacerbated by soil depletion. There is even concern that genetic tinkering may escalate to the point where breeders can manipulate fruit flavors in much the same way that food technologists manipulate flavor now.

Fresh fruit can also be sprayed with chemical coatings to retard shrinkage and hinder spoilage. These invisible films are designed to remain on the fruit while eaten and may trap in contaminants while cementing the illusion that the product is fresh.[6] These coatings lack taste and odor, eluding sensory detection, and typically cannot be removed by scrubbing. In some countries, such coatings are even approved for use on organic fruit. Similarly, the United States Food and Drug Administration allows fresh oranges to be dyed a more intense color[7] to simulate riper fruit. Manufacturers may also infuse fresh or dried fruit with artificial flavors, with creations such as grape-flavored apples or blueberry-flavored cranberries.

Despite these problematic practices – and the increasing advantage of growing your own produce or buying from local suppliers you know and trust – almost all fresh fruit available today delivers reliable flavor-nutrition relationships. It is only when fruit flavors are mimicked and applied elsewhere that problems arise.

What about fruit juices? Some people worry that the concentration of natural sugars and the ease of drinking juice compared to eating whole fruit make juices unsuitable for those with weight loss goals. Yet 100% freshly squeezed juice delivers a wealth of nutritional benefits. For example, fresh citrus juice contains vitamin C and many other nutrients such as potassium and folate. Furthermore, drinking pure orange juice has *not* been found to correlate with obesity.[8] Those undertaking fresh juice 'fasts' (restrictive diets in which only freshly squeezed juices are consumed) typically report weight loss as a side effect.

As an interesting example, the movie *Chimpanzee* (2012) depicts footage of chimpanzees popping handfuls of fruit into their mouths, chewing rapidly to release the juice, before spitting out an enormous wad of fibrous remains. This allows the chimpanzees to quickly access the sugar, vitamins, and other beneficial plant compounds without wasting hours chewing mouthfuls of fiber.

Much of the uncertainty around modern juices exists because there is a wide variety in what constitutes 'juice.' Juice in the grocery store is often heat-treated, with preservatives added to extend shelf life. Additionally, many juices are made from concentrate (making storage and shipping cheaper), which further depletes flavor, vitamins, and phytonutrients[9] (this is why vitamin C is often added back to manufactured juices;

however, the many hundreds of other beneficial compounds naturally occurring in fresh juices are not). Finally, colors and flavoring agents are added to disguise the fact that one is consuming old, cooked juice.

If you boiled a pot of juice on the stove and sealed it within an air-tight bottle, it would indeed be drinkable many months later as a pale, dull liquid (after all, you can preserve fruit in a similar manner). Yet, this old juice would not have the same nutrition, tang, and vitality as freshly squeezed juice.[10] Thus, to compete with the chilled juices available in the refrigerated section of the supermarket (which are far more expensive to ship and sell), manufacturers manipulate the color and flavor of shelf-stable juices, so taste and smell receptors cannot tell the difference.

In retaliation, many fresh juice sellers now add flavors to *their* juices. Luckily, in response to consumer concerns, refrigerated, cold-pressed, genuinely 100% fruit juice is becoming more widely available in some parts of the world.

To understand why freshly squeezed juice is an acceptable addition to the diet, consider a slice of fresh orange versus freshly squeezed orange juice. The flavor of these two items is recognizably different. This is partly due to the change in texture, but it is also because many of the flavors present in the skin, pith, and fibrous membranes of the whole fruit are less prevalent in the juice. The change in flavor thus occurs in a way that is logical, predictable, and consistent across time, directly correlating with the expected change in nutrition. Consequently, the body can learn such flavor-nutrition relationships. At least, it *could* if other juices were not regularly tampered with by manufacturers.

Sun-dried fruit, loaded with natural sugars, is also beneficial and offers a wealth of vitamins, antioxidants, and phytochemicals. Some researchers recommend daily consumption of dried fruit.[11] Raisins, for example, have been found to "lower the postprandial insulin response [...] and promote satiety via leptin and ghrelin."[12] Raisins also provide an excellent source of boron – a micronutrient that plays an important role in bone health.[13] Dried dates provide potassium, magnesium, vitamin B6, boron, and iron – and are a rich source of copper, a trace mineral essential for many bodily functions, including the synthesis of collagen. Much dried fruit available today, of course, is contaminated with sweeteners, flavoring extracts, sprays, and preservatives. However, the genuine foods on their own are beneficial.

Even the most potent natural sources of fructose, such as raw honey, have an extensive body of traditional lore behind them, as well as contemporary science supporting their dietary and medicinal use. Many traditional populations consume liberal quantities of honey. Mbuti pygmies, for example, were described in 1983 as consuming *80% of their diet as honey* for two months of the year.[14] Raw honey is brimming with beneficial compounds,[15] such as pollen, propolis, and other substances that contribute to its antimicrobial and anti-inflammatory properties. Honey is also rich in antioxidants like flavonoids and phenolic acids that help combat oxidative stress.

Similarly, maple syrup is believed to offer numerous benefits,[16] containing minerals like manganese and zinc, as well as antioxidants. Some studies have found that maple syrup has antibacterial compounds that benefit the immune system.[17]

Coconut sugar, made from the sap of coconut palm flowers, also retains nutrients such as potassium, magnesium, and zinc, as well as short-chain fatty acids, polyphenols, and antioxidants.

Jaggery (made from unrefined sugar cane sap – with vitamins and minerals intact) is also believed to deliver numerous health benefits.[18] [19] Cane honey (boiled sugar cane juice, with nothing extracted or added) is lighter and thinner in consistency than molasses and, like jaggery, has abundant phenols (known for their antioxidant properties), which are absent in white sugar.[20] Brown sugar (which is merely white sugar with a small amount of molasses added back in) has a significantly lower phenol count.

Despite recommending that refined sugar be substituted with unrefined sweeteners, one study notes that this has a downside for manufacturers:

> Full replacement of white sugar for the non refined alternatives may not be realistic since, among other reasons, significant changes in the food characteristics such as colour or flavour may be expected.
>
> — LUCÍA SEGUÍ, LAURA CALABUIG-JIMÉNEZ, NOELIA BETORET, AND PEDRO FITO, *PHYSICOCHEMICAL AND ANTIOXIDANT PROPERTIES OF NON-REFINED SUGARCANE ALTERNATIVES TO WHITE SUGAR* (2015)

This quote spells out why refining sweeteners into their molecular building blocks makes them much more useful for manufacturers as a deceptive flavoring agent. If unrefined sweeteners (such as honey or maple syrup) are added to a mixture, a large number of flavor molecules are added (rather than merely glucose, fructose, or sucrose alone). The presence of any natural, unrefined sweetener can thus be *detected by the taste and smell receptors*, with intake guided appropriately.

As Joanna Blythman explains in *Swallow This* (2015), naturally sweet ingredients, like maple syrup or honey, “taste too much of themselves, so they don’t have the neutrality to work in a wide range of products.”

To understand this more clearly, imagine you peel, slice, and cook fresh apples in a little water, serving the freshly stewed fruit in two bowls. In one bowlful, you mix in a spoonful of honey; in the other, you mix in a spoonful of white sugar. Assuming you like and desire stewed apples, both bowlfuls will taste great. However, the first bowlful will also have the *faint taste of honey.*

Adding honey involves not only the addition of sugar but also the many naturally occurring flavor molecules and nutritional elements within honey. As such, the presence of both the apple *and* the honey can be detected by the mouth and nose – with the intensity of each flavor in direct proportion to the volume of each ingredient. The body can thus *accurately predict the incoming nutritional content* and guide you toward consuming the optimal amount from the honey-sweetened bowl.

In the second bowl containing sucrose, however, you now have what appears to be a serving of extra-ripe (and thus extra-nutritious) stewed apple. As the added sucrose is unaccompanied by any other flavor signals, the increased sweetness *appears to be coming from the apple.*

The problem is not with the chemical property of sucrose (or fructose). After all, natural sugars are found within an enormous array of nourishing foods that have been part of the human diet for millennia. The problem comes with *isolating sugar from its source.*

Remember, humans experience flavor as a *pattern*: a memorable combination of molecules – just as a song is a memorable pattern of notes. Sucrose, on its own, means very little – just as a single note or an individual letter of the alphabet means very little on its own. It is only the *pairing of sucrose with other recognizable flavor molecules* that tells the brain: *Ah, I'm eating apple.*

Traditional processing methods are relatively basic and

result in something akin to extracting a verse from a song. Even after squeezing juice from an orange, you are still left with a recognizable flavor pattern. But disassemble those flavor molecules down into their individual notes? You are not left with music. You are left with isolated building blocks that are only useful for *recrafting into something new*.

Refined sugar is not used as an ordinary ingredient but as a flavor-manipulation agent. Sugar itself is not inherently toxic to your cells.[21] But just as water kills you if you drink too much, sugar kills you if you siphon it off and add it to other items on a haphazard basis, making all methods of identifying and discerning reliable flavor patterns impossible.

Refined sucrose was humanity's first deceptive flavor molecule and is likely responsible for the uptick in obesity among wealthy populations in historical times. However, it was not until sucrose was joined by the full cast of other flavor molecules that food-based illusions really got out of hand.

Other refined sweeteners such as aspartame, acesulfame potassium, refined stevia, and sucralose have joined the fold, as have an enormous array of other isolated flavoring chemicals.[22] There is now an endless supply of potential refined sweeteners from countless sources. To be clear, no refined sweetener will ever be 'safe' because the danger comes not from the molecule itself but from the process of *isolating and extracting this from its source*.

Any refined chemical that is added to a food for flavoring purposes deceives the sensors. *All refined sweeteners provide a misleading flavor signal* that attempts to convince the consumer that the modified product is more nourishing than it really is.

Grains, Nuts, Seeds, and Legumes

The seeds of plants have played a fundamental role in human history, with archaeological evidence suggesting that we have eaten grains for a very long time.[23] [24] In some parts of the world, stored grain was the only food available during long winters or famines, hence the proverb that bread is the "staff of life."

But might modern refined grains be problematic? If refined sugar deceives, surely refined white flour is equally deceptive? To understand why this is not the case, consider several key differences between refined sugar and refined flour.

Firstly, refined sugar makes up a tiny percentage of the original cane or beet, whereas white flour comprises 72-75% of the original whole grain.[25] In other words, *most of the grain remains* at the end of the refining process.

A wheat kernel consists of three main elements: the germ, bran, and endosperm. The germ is the part that sprouts and is rich in concentrated fats, vitamins, and minerals. The bran is the protective outer layer of the grain and contains fiber, fats, minerals, vitamins, and other compounds. The endosperm is the middle part of the grain, and it is this that is ground up into white flour.[26]

In contrast to white sugar, which is almost entirely sucrose, white flour contains many substances. In addition to glucose, it includes approximately 12% water, 10% protein (comprising of "many hundreds of individual proteins, which may have structural, metabolic, protective or storage functions,"[27] including gluten), 3% fiber, 1% fat, and trace amounts of other micronutrients. Although this nutritional profile is far less impressive than that of whole grains, white flour is *not* an isolated substance like white sugar.

Secondly, white flour is not useful as a flavor enhancer. Rather than *strengthening* a flavor, adding white flour *dilutes* flavor and makes things blander. Although white flour is a significant ingredient in many deceptive foods – and is found at the scene of the crime, so to speak – its role is as a *cheap calorie substrate* that is flavored and enhanced using *other* things.

If you are unsure about this point, try an experiment: mix up a batch of cookies and divide the dough into two. Mix extra flour into one batch (adding a little water as necessary to keep the moisture level consistent). Once baked, it will become clear that the batch with additional flour tastes inferior – with the concentration of flavorsome ingredients diluted.

Furthermore, while animal studies have shown that refined sugar can cause withdrawal symptoms, such as chattering teeth in rats,[28] the same has *not* been found for white flour.

Although white flour and white rice are poor sources of nutrition compared to many other foods, their *bland flavor accurately reflects this*. In other words, white rice and white flour do not mislead the body about what they contain. When calorie needs are reliably met, bland white flour products lose their allure...*unless they are deceptively flavored.*

There is no doubt that people often lose weight while avoiding wheat; however, it is important to remember that, in such cases, the individual simultaneously excludes the vast majority of flavor-manipulated cakes, cookies, pizza, and so on, making it very difficult to pinpoint whether the weight loss is due to the absence of wheat alone. Even plain wheat products like white bread are often sweetened and manipulated with additives so that the resulting product is fluffier, spongier, and sweeter than it ever would be if made solely with genuine ingredients.

It is also important to remember that white flour is often mixed with far more nourishing ingredients. For example, when eating cookies made from free-range eggs, grass-fed butter, freshly ground organic flour, honey, and ginger, an individual may eat slightly more than they would have done if these ingredients were served on their own. When separate ingredients cannot be *easily disentangled*, accessing the nutrition from a single ingredient is challenging and requires simultaneously consuming those ingredients with which it is mixed. Of course, if such items are only eaten occasionally, this is not a problem, as intake can adjust accordingly over subsequent meals.

However, if someone *constantly* consumes white flour products, where ingredients are pre-mixed with other more nourishing ingredients, a higher calorie intake is likely to result, just as animals who consume pre-mixed feed grow fatter than those who can sort through individual ingredients and navigate toward precisely what they need.[29]

However, this doesn't mean there is anything *addictive* about white flour. No deception has taken place. Sensory mechanisms do not recalibrate; hunger does not climb over the days and weeks to come.

Although some might accept that refined grain is not in the same category as white sugar, isn't it nonetheless advisable to consume *whole grains* due to their higher nutritional content? After all, studies show that rats die more frequently when consuming a diet that is predominantly white rice.[30] Similarly, outbreaks of beriberi (a lethal condition caused by thiamine deficiency) in human prison populations in the early 20th century were reduced when brown rice was substituted for white.[31] [32] [33] [34]

In light of these findings, it might seem obvious that whole grains are superior in every case. Yet, compare the process of removing the bran and germ from a wheat grain with peeling a potato to leave only the white interior. There is nothing inherently wrong with discarding parts of natural foods, *even if these parts are nutritious*. Many fruits and vegetables are peeled before eating, such as bananas and oranges, despite there being many nutrients in these outer layers (and some people *do* eat these peels).

Even rats and mice often pick up individual wheat grains in their paws (holding these in much the same way as humans hold a cob of corn), gnawing through the bran to get at the interior before discarding the remainder with a significant portion of the bran uneaten. If the grain is soaked in advance so the outer layer can be easily peeled off, the mice and rats often do so, discarding even *more* of the bran. When rats eat freshly ground wheat, they sometimes feed almost entirely on the white flour portion, leaving the wheat germ behind. However, *other* colonies of rats (of the same breed) have, at other times, eaten *only* the wheat germ.[35]

This implies that different nutrients are available in each part of the wheat grain, just as there are different nutrients in the skin of an apple compared to the flesh. Depending on your current nutritional needs, these elements may or may not be optimal in different circumstances.

It is also worth noting that, in some people, the high roughage content of wheat bran can cause digestive issues. Whole grains also contain higher amounts of antinutrients, such as phytic acid, which are far more prevalent in the germ and bran and are significantly reduced in white flour.

Antinutrients are named such because they bind to specific nutrients in the digestive tract, reducing absorption. In other words, although whole grains contain many more nutrients than white flour, they simultaneously *lower* the absorption of certain minerals, like calcium, iron, and zinc, by binding to these within the gut. These minerals are then excreted along with the fiber and cannot be used by the body. In his book *Cure Tooth Decay* (2007), Ramiel Nagel makes a compelling case that the antinutrients in whole grains may play a critical role in tooth decay. If sufficient volume is consumed, antinutrients can inhibit digestive enzymes, irritating the gastrointestinal tract.

Oxalates – a particular type of antinutrient present in whole grains, as well as nuts (particularly almonds), seeds, legumes, cocoa, and specific vegetables, such as spinach and beetroot – can contribute to kidney stones, joint pain, and a host of other health complications. Oxalates can pose a surprising threat for dieters who may consume high amounts of almond flour, almond milk, and so on in the name of 'health' – ingesting far higher oxalate volumes than would ever ordinarily be consumed.[36]

Despite the downsides of excessive antinutrient consumption, other studies suggest that antinutrients are *beneficial* in certain doses. For example, wheat germ agglutinin (WGA) – a lectin naturally occurring in wheat and other grains to protect against insect infestation – may have anti-tumor properties.[37] Other studies suggest that phytic acid might have medicinal effects, such as protecting against certain diseases and cancer.[38] It is also worth noting that these antinutrients are present in *almost all plant foods* and have been part of the human diet for millennia.

Legumes, such as beans, lentils, and chickpeas, are also high in antinutrients yet deliver protein, magnesium, potassium, and various B vitamins. The antioxidants and phytonutrients in legumes are linked with lower risks of chronic diseases such as heart disease and certain types of cancer. Many traditional populations consumed diets rich in legumes, such as the Tarahumara Indians, who thrived on a diet heavy in corn and beans.[39]

It is also important to consider that traditional methods of preparing grains and legumes, such as soaking, boiling, and fermenting, often deactivate or reduce these antinutrient compounds.[40] John Douillard notes in *Eat Wheat* (2017) that slow-fermenting sourdough can also break down gluten, making it more digestible.[41]

Many problems attributed to modern wheat consumption may, in fact, stem from harvesting and processing procedures. Modern flours are often bleached using chemicals like chlorine gas and benzoyl peroxide.[42] Bran flakes can also be whitened and pulverized to mimic the texture of white flour.[43] [44] Other manufacturing methods acidify the bran before oxidizing the naturally occurring ferulic acid, so this bitter compound is transformed into vanilla flavor, providing "better flavored bran."[45] Manipulated bran of this type is used to create misleading whole wheat products that appear to be made with white flour. These are often marketed as a cunning way to entice young children to consume whole grains. Of course, young children, like all humans, may have a very valid reason for minimizing intake of these bitter compounds.

Many modern flours are also 'enriched,'[46] whereby some (but not all) of the nutrients lost during the refining process are added back in.[47] In populations with a particular deficiency, enrichment may help in the short term. The difficulty is that (as described in chapter 4: *Supplements and Fortification*) this directly interferes with the learned relationships between flavor and nutrition, and those who are *not* deficient may receive an excessive amount.

Commercial bakeries may also add refined gluten to baked products, particularly those marketed as high-protein. This alters the texture and elasticity of the dough and likely increases the issues for those with gluten sensitivities.

With such a wide range of flour treatments, 'white flour' becomes many different products that often look and taste the same: sometimes ordinary flour, sometimes enriched flour, sometimes high-gluten flour, sometimes whole grain flour disguised as white, and so on. In other words, the relationship between the flavor of white flour and the nutritional outcome becomes intermittent.

Luckily, other grains, such as oats and barley, are not yet manipulated to the same degree. However, another serious issue affects almost all grain crops: glyphosate absorption.

Glyphosate, the active ingredient in common herbicides, works by inhibiting an enzyme pathway essential for plant growth, killing the plant to which it is applied. Ordinarily, herbicides are sprayed onto a field to eliminate weeds prior to planting. However, in the case of grains, glyphosate is used as a desiccant. This means it is often applied *directly to the crop* before harvest. This is a useful strategy for the grower because when a plant detects that it is dying, it *immediately ripens all seeds* in a last-ditch attempt to get its genes into a new round of the game.

If a crop ripens naturally, each grain matures at a slightly different rate. As individual grains are tiny and threshing machines are enormous, harvesting only the mature grain and leaving behind the rest is impractical. Applying a desiccant solves this problem and ensures that *all grains ripen in unison*, significantly increasing crop yield.

Unfortunately, dousing an entire crop with glyphosate just prior to harvest leads to the individual grains soaking up the herbicide "like a sponge."[48] Because glyphosate is absorbed predominantly by the outer layers of the grain, whole-grain products are far more problematic in this regard.

Tests routinely find glyphosate contamination in grain products. *The 2015/2016 Report on Pesticides in Fresh and Frozen Produce*,[49] carried out by the Ministry for Primary Industries in New Zealand, for example, found that 20 out of 60 wheat samples tested had glyphosate levels exceeding permitted amounts. This may be one reason why a growing percentage of people appear to be developing wheat allergies.

Organic food is expensive, but grains are one area where this is very wise. Bear in mind, however, that not all products sold as organic actually are. A 2019 research report by *Consumer*, for example, found that a New Zealand grower of 'organic' barley was contaminated with glyphosate and had their organic status revoked.[50] Even organic growers with good intentions may find it difficult to ensure their products are herbicide-free due to the drift of spray from other farms.

Herbicides are not usually applied to rice as a desiccant; however, rice is grown in water-saturated conditions and may be irrigated with arsenic-contaminated water, which is then absorbed by the rice plants.[51] Because arsenic is stored primarily in the outer layers of the grain, white rice may also be safer in this respect.

After all of this information, you may remain very uncertain about whether eating whole grains or refined grains is best. This is because the situation is fraught with conflicting data.

Eating is complicated. Foods can be beneficial in one way while delivering harm in another. The *net gain* is ultimately what matters. With so many variables and individual differences in nutritional needs, the best solution is to let your taste buds guide you. If you *like* whole grains, eat them. If you do not, do not. But remember that the body can only make these distinctions accurately when flavor signals are reliable.

Freshly milled organic flour is a genuine food – whether it is white or whole grain. So, too, is white rice, brown rice, oats, legumes, nuts, and seeds – as long as these have not been chemically interfered with or tainted with added flavors.

Humans have been successfully eating grains, nuts, seeds, and legumes for thousands of years. The issue arises when these foods are altered with isolated chemicals, introducing misleading molecular signals.

Vegetables and Tubers

There are no known traditional human populations that completely avoid all plants. Even the Inuit, who traditionally consume a diet heavy in meat and fat, eat more plants than was previously thought, including kelp, Arctic sorrel, willow leaves, lichen, and the stomach contents of herbivores.[52]

As with grains and legumes, starch-rich vegetables, such as corn and potatoes, played a critical role in human history. Kumara, a sweet potato, was a traditional dietary staple of the Maori people in New Zealand.[53] Many other traditional populations, such as those in Europe, relied heavily upon potatoes.[54] A study in 1928 noted that potatoes and bread were the main foods consumed by rural populations in Poland and Russia and described these people as healthy and hard-working.[55]

Like grains, tubers store well for a long time. Whereas grains are seeds, potatoes and kumara are the living roots of plants. When stored in their whole form, these foods remain *alive* – and are hence rich in many vitamins and minerals.

With the uptick in ketogenic and carnivore diets, fears about plant foods abound. Nightshades – which include tomatoes, potatoes, eggplant, capsicums, and peppers, as well as spices like paprika and cayenne – are sometimes avoided due to fears about alkaloid content, which, when consumed to excess, may contribute to inflammation, arthritis, and autoimmune disorders. Other individuals report digestive discomfort when consuming nightshades.

When evaluating this category of food, however, it is important to realize that nightshade vegetables are repeatedly consumed alongside deceptive ingredients. Tomato-based pasta sauces or ketchup, for example, frequently contain added flavoring agents and extracts, as well as refined sweeteners.

Many people have never tasted a sun-ripened tomato directly picked from a garden – nor experienced the difference between the tasteless, bland varieties available in supermarkets and those that are grown in natural conditions. Even canned tomatoes often contain an acidity regulator – a broad category of chemicals that are added to foods to adjust the "sour or sharp taste"[56] and to inhibit the growth of certain bacteria. A tiny amount of acidity regulator within a can of tomatoes is likely a minor issue in the larger scheme of things. However, organic cans of tomatoes (containing only tomatoes) often cost only a few cents more, making these products a logical and obvious choice when budget allows.

Many vegetables are also feared for their starch content and impact on blood sugar levels. Yet, recall how followers of potato-only diets (as discussed in chapter 7: *Insulin Resistance*) often report the opposite effect: a lowering of insulin levels.

It is also interesting to discover that modern humans have much more amylase in saliva than chimpanzees (this protein helps digest starch, which is coded for by the AMY1 gene). Whereas chimpanzees have two copies of this gene, humans have between 5.5 and 15 (the variation depends upon ethnicity – and whether one's ancestors consumed a starch-rich diet).[57] The implication is that humans are well-suited to consuming starchy foods. (A chimpanzee diet, by comparison, primarily consists of fruit and young tree leaves supplemented with insects, eggs, and meat. Chimpanzees may spend up to 80% of each day eating in order to obtain sufficient nutrition from this diet.)[58]

Fresh potatoes are a powerhouse of nutrition. They are rich in vitamin C and contain potassium, B vitamins, antioxidants, and even some protein.[59] They are also rich in copper. Despite this, dieters often condemn potatoes – sometimes because they are a nightshade, sometimes because they are high in starch, sometimes because they are a source of carbohydrates, and sometimes because they are the same color as white flour, white rice, and white sugar. Yet, the problem is not with genuine potatoes but with what manufacturers *do* to these things.

Some might suspect that the primary issue with manufactured potato products is that they are drenched in refined seed oils, but the problem goes far deeper than this. A growing number of potato products are reformed from dried potato flakes or dehydrated powder that is mixed to form a sludge that is extruded, fabricated, and shaped. This dehydrated potato mix is used to create a variety of 'composite potato products,' such as croquettes, dumplings, and so on. These creations often include binding agents and "fibrous cellulosic material" to increase the perceived crispiness.[60]

After a lengthy manufacturing process, dehydrated potato tastes nothing like fresh potatoes. The resulting mixture is bland and may have unpleasant off-flavors.[61] This is particularly a problem when using offcuts that don't make the premium potato product grade (and hence go through a much longer processing journey). These aged potato derivatives are in dire need of flavor-enhancement, with the resulting items described within industry patents as "relatively flavorless particles that are bound together in a watery mass" with "only passing resemblance to real potato..."[62]

The solution? Trusty flavor molecules are brought out once again. These ensure that the aged potato product does not develop "an objectionable flavor totally unrelated to natural potato flavor." Unlike a fresh potato, which is rich in nutrition, the flavor of these deficient products must be masked and disguised so that taste and smell receptors do not detect the substitution.

Favoring agents can even be isolated from potatoes themselves. For example, one patent, first filed in 1973, describes the process of extracting potato flavor from potatoes using a water and alcohol solvent. A resin attracts and absorbs the flavoring compounds before another solvent releases the flavor from the resin.[63]

Some individuals really *are* intolerant or allergic to various plant compounds. But consider how your genes would have navigated this scenario historically. Your ancestors could not read a book to inform them about the presence of antinutrients or nightshades. All they had to operate with was food-based traditions and wisdom passed down through the generations. How would an individual know if they were intolerant to a commonly consumed food?

They would know the same way that all living creatures know: by associating survival outcomes with the prior ingestion. In other words, they would develop flavor preferences – *likes and dislikes* – based on learned experiences with a particular flavor. Parents quickly discover that despite being raised in the same household and exposed to the same food traditions, individual children often acquire quite unique food preferences, which may morph and change with time. One child may love sweet potatoes; another may despise them. Some may hate peas so much that they are picked out of a dish one by one. Another may ravenously swallow green vegetables without a speck of complaint.

Potatoes, tubers, and all other vegetables, whether peeled, unpeeled, mashed, boiled, fried, or baked, are genuine, nourishing foods that deliver reliable flavor-nutrition relationships. These foods have nourished humans for thousands of years. In almost all cases, the problem is not with the genuine item – but the *distorted flavor-nutrition patterns* that are prevalent in the modern food environment.

Animal Products and Saturated Fat

Just as no known human populations consume a diet totally devoid of plants, no traditional human diet is totally devoid of animal products. In fact, many cultures revere animal foods, with every part of the animal used, including the hide, horns, organs, and offal – so nothing is wasted.

Nowadays, animal products are often surrounded by controversy. Part of this controversy relates to saturated fat, which is prevalent in a great number of animal foods.

Since the mid-1970s, saturated fats have been linked with heart disease,[64] with officials suggesting people limit their intake of fatty meat, eggs, and dairy. However, a growing number of studies indicate that this fear of saturated fat is unfounded.[65] [66] [67] Despite this new evidence, the field remains rife with opposing viewpoints, and outspoken experts continue to promote the idea that saturated fat is detrimental to health.[68]

Why such conflicting viewpoints? One possibility is that saturated fat might be beneficial in certain amounts but detrimental when consumed to excess (as with almost every other survival reward). Another possibility is that the heavy prevalence of saturated fats within *manufactured foods* might confound the data.[69] In other words, perhaps saturated fats are condemned by association.

It is well-known, for example, that many mass-produced foods contain high amounts of *trans fats* in addition to saturated fats. Trans fats are found within partially hydrogenated oils. Hydrogenation is a chemical process[70] in which hydrogen is added to refined, bleached, and sometimes deodorized plant oils in the presence of a metal catalyst[71] so that the liquid oil turns into a solid fatty product containing trans fats.[72] Trans fats have commonly been used within margarine, table spreads, pies, cookies, cakes, bread, ice cream, frosting, confectioneries, and fast food, often replacing or accompanying traditional fats, such as butter and lard. Many manufacturers prefer partially hydrogenated plant oil because it is inexpensive, offers increased shelf life, and has reduced refrigeration needs. Trans fats can also be used for deep-frying for long durations without turning rancid.

Once trans fat is added to processed foods, flavorings, such as those that impart the fragrance of butter,[73] help to disguise the substitution.

Although trans fats are being phased out in some countries due to health concerns, the integration of these manmade fats has complicated the interpretation of saturated fat studies. One study that attempted to separate the effects of saturated fats from trans fats, for example, found that there was "no convincing association" between saturated fat and death from cardiovascular disease but that there *was* an association between *trans fat* and cardiovascular death.[74] [75] In monkeys, trans fat consumption increases abdominal fat, even without caloric excess.[76]

Almost all experts now agree that trans fats are detrimental to human health. According to the FDA, partially hydrogenated oils are no longer recognized as safe, and American food manufacturers have been instructed to remove these from the food supply.[77]

Another variable that complicates the saturated fat argument is that those who examine 'high red meat intake' often do not distinguish between meat that is minimally processed versus meat products that are combined with numerous fillers, preservatives, and flavoring agents.

Animal products may also be demonized because they are often high in calories in general. However, it is critical to note that calories, in and of themselves, are not the enemy. All lifeforms *need* energy. No one can survive on protein, vitamins, and minerals alone. The issue is not whether an individual food is high in calories but whether it *satiates appetite, rather than escalating it*. Eating a food that is higher in calories is thus not a problem if it causes overall food intake to stabilize at an optimal level.

Abandoning high-calorie food sources is particularly problematic if these provide essential nutrients that are difficult to source elsewhere. There is no point in consuming a light salad as a dinner meal, for example, if doing so leaves the individual aggravated with hunger and more likely to overeat later. Satiation only occurs when the body *has what it needs.*

Fred Provenza describes what happened to early Arctic explorers who found themselves with only lean rabbit to consume:

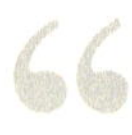

> No matter how much they gorged on rabbit, they were unremittingly hungry. After just seven days, explorers were eating three to four times more rabbit than at the beginning of the week, and by day ten the swelling of their distended bellies was visible through layers of clothing. When they ate only lean meat, they became ravenous for fat. They were attempting to eat enough fat, present only in low amounts in rabbit, by overeating rabbit. Given a chance, they'd eat a large quantity of pure fat, even oily fat, without nausea. Without fat, they died a few weeks later.
>
> — FRED PROVENZA, *NOURISHMENT: WHAT ANIMALS CAN TEACH US ABOUT REDISCOVERING OUR NUTRITIONAL WISDOM* (2018)

In his book *Nutrition and Physical Degeneration* (1939), dentist

Weston Price analyzed the teeth, jaws, and facial bone structure of isolated populations around the globe. His work was particularly valuable because he conducted this analysis just as modern 'store' foods (such as refined sugar, jams, canned goods, and vegetable fats) were reaching these parts of the world. Price could thus contrast people consuming traditional diets with their relatives in nearby villages who consumed a Westernized diet.

Price found, time and time again, that those consuming their original diet were in robust physical health with cheerful, smiling natures and strong, white teeth that were largely absent of decay (despite not owning toothbrushes or having access to dentists). In contrast, those who ate store food had rampant cavities, narrow facial structures, and crowded teeth, with poor resistance to disease. (His findings are accompanied by photographs that communicate these striking changes in ways that words do not.)

Shockingly, Price found that dramatic dental and bone structure changes often occurred *within a single generation* after parents abandoned traditional foods.

If children were born before the introduction of Westernized foods they had good teeth and wide jawbones, whereas younger siblings, born to those same parents after the introduction of modern foods, had far more cavities, narrower faces, and crowded teeth.

Price concluded that an important "vitamin-like activator" was present in the full-fat milk, butter, cheese, fatty fish, and fatty meats that the traditional populations consumed and that this factor was missing in store foods. This crucial nutrient is now believed to be Vitamin K2, which is different from the Vitamin K1 present in plants such as spinach, kale, and broccoli. (The human gut microbiota can convert some vitamin K1 into vitamin K2; however, vitamin K2 – available predominantly from animal foods – is considered more bioavailable.)[78] Vitamin K2 is also present in some fermented plant foods like sauerkraut (fermented cabbage) and natto (fermented soybeans).

Nowadays, adequate vitamin K2 intake is understood to be associated with reduced cardiovascular risks, including lower rates of aortic calcification,[79] while also promoting calcium retention in teeth and bones.[80]

When Price returned home, he treated his patients with mineral-rich bone broths (including bone marrow), cod liver oil, and "high-activator" butter oil from grass-fed cows. He found that many of his patients reversed dental cavities. In other words, once an optimal diet was consumed, the teeth naturally resealed and remineralized. These findings are echoed by Steven Lin in his book, *The Dental Diet* (2018).

Price also conducted studies on saliva and found that consumption of Vitamin K2 altered the saliva and bacteria count (the oral microbiome) so that it helped to protect against tooth decay. This may explain why a common complaint from long-term vegan dieters is sensitive teeth and dental decay.[81]

When people consider a 'nutrient-dense' diet, they often think of fruit and vegetables, but animal products are also very nutritionally dense.[82] Not only are these foods rich in protein and essential amino acids (critical for cell function, as well as repairing and building the body),[83] but nutrients found in animal foods are often far more bioavailable than their equivalent in plant foods. Heme iron, for example, abundant in red meat, fish, and poultry (but not dairy products and eggs), is much more readily absorbed than the non-heme iron in plant foods.

Chicken skin, pork crackling, salmon skin, beef tallow, pork lard, duck fat, and dairy fats are laden with essential fatty acids, vitamins, and minerals. Along with bone broth and bone marrow, these foods are rich in collagen, supporting skin elasticity[84] – something that may be of particular benefit for those aiming to lose weight. (Vitamin C-rich fruits and vegetables also help with the body's natural collagen production.)

Animals raised in their natural habitat contain the most nutrients of all, such as grass-fed meat, free-range chicken, and wild-caught seafood. For example, pigs raised in the sunshine have much more vitamin D in their lard. Vitamin K2 is also higher in cheeses and butter from grass-fed cows (the more naturally yellow/orange the butter is, the more vitamin K2 it has). Similarly, free-range eggs, with bright orange yolks, are higher in nourishment. The animal's diet also influences the nutritional profile and perceived flavor of the meat,[85] as does the breed of the animal (heritage chickens are reported to have superior flavor, for example).[86]

Because some humans are lactose intolerant, it is often argued that cows' milk is not an optimal food. However, this should be considered from the alternative perspective. The ability to digest lactose would only have spread so rapidly through the human population *if it conferred a distinct survival advantage*. In other words, those who *can* digest milk should embrace this awesome capability.

Over 90% of people from the British Isles and Scandinavia and over 30% of the population worldwide can drink cows' milk without difficulty.[87] (Interestingly, those who cannot digest milk from ordinary cows may tolerate milk from 'A2' cows, which have a different gene set – *Devil in the Milk* (2009) by Keith Woodford offers more information about this fascinating topic.)

Dairy products are not just good sources of vitamin K2 but are rich in calcium, fats, and protein, as well as numerous other vitamins and minerals. Dairy fats, like other animal fats, are beneficial for skin elasticity and hydration, as well as for supporting the structural integrity of skin and nails. Butter provides essential nutrients like Vitamin A, as well as beneficial fatty acids, including conjugated linoleic acid and butyrate, which can promote gut health. Like other natural fats, butter also helps with the absorption of fat-soluble vitamins from other foods.

The issue is not with the genuine versions of these things but with the manufactured counterparts. Let us contrast and compare just a few.

We have already touched upon how butter can be made more buttery by adding diacetyl (see chapter 4: *Strengthening Flavor*). Margarine and other fatty table spreads also contain yellow colorings and fake butter flavors,[88] so the thickened white plant fat more closely resembles its genuine counterpart. If people could detect what these substances really tasted like, they would likely never be consumed.

Genuine cheeses are highly nourishing and have been enjoyed by humans for thousands of years. Modern varieties available in supermarkets are often made in the same way – from a handful of ingredients: milk, salt, and rennet (an enzyme to coagulate the milk, originally sourced from the stomach of animals), with specific cultures or bacteria added to aid fermentation. Other cheeses, however – particularly those that are pre-sliced – include an assortment of extracts, emulsifiers, preservatives, colors, and unspecified flavor enhancers.

Yogurts that are traditionally made from milk fermented with a live bacterial culture are also highly nourishing. Unfortunately, as with flavored milk and many milk substitutes, yogurts are often spiked with refined sweeteners, emulsifiers, synthetic vitamins, flavors, and flavor-masking solutions.

Assorted dairy flavorings can also be used to strengthen a product's sweetness and milk-like fragrance. For example, one patent notes that a milky flavoring is useful for disguising "imported raw materials that are cheap and inferior in quality" and compensating when natural dairy ingredients are reduced.[89]

Whereas traditional bone broths – created by simmering meaty bones and joints in water – create nourishing bases for slow-cooked soups and stews (particularly beneficial for the natural gelatin and collagen content), most modern stocks and bone broths – typically sold in liquid, pill, cube, or powdered form – contain heavy doses of added flavor, colors, and extracts.

In a similar vein, protein powders, such as those marketed toward bodybuilders, are isolated from their original source and create an enormous raft of unpredictable flavor combinations – such as blueberry-flavored protein powder.

Refined proteins are also used to create plant-based 'meats,' simulating the texture, appearance, and flavor of animal flesh. Unlike a traditional chickpea patty, these are counterfeits in the true sense of the word. Engineered within a laboratory, these plant-based deceptions use advanced technologies and biochemistry to mimic the taste, aroma, and fibrous structure of meat. Numerous patents detail the lengths undertaken to achieve an appropriate mouthfeel and to replicate characteristics such as 'brothy' and 'bloody' in a wide range of products, mimicking a broad range of flavors from beef to bison.[90] These plant-based 'meats' are designed to mimic the sensory characteristics of both raw and cooked meat and sometimes even mimic the "red-to-brown" transition while cooking.[91] This deception is cemented at every level, with numerous added flavorings.

These patents make it blindingly clear that these products are not traditional recipes whipped up by a passionate plant-based cook but are the result of complex chemical reactions and molecular wizardry. These mass-produced counterfeits isolate refined plant proteins from their source, "resulting in pure, de-colored, de-odored protein."[92] These imitation products are created from the ground up by "breaking down non-animal materials into their constituent parts and reassembling those parts."[93]

One patent that details a method for creating plant-based mince notes that the "meat dough" can be boiled in a broth of "flavors and off-flavor masking agents," which absorb into the dough. This patent also describes using "solution spun protein fibers" to create "connective tissue replicas."[94]

Manipulation of this type leads to intermittent reinforcement at an extreme scale. Unsurprisingly, preliminary studies investigating the impact of plant-based 'meat' consumption on rats suggest concerning outcomes.[95]

Animal products are a vital part of the human diet. It is not the genuine meats, fish, animal fat, or dairy products that are the problem, but the distortion and mimicry of these foods.

Herbs, Spices, and Condiments

Let's now discuss how modern flavor manipulation differs from adding herbs and spices to a meal. Whereas commercial flavoring techniques involve the addition of isolated chemicals, herbs and spices are minimally processed pieces of plants. For example, garlic and ginger are roots; coriander and cumin are seeds; oregano and chives are leaves; and cinnamon is bark from a tree. Adding these items to meals is not the addition of a single chemical alone but the addition of many hundreds of chemicals that naturally occur in that part of the plant, many of which have nutritional and medicinal properties.

Joseph Henrich, professor of human evolutionary biology at Harvard University, explains in his book *The Secret of Our Success* (2015) that many spices, along with onions, chili, and garlic, have antimicrobial properties and act as natural fungicides, killing food-borne pathogens. In her book *This is Your Brain on Parasites*

(2017), Kathleen McAuliffe describes how every single one of 30 spices tested by scientists was found to inhibit the growth of various bacteria – with the most common spices (including oregano and allspice) being so potent they killed every bacterium they were exposed to. McAuliffe notes that common combinations of spices – such as curry powder – are particularly powerful in this regard.

As discussed in chapter 3: *The Role of Flavor*, human food preferences are shaped and molded by experience.[96] Flavors that reliably lead to positive outcomes (such as the absence of pathogens) are more likely to be preferred. This wisdom is subsequently embodied within traditional recipes and food customs,[97] explaining why cultures in hotter climates often feature more heavily spiced foods, as this helped to protect against the consequences of food spoilage in times before refrigeration.

Other common condiments, such as fresh citrus juices, are gaining recognition for their potential health benefits. For example, the citric acid in lemon juice helps to deactivate oxalates (oxalates are a common antinutrient found in plant foods – see chapter 8: *Grains, Nuts, Seeds, and Legumes*). Similarly, raw unfiltered fermented vinegars, such as apple cider vinegar, contain the 'mother' – a cloudy substance that contains beneficial live bacteria and enzymes. The acetic acid in vinegar may also help regulate blood sugar levels, aid digestion, and act as an antimicrobial.

Salt is another common seasoning. Unrefined salts, like pink Himalayan salt or Celtic sea salt, contain sodium chloride (the main constituent of salt) as well as numerous trace minerals, such as calcium, magnesium, and potassium[98] (and occasionally pollutants from marine environments).[99] Many of these trace minerals are removed during the modern refining process to create common table salts.[100] Modern table salts may also include additives, such as anti-caking agents, and are commonly iodized through an industrial process. While Himalayan salt contains some natural iodine, unrefined sea salts can have added kelp (a rich iodine source).

Salt is essential for humans[101] and is so vital that it is provided to infants via breastmilk. Like all essential nutrients, there is an optimal intake, above and below which complications occur.

Modern dietary recommendations focus heavily on the dangers of overconsumption – noting that excessive salt intake is associated with high blood pressure (a risk factor for cardiovascular disease) and, at the extremes, salt poisoning.[102] Yet cardiovascular research scientist James DiNicolantonio argues in his book *The Salt Fix* (2017) that modern low-salt recommendations are misguided and that salt is not the villain it is made out to be. He reminds readers that salt is essential for various aspects of human health, including blood pressure regulation and overall metabolic function. DiNicolantonio contends that many people actually consume insufficient salt.

Low sodium levels in the blood lead to attention deficits and a tendency to stumble or fall. Extremely low sodium concentrations can lead to swelling of fluid in the brain and death.[103] In other words, although we are commonly advised to *reduce* our salt intake, having too little salt is also dangerous and problematic.

As we might suspect, the body has a clever system for ensuring the correct salt intake. The learned relationship between salty flavors at the mouth and the amount of salt that arrives in the gut influences the desire for salty flavors going forward. At each meal, the amount of salt is perceived as tasting just right, too salty, or not salty enough,[104] guiding an individual toward the optimal salt intake.

Two separate types of salty taste receptors have so far been identified. When sodium chloride enters the mouth, it dissolves in saliva and breaks down into sodium ions and chloride ions. The sodium ions slot into the first kind of salt receptor, sending signals to the brain that sodium is entering the body (the presence of the chloride ions also plays a role in a way that isn't yet understood).[105] We experience this as a *salty taste.*

Little is known about the second type of salt receptor. It appears that sodium ions trigger this receptor, as does potassium chloride[106] and calcium.[107] These molecules may hence trigger the perception of a salty taste, even if the first salt sensor type is blunted. Interestingly, all three of these elements are naturally present in unrefined salt, as well as in many animal foods. MSG (which contains glutamic acid and sodium) also results in an increased perception of saltiness.[108]

Like herbs and spices, salt has strong antimicrobial properties. This leads to refined salt being used heavily in processed foods. Combined with fears about high-salt intake, manufacturers set about devising strategies to deliver a salty flavor while reducing the amount of salt. This task initially proved very challenging. Unlike sweet flavors, which can be easily mimicked,[109] it was difficult to locate another substance that could communicate a salty taste (lithium fits into the same receptor but is not useful due to its harmful pharmacological effects). MSG is now frowned upon by consumers – and, because of its affinity with savory products, is generally unsuitable for sweet products. Potassium chloride, as noted above, also tastes salty, but this can result in the product tasting too bitter, so has limited usefulness.

Undeterred, manufacturers went to spectacular lengths to create 'mock salts.' For example, one approach involves coating starch particles with salt so the outside appears to be an ordinary salt crystal, but the inside is not. Another approach, detailed within *Strategies to Reduce Sodium Intake in the United*

States (2010) by the US Institute of Medicine, involves low-salt emulsions that consist of "water droplets dispersed in fat droplets that are then dispersed in another outer layer of water that contains salt."[110] Such tactics boost the volume of the salt product, yet only the outer layer – the bit that interacts with taste receptors – contains salt. Companies have also filed patents detailing how "saltiness enhancers"[111] can exaggerate or magnify the flavor of salt.[112]

The aim of these strategies is to fool the taste buds into believing that a higher volume of salt is incoming when it is not. As with all forms of deception, this creates a confusing and intermittent relationship between salty flavors and the amount of salt that arrives in the gut. This deception is immediately revealed when the food is digested, whereupon the relationship between salty flavor and salt is recalibrated, encouraging the pursuit of ever more salty flavors. In other words, like every other form of sensory manipulation, deceptive low-sodium products drive engagement higher.

Special Occasion Foods

Across the course of history, humans have celebrated with extravagant meals. These celebratory feasts often mirrored the natural rhythms of agricultural cycles. For example, a traditional Thanksgiving feast celebrates a bountiful harvest. Traditional feasts often involved an array of genuine foods, incorporating seasonal or rare ingredients that were only available at specific times of the year or expensive ingredients that were too costly for everyday use. These celebrations also featured decorative or complicated dishes, crafted using specialized cooking methods reserved for special occasions due to their labor-intensive nature. They also included a greater number of dishes, with families and communities pooling resources and catering for a larger number of guests.

Although traditional celebrations typically included a wider range of food than usual, what they didn't include was factory-made products with precision-engineered flavor profiles.

Consider the difference between a packaged cookie made from partially hydrogenated vegetable fats, chemically bleached flours, dried-fruit-like solids, sucrose, emulsifiers, and a range of unspecified flavoring solutions...versus a home-baked cookie made from free-range eggs, grass-fed butter, freshly ground organic wheat, honey, spices, and sun-dried fruit. The former is a pale charade of the latter.

Similarly, contrast a bowl of manufactured ice cream made from sucrose, 'milk solids-non-fat,'[113] trace berry fragments that are artificially strengthened in flavor and volume, emulsifiers, vegetable gums, acidity regulators, colorings, and an assortment of unspecified flavorings...versus a bowl of freshly whipped cream, freshly picked berries, and a drizzle of raw honey. The former is an empty mirage: an illusory, sensory façade.

These modern mass-produced counterfeits are not only cheap, readily available, and consumed with little (if any) preparation, but are marketed aggressively via pervasive advertising campaigns that seek to reassure society that the consumption of these counterfeits is an ordinary part of human life. Though our ancestors never once encountered such phenomena, it can seem that consuming these misleading delicacies is the normal way for humans to celebrate.

Luckily, it is very straightforward to create nourishing flavor-honest cakes, cookies, and other special occasion foods using authentic, genuine ingredients – for example, using honey or coconut sugar for a sweetener. It is more than possible to spread a table with a wide range of delicious, flavor-honest fare – sweet fruits, grapes, watermelon, cheeses, unsweetened pickles, salmon, crispy chicken wings, little homemade mince pies, homemade pizza, and so on. Peer expectations for heavily manufactured items at children's birthday parties may complicate things; however, it is still possible to ensure that celebrations involve predominantly nourishing, flavor-honest food.

Something else must be understood about many modern celebratory food products – something important. Many modern party foods are chocolate-flavored. These items not only include potent flavor manipulation but introduce another form of molecular mimicry.

Neurochemical Mimicry

Thus far, we have looked in detail at the intermittent reinforcement that arises in response to the manipulation of flavor. However, a growing number of deceptive foods also contain molecules that mimic neurotransmitters, such as caffeine. Manufacturers view 'energy drinks,' soft drinks, and various chocolate and coffee-flavored products as particularly suitable for this type of manipulation.

> It would be appealing to many consumers to eat chocolate to enhance their mood rather than, for example, to take prescription medicines.
>
> — CONOPCO INC PATENT APPLICATION US20090285947A1, *FROZEN CONFECTIONERY PRODUCTS* (2009) [TRANSLATED FROM PORTUGUESE]

Although many people are aware of the effects of drinking coffee and take care to minimize intake, far less is known about the inclusion of caffeine within food. In high doses, caffeine can induce jitteriness, irritability, hostility, anxiety, headaches, tremors, rapid or erratic heartbeats, blood pressure changes, liver and kidney injury, psychotic symptoms, disorientation, vomiting, diarrhea, seizures, and even death.[114] [115] [116] [117] Hospital visits provoked by caffeine are increasing[118] [119] due to the growing use of refined caffeine within the food supply and sports supplements, prompting a tightening of regulations in some countries.[120] Despite these regulatory changes, there often remains a lack of clarity due to the blurry boundaries between medicine, supplements, sports drinks, and food. This confusion allows companies in some jurisdictions to classify products as 'dietary supplements' despite being sold alongside virtually identical items that are classed as 'food.'[121]

It is also critical to note that rules regarding caffeine disclosure typically apply only to products with *added* caffeine.[122] For example, a chocolate-flavored product that includes cocoa (a powder made from cacao beans, which naturally contains caffeine) does not need to declare the presence of caffeine on the label – only the ingredient itself, cocoa, must be specified.

At first glance, this does not seem to be a problem. After all, the amount of caffeine naturally occurring within cacao beans is low. In normal circumstances, someone would have to consume a copious amount of dark chocolate to come close to matching the caffeine intake from coffee. However, as is no doubt becoming obvious, ingredients can be refined, strengthened, and reformulated in a myriad of different ways that escape general consumer detection.

Before we discuss strategies for strengthening the concentration of caffeine, we need to examine another active component within cocoa: theobromine. Theobromine is chemically similar to caffeine and, like caffeine, slots into adenosine receptors but occupies a different sub-type (there are four known types of adenosine receptors).

Theobromine is often described as having a 'milder' effect than caffeine, but it is more accurate to say theobromine has a different and partially unknown effect. For example, theobromine affects blood pressure in a different way than caffeine, but the reason for this is unknown.[123] It is also worth noting that theobromine is chemically similar to pentoxifylline,[124] a synthetic drug used to improve blood flow in certain medical conditions.

One study found that when people consumed theobromine, heart rate increased in a dose-dependent fashion.[125] Another study suggested that while caffeine temporarily increases alertness and blood pressure, theobromine *decreases* blood pressure. Hence, when caffeine and theobromine are consumed in tandem (as often occurs with manufactured chocolate products), these blood pressure effects may cancel each other out.[126] One patent describes how the amount of theobromine in foods must be carefully balanced with caffeine to counteract the "significant but transient increase in blood pressure."[127]

Theobromine makes up approximately 2% of cocoa powder by weight on average (and caffeine 0.2% by weight). To increase the amount of theobromine in a product would ordinarily involve adding more cocoa. However, because only so much cocoa can be incorporated before a mixture becomes too stiff to stir, aerate, or pour,[128] there is an incentive for manufacturers to find inventive ways to concentrate these molecules to achieve the desired effect.[129]

One patent details a process by which manufacturers can increase the amount of caffeine and theobromine in frozen desserts without needing to increase the volume of cocoa. Strategies include concentrating these stimulants within potent chocolate-like coatings, wave or spiral sauces, toppings, nuggets, or gritty elements, which can be offset and masked by the sweetness of surrounding areas. This patent explains that if the gritty parts within the ice cream are small enough, many of these are swallowed whole, so the unpleasant flavor is undetected. The textural contrast of the gritty elements may also distract consumers from the bitter taste.[130] These tactics allow manufacturers to increase these stimulants within a product without consumer detection.

Another patent describes a taste comparison between stimulant-strengthened ice cream and chocolate bars containing a similar level of concentrated theobromine and caffeine. The patent notes that only half of the volunteers could finish the chocolate due to its extremely bitter taste. Yet, 100% of those who consumed the stimulant-strengthened ice cream rated its flavor positively.[131] This is because while the bitterness of caffeine and theobromine ordinarily curtails intake, when these chemicals are concealed within textural pellets within ice cream, there are no such issues.

Whereas chocolate-flavored ice cream might ordinarily contain 70mg of theobromine and 3mg of caffeine per 100g, the methods described above allow the creation of frozen desserts that contain up to *700mg of theobromine and 70mg of caffeine per 100g of product*[132] – an increase of over ten-fold.

To put this in perspective, the FDA says that, on average, one cup of coffee contains 80-100mg of caffeine (though some brands contain much more than this). A cup of this stimulant-strengthened ice cream thus has more caffeine than an average cup of coffee. It also contains over *1,400mg of theobromine* (adverse mood effects have been found above 500mg,[133] and there is very little known about toxicity levels or consequences of long-term usage).

How widespread is this kind of manipulation? We can only speculate. It is impossible to tell because there is no legal requirement to declare substances that are naturally derived from an ingredient that appears on the label, as long as these are delivered within that same ingredient.[134]

These products deliver a double whammy of deception – both flavor deception and neurochemical deception. It is no surprise at all that chocolate and ice cream rank near the very top of the list in surveys about the most addictive foods.[135] [136] These goods are openly designed to be "mood-enhancing."[137] The unfortunate reality, however, is that, like all so-called artificial mood-enhancing substances, they systematically degrade mood as the bodily recalibration kicks in.

Is it sensationalist to describe derivatives of cocoa and coffee beans in this way? Surely there are benefits to consuming caffeine and theobromine in small doses? After all, some studies have found associations between caffeine use and reduced cognitive decline. Other research suggests that cocoa is anti-inflammatory, rich in minerals,[138] and has a high antioxidant count, providing an abundant supply of dietary polyphenols. Some studies propose that cocoa might positively impact the cardiovascular system, improving "blood pressure, insulin resistance, and vascular and platelet function."[139] Another study found that the consumption of dark chocolate reduces platelet aggregation,[140] the process by which blood cells clump together to form blood clots. (Excessive platelet aggregation can lead to unwanted clotting in blood vessels, causing heart attacks and strokes. However, platelet aggregation is also a crucial mechanism for stopping bleeding when you get injured – hence, a delicate balance is required.) Another meta-analysis found that reductions in blood pressure following cocoa administration were akin to that achieved by blood pressure medication.[141]

These effects might all sound positive, but think about what this means. *Something in these foods is acting like a drug.* In fact, as the information about caffeine and theobromine might suggest, *like* is probably not quite the right word.

It is important to remember that scientists can be funded by those with commercial interests, and marketers of these products have a tremendous incentive to reassure people that small doses of these things are beneficial. If the public can be convinced that these items are harmless in low doses, manufacturers immediately escape culpability and place the burden of responsibility upon the individual – who, for some inexplicable reason, struggles to keep intake to the recommended minuscule amount.

One study proposed that the optimal maximum intake of chocolate was 45g per week, noting that any more than this might negate these supposed benefits and deliver a risk. This study also pointed out that the top fifth of chocolate users under age 65 have an increased risk of coronary heart disease and stroke.[142]

Those who are convinced that dark chocolate is beneficial may wish to test consuming plain cocoa powder mixed with water or plain cacao nibs (small pieces of crushed cacao beans) without any sugar or added sweeteners. This approach is unlikely to last long because cocoa on its own is very bitter. Of course, with persistence, the individual will acclimatize, just as the smoker acclimatizes to breathing toxic smoke into the lungs.

As noted in chapter 6: *Addiction*, regular caffeine consumption leads to an increased number of adenosine receptors, increasing fatigue. The primary 'benefit' of caffeine is thus the avoidance of withdrawal caused by the previous dose.[143] [144]

In fact, adenosine receptors are implicated not just in caffeine and theobromine withdrawal but in withdrawal from opiates,[145] as well as in many psychiatric disorders.[146]

Caffeine is now included in a wide range of unexpected

items, such as candies, baked goods, yogurt, chewing gum, chips/crisps, jerky, and waffles.[147]

Why are food manufacturers so keen to add an extract from a bitter bean to so many products?

Why do you think?

This mimicry adds another layer of potent deception to foods. These products promise alertness, energy, and an elevated mood while delivering the opposite and introducing multiple streams of intermittent reinforcement within one product.

Lest you think that caffeine and theobromine are the only culprits to be alert for, rest assured there are many others. One patent outlines a process for producing chocolate-flavored products that are high in gamma-aminobutyric acid (GABA).[148]

GABA is a neurotransmitter that reduces neuronal 'excitability' (the rate at which cells in the nervous system 'fire' and send signals to one another). Increasing GABA leads to a calming and tranquilizing effect, playing a crucial role in regulating muscle tone and mood. All benzodiazepines amplify the effects of GABA in the nervous system, introducing an artificial sense of calm. Of course, this interference soon leads the body to reduce the sensitivity of GABA-A receptors, ensuring that the correct calmness signal once again gets through. Higher and higher doses of medication are thus needed to achieve the same effect. Consequently, as the influence of each dose wears off, the individual is likely to experience far more agitation than before.

Dietary sources of GABA are relatively rare (it is found in small quantities within some types of tea and fermented foods). There is also debate about the bioavailability of dietary GABA – which is less potent than synthetic substances, such as benzodiazepines. However, concentrated versions of dietary

GABA are readily available as supplements, and chocolate "can be produced by simply mixing GABA into the composition."[149]

As with chocolate and coffee-flavored products, manufactured beverages (including soft drinks, flavored caffeinated waters, sports drinks, and a wide assortment of 'energy' drinks) present some of the most deceptive dining experiences available. These beverages may contain other psychoactive herbal derivatives, such as guarana, in addition to caffeine and theobromine – not to mention copious flavorings, sweeteners, and synthetic vitamins, which disturb flavor-nutrition relationships further.

Deceptive beverages have a long history. Coca-Cola originally included cocaine isolated from coca leaves and was first described as a "brain tonic and intellectual beverage."[150] [151] Although cocaine is no longer an ingredient, the drink still includes a decocainized extract from coca leaves, along with caffeine. Red Bull Cola also purportedly uses a coca leaf extract as a flavor.[152]

When discussing the benefits of investing in soft drink companies, Warren Buffett described the advantages of what he called "*no taste memory.*" Buffett went on to explain how most foods and drinks "accumulate" on you (in other words, trigger satiation), yet this does not seem to happen with drinks such as Coca-Cola, leading to "incredible per capita consumption."[153]

Many of those who regularly consume such beverages believe they do so to combat tiredness and give themselves a 'lift.' But when tiredness is dulled by artificially blocking adenosine receptors, energy is not recouped, nor is the body rested. Instead, the true state of exhaustion is temporarily masked, and an inaccurate bodily signal received. Because the human body cannot stand for such tomfoolery, it sets about adjusting receptors so that the accurate signal once again gets through, resulting in far more exhaustion overall.

During the beta reader phase of this book, many readers wondered whether regular coffee consumption should also be avoided when breaking free from deceptive foods.

Like all deceptive substances, caffeine offers the illusion of a benefit while stealing the very thing it pretends to deliver. While a full discussion of this topic is beyond the scope of this book, it is worth noting that although caffeine is detrimental, normalizing food intake does not require discarding every other deceptive substance. People do not always choose to quit nicotine, alcohol, and hard drugs all at once; sometimes people prefer to tackle one thing at a time.

In other words, if an individual chooses to continue drinking coffee while avoiding deceptive food, that is surely a whole lot better than continuing to pursue both.

Genuine vs. Deceptive Foods

This book has thus far described many genuine and deceptive items to illustrate the wide range of manipulative techniques and strategies used by modern food manufacturers. Unfortunately, it is not possible to detail every deceptive item that exists or to document a long list of dubious ingredients, additives, and problematic manufacturing processes. Even if someone undertook such an exhaustive project, manufacturers would soon generate new products and devise novel strategies for evading inclusion upon this list. Rather than an ever-changing description of the counterfeits, what is needed is a broad-brush strategy for identifying the deceptive item in all its various guises.

A simple rule of thumb is that *genuine food tastes like it should* – delivering nutrients in a reliable, predictable, flavor-honest way. *Genuine food is grown of the Earth* – not created by man. Genuine foods can be prepared and consumed using any traditional processing method – chopping, peeling, squeezing, grinding, cooking, and so on. *But we cannot play God and reformulate items from the ground up.* We cannot disassemble substances into their individual molecular building blocks and recraft something new.

Deceptive food, on the other hand, *is any edible item that contains an isolated chemical additive* (including added refined sweeteners, flavors, and extracts) or that naturally contains high concentrations of molecules that mimic those within the human body (such as caffeine and theobromine).

Even if an additive does not directly impact flavor or mimic a neurochemical, its presence still sets up the potential for intermittent reinforcement. For example, if one brand of bread contains added folic acid, whereas another does not, the two loaves may be indistinguishable in taste and appearance yet lead to differing nutritional outcomes. Something similar happens when chemicals are added sporadically to foods as preservatives. For example, a preservative that works by killing bacteria may also compromise the beneficial bacteria in the gut (as discussed in chapter 7: *Disruption of the Microbiome*). Yet if this additive is flavorless (as many preservatives are) and is added only to some foods, the presence of this potential threat cannot be reliably detected at the mouth, and intermittent reinforcement may result.

All refined and isolated chemical additives can create intermittent reinforcement. Using isolated chemicals confuses flavor-nutrition relationships and misleads sensory receptors about what is entering the body.

The danger within modern foods is the *manipulation of sensory signals* caused by isolating and reassembling molecular building blocks into new nutritional patterns.

Many of these isolated chemical additives are not inherently harmful. In fact, many occur naturally within plant and animal foods – such as sucrose (refined white sugar). How can something be good in its natural form yet problematic when transported elsewhere? The danger arises because the *value* of a survival reward depends not just on the item itself, but on *being able to find it when you need it.*

If oxygen could burst into your bloodstream without warning, the body would not know how much air to breathe, and you would run the risk of oxygen toxicity – leading to spontaneous convulsions, seizures, and death.

What would you prefer? Erratic love and hatred from random individuals or a few people you can rely on to offer love, kindness, and assistance when you need it?

To thrive, lifeforms must have a *reliable supply of nutrients in predictable quantities*. Too much or too little of any one nutrient becomes a threat. It is *dangerous* to have survival rewards appear or disappear spontaneously.

Lifeforms need a reliable strategy for finding and sourcing nutrition. Humans achieve this by monitoring the patterns between flavor stimuli and nutritional outcomes. Incoming flavors are analyzed via an automated chemical sampling process carried out by the sensory cells within the mouth and nose. Chemicals that are subsequently detected in the gut are then associated with the flavors that precede them.

Intermittent reinforcement causes the average predicted nutritional value per unit of flavor to fall. Consequently, taste and smell receptors downregulate, combined with a corresponding upswing in hunger – and a tendency to seek out that flavor again.

The problem is not just that these deceptive items don't offer what they promise but that the resulting intermittent reinforcement causes sensory systems to recalibrate.

As flavor-nutrition relationships weaken, the pleasure experienced per unit of flavor declines while appetite increases.

You don't need another expert to tell you what to eat. You could spend a lifetime researching and still be unsure. A staggering number of biochemical reactions occur within each cell of the human body (diagrams of these known chemical reactions provide a sobering illustration of just how complicated the task of keeping us alive really is).[154] [155] Biochemist Rhonda Patrick explains that each of these biochemical reactions requires vitamins and minerals in specific quantities and combinations,[156] with the byproducts of each reaction influencing the next.

The human body is unbelievably complex. The change of one variable impacts another across multiple pathways. If the intake of one nutrient goes up or down, another rises or falls to compensate – and the body excretes a little more of this or a little less of that.

Even if, by some miracle, the experts could put their heads together, stop arguing, and settle on the optimal intake for the average human being, *you* are not the average (no individual ever is). Even if someone invented a machine capable of tracking nutrient status alongside the live analysis of biochemical pathways, it would not come close to the sheer wisdom of the genes within your body – genes that have competently managed this task since the dawn of time.

You don't need an arbitrary external system to determine precisely what or how much to eat. You already carry the perfect system within you – a system that operates flawlessly...*unless it is misled.*

When the raw materials needed to carry out this great biological dance are *falsely labeled* and *mislead the very apparatus tasked with regulating these items*, the body is faced with a critical error.

This critical error often first presents as *disordered eating patterns.*

9

EATING DISORDERS: THE COMMON PATH

The conventional viewpoint is that an eating disorder is caused by a complex combination of psychological, biological, and environmental factors. Associations are made with childhood trauma and low self-esteem, as well as hereditary traits, such as 'perfectionism.' In other words, although food intake and body weight concerns appear integral to the disorder, they are not considered to be the root cause.

Let us contemplate a new possibility: that eating disorders are not only directly related to food but are the expected and normal outcome of encountering a misleading and unpredictable food supply while experiencing extreme hunger.

It might seem that someone who persistently overeats – such as a chronic grazer, binge eater, or 'compulsive' eater – has nothing in common with someone who is anorexic, underweight, and eats very little. Yet, a growing number of specialists believe that eating disorders of all types, including Eating Disorder Not Otherwise Specified (EDNOS), have many things in common.[1]

Those diagnosed with different types of eating disorders

often exhibit similar thought patterns, and many morph from one diagnosis to another (with a large percentage of individuals not neatly fitting into a single set of diagnostic criteria – hence the necessity for the EDNOS umbrella). For example, approximately one-third of people with anorexia later develop bulimia, and 62% of those with restricting-type anorexia subsequently exhibit binge/purge behaviors.[2]

> “Diagnostic migration” is the norm, rather than the exception. In my clinical practice I have encountered innumerable people in their 20s or 30s who have had an eating disorder since their teens, but at one stage it would have been called anorexia nervosa, later on bulimia nervosa, and most recently an atypical eating disorder. Have they really had three separate mental health disorders, one after the other? No, they have had a single eating problem that has evolved in form over time.
>
> — CHRISTOPHER FAIRBURN, *OVERCOMING BINGE EATING, SECOND EDITION* (2013)

In fact, not only is progressing from one eating disorder diagnosis to another commonplace, but the progression often happens in a very predictable sequence.

Let us now look at this situation with fresh eyes, considering these behaviors in light of deceptive food.

The Charm of the First Encounter

Many modern children begin life eating a variety of nourishing, genuine foods, as well as some deceptive items – such as cakes and sweets on special occasions, with take-out and flavor-manipulated dressings and sauces consumed now and again. If the ingestion of such items is relatively rare and offset by the consumption of a predominantly nourishing and genuine diet, these deceptive foods cause only minor, undetected blips in learned flavor-nutrition relationships. As such, the downsides are correspondingly slight and typically remain undetected. The child's weight does not balloon. Appetite does not climb. Health does not deteriorate in any noticeable manner.

From the child's perspective, these items only seem extra delicious, extra wonderful, extra good. In fact, the child may perceive special occasions to be special *precisely* because they are accompanied by a spread of artificially flavor-strengthened foods.

Even if surrounding adults are dieting, obese, or openly struggling with their weight, the child is very unlikely to detect a personal problem with consuming these delicacies.

This honeymoon phase occurs with all deceptive substances and is the period of innocence during which the danger of the situation remains concealed, unseen, unknown.

Of course, some modern children skip straight over this phase. The infiltration of deceptive flavors has reached such dizzying proportions that a growing number of youngsters are no longer raised in a predominantly flavor-honest environment at all. These children may be overweight from a very young age and launch rapidly into the next predictable phase.

The First Diet

Teenagers, like all other creatures approaching breeding age, preen and groom themselves to entice a high-quality mate. The pursuit of an attractive figure during this period is not only expected but normal and healthy behavior. No lifeform wishes to select a low-quality, unappealing, dimwitted mate when better options are available; hence, teenagers often take action to ensure they compare favorably in this competitive mating game.

Across history, demonstrating some form of proficiency or prowess in relation to one's peers was readily achievable for many. For example, a youngster might not have been the most attractive in their small tribe, but perhaps they could be the best at catching fish, weaving baskets, or telling hilarious stories around the campfire. Furthermore, the small pool of competing young men and women in a local tribe was very unlikely to include an airbrushed, top-model lookalike.[3]

In modern times, however, teenagers gauge their performance against a sea of seemingly spectacular specimens, sourced from the global population of celebrities, 'influencers,' and movie stars – many of whom pursue extreme diets and exercise regimes to achieve a physical state that is only fleetingly maintained.[4] Surrounded by a stream of meticulously composed and digitally enhanced imagery, with physiques appearing far more flawless than they ever would in reality, it is easy to see how even teenagers of normal weight might conclude they are *a little too fat*.

This outcome is even more likely when the youngster grows up in a society that is openly struggling with an obesity crisis. In this environment, becoming *too fat* can seem an entirely realistic possibility. It is no mystery why a great number of teenagers (even those who are not overweight at all) decide that weight loss might be wise.

Unlike other aspects of appearance, which are not so flexible, body weight is rightly perceived as *changeable*. As such, the teenager launches enthusiastically into action. Quick research – or even a basic guess – provides what appears to be an infallible solution: *eat less*.

A meme is an idea that spreads through a population via a kind of non-genetic evolution (as per the conceptual illustrations shared on social media). Some memes offer survival benefits and replicate across time and space as a consequence. Others *seem* to offer a benefit and spread like viruses, each infecting the host just long enough to infect the next.

Calorie restriction – the idea that weight loss depends upon deliberately consuming fewer calories than appetite dictates – is one such meme. It spreads like wildfire because the concept sounds so logical from a mathematical perspective and because, initially, it seems to work.

Because an attractive physique is a clear survival asset, many teenagers summon immense willpower to achieve this goal.

Although food restriction is unpleasant, after initiating a diet, other areas of life often begin to look up. You may feel more energetic and alert (this is part of the starvation response, ensuring you can hunt out food whenever the opportunity arises). If the scale shows results, you may feel uplifted and excited, knowing you are progressing toward an important goal. Furthermore, physical changes may be encouraged and rewarded by peers, providing social validation, attention, and praise. These benefits can initially outweigh the quiet aggravation of hunger.

As time passes, however, hunger becomes more obtrusive and begins to monopolize thoughts.[5] The energy experienced at the outset may fade, replaced with exhaustion and irritability, as the body adapts to the reduced energy supply by burning fewer calories.[6] Sleep may become compromised because hungry individuals must remain awake longer so as not to miss out on feeding opportunities.

As the diet progresses, these downsides accumulate...until, one day, the prospect of *continuing the diet* seems slightly less appealing than *taking a break*.

Extreme Hunger and Anorexia

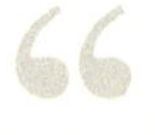

> "*Come with me*," Socrates replied. He took the lad to a river and shoved his head underwater. He held it there until the boy struggled for air. Then he let him go.
>
> Once the boy regained his composure, Socrates asked him, "*What did you desire most when your head was underwater*?"
>
> "I wanted air," the boy told him.
>
> — JOSEPH MURPHY, *THE POWER OF YOUR SUBCONSCIOUS MIND* (1963)

Eating a large volume of food following a restrictive diet is a logical attempt to recoup lost nutrition and restore the body to health. After the Minnesota Starvation Experiment (a clinical study in the 1940s that examined the effect of a calorie-reduced diet upon healthy men), one man consumed so much food that he had to have his stomach pumped. Another found he was unable to satisfy his cravings for food, no matter how full his stomach became. Another described his stomach as having a "year-long cavity."[7] While refeeding, these men sometimes consumed up to 10,000 calories per day.

Although eating a lot is a normal response to food deprivation (and ensures an underfed individual returns to health), binge eating increases enormously when deceptive food is encountered at this time.

In a hungry, starving state, the brain prioritizes *high-concentration flavor cues* because these are predicted to provide the necessary nutrition with the urgency and volume required.

Whenever a diet is broken, therefore, the tendency is to gravitate toward deceptive food like a moth toward a flame.

In contrast to the gnawing pain of hunger, concentrated flavor molecules appear to offer salvation. As the misleading chemical signals lock into taste and smell receptors, it seems as though the nutritional crisis is over, and a correspondingly high dose of pleasure is issued.

Unfortunately, when eating deceptive food, very little of the promised nutrition arrives. Despite a stomach filled to exploding capacity, insufficient nutrition is often received. As such, satiation does not kick in, and it feels as though you cannot *get enough*.

In this scenario, the individual is sham eating. There is a mismatch between the signal at the mouth and the contents arriving in the stomach, increasing the likelihood that the individual will binge eat an enormous amount of food.

As bodily systems recalibrate, the binges grow in intensity and duration, seeming to take on a life of their own. It may feel as if hunger and satiety mechanisms are well and truly broken.

Without understanding how deceptive flavors distort and exaggerate hunger, repeatedly binge-eating enormous amounts of food appears utterly nonsensical. It suggests that something is horribly wrong; that dieting has cultivated an insatiable monster.

The shock of these bottomless-pit eating experiences – partly brought on by starvation and partly brought on by the effects of deceptive food – is terrifying. It not only threatens weight loss progress but prompts a 'doubling-down' effect – the initiation of tighter rules and stricter dietary guidelines in an effort to close off loopholes that might lead to such disastrous outcomes in the future. This can eventually lead the dieter to consume only a few 'safe' foods. If these restrictive behaviors are maintained for long enough, a diagnosis of *anorexia nervosa* may result.

As with other eating disorders, anorexia is believed to be influenced by numerous genetic, psychological, and environmental factors. However, a 2023 paper summarizes the official understanding of anorexia more accurately and succinctly than most: as a condition with "*unknown etiology*."[8] In other words, the experts do not really know what causes this condition.

Those diagnosed with anorexia are typically high-achieving, intelligent,[9] and well-articulated.[10] This outstanding skill set – which leads to success in many other areas of life – also helps an individual *excel at dieting*. Yet, despite possessing these positive traits, the anorexic is viewed as behaving in a way that is highly irrational. Whereas other forms of voluntary food restriction (such as hunger strikes, religious fasting, and extreme weight loss regimes) are believed to be selected for logical reasons, the anorexic alone is construed as suffering from a distortion of the truth. While it is acknowledged that anorexia may *start* with an ordinary diet, it is thought the individual somehow "loses control" and "spirals down in the grip of the anorexia."[11]

In fact, some hypothesize that anorexia is precisely about *regaining control*. Many sufferers of this condition indeed report feelings of powerlessness, with food avoidance behaviors selected specifically to "retain control over the self."[12]

But why does someone feel the need to exert control over this particular aspect of their behavior? The answer is simple: encountering deceptive food while in a state of extreme hunger leads the individual to believe that appetite is very much *out of control*. As one paper suggests, "restrictive eating behavior in anorexic patients could be implemented to suppress the hunger impulses and the loss of control over food."[13]

After all, if appetite appears demonstrably obscene, and

giving in to this appetite results in dramatic weight gain (as it certainly does when binge eating deceptive food), limiting access to food is, in some manner, *a rational response*.

Trained nurse and eating disorder specialist Jean Antonello argues that beliefs about appetite and food are *central to the anorexic's problem*, with their appetite being "so extreme that it frightens them."[14]

> Their intense fear of weight gain, coupled with their adapted monster appetites, which also provoke fear, leaves anorectics without much choice but to maintain control, or die, some of them say. And control at the absolutely thinnest weight possible adds some insurance against the possibility of ever losing their grip on that huge appetite lurking within.
>
> — JEAN ANTONELLO, *BREAKING OUT OF FOOD JAIL* (1996)

In other words, Antonello suggests that anorexia is not so much a fear of food or of being a normal weight but *a fear of what might happen if one gives in to the out-of-control appetite*.

In this situation, it can truly seem that allowing appetite free rein would lead to rampant, out-of-control obesity. If an individual started dieting because they felt their original weight was unsatisfactory, it is easy to see how it can seem that, even in the best-case scenario, returning to 'eating as normal' would result in the return of an unsatisfactory weight. In fact, the situation now feels very much worse than this because by initiating a strict diet, an out-of-control monster appears unleashed.

In a haunting essay about her experience of anorexia, Lea

Muldtofte describes the fear of "not being able to master the organism." She explains how the perception of anorexia often centers around the patient's refusal of food and their apparent disgust of eating, but she notes this is "a common lie that the anorexic tells people around her in order to deliver a logical explanation for saying no."[15]

Muldtofte describes her own *obsession* with food and notes that another anorexic patient hospitalized alongside her consumed copious quantities of sugar-free sweets.

This quote shared online at 'pro-anorexia' websites perhaps says it all:

> If I eat anything, I'll eat everything, so I eat nothing.
>
> — SOURCE UNKNOWN

Anorexia is best understood as the stalemate between two competing survival drives. Is it better to be full, yet fat and rejected, or hungry and loved? There is no correct answer to this question because neither option leads to winning the game.

Eating fewer calories than the body needs to survive is a clear survival threat. Fearing fatness in comparison to the *risk of dying from starvation* seems utterly unreasonable. But being unfavorably judged by society (particularly at an age when you are entering a highly competitive mating game that *directly influences the propagation of your genes*) is also a survival threat.

Being fat is no joke. Modern society disdains voluptuous flesh. It is no surprise at all that young humans take this possibility very seriously. Who wants to be fat when it results in isolation, stigmatization, and social judgment?

If you face an unruly appetite that does not seem to subside, it can feel like being stuck between a rock and a very hard place. It can appear as though you are forced to choose between two kinds of hell – the hell of hunger or the hell of societal rejection. There does not seem to be a sensible middle ground. Although it can appear unfathomable from an outside perspective, the nightmare of starvation can initially seem more tolerable.

After all, someone who is thin receives far more care and attention than someone who is obese. Whereas the anorexic has a 'tragic mental disorder,' the overeater is a 'lazy glutton who cannot control themselves.' Of course, both are captured by the very same deception, and neither has yet reached the accurate understanding about *what to do.*

A *fear of appetite* is the predictable outcome of encountering deceptive foods while in a state of extreme hunger. Sadly, the food avoidance strategies employed in the face of this elevated appetite only exacerbate the problem.

Complicating matters further, when starvation is the chosen dietary approach, it is never clear when a satisfactory physique has been 'achieved.' When subjected to chronic malnourishment, the body morphs from plump to skinny-fat to emaciated, without a beautiful phase in between. Pockets of residual fat may remain on even the most skeletal of frames, clinging in desperate reserves of energy while muscles atrophy, bones jut out, and internal organs degrade.

If low-nutrition is the chosen weight loss strategy, the dieter never reaches a day when an optimal physique stares back from the mirror. Sometimes, it seems as though you might *almost* be there, but the state always feels so intangible, just out of grasp.

And the worst thing is, you don't know how to maintain it, how to keep it, without an enormous appetite re-emerging and flinging you savagely off the rails.

After initiating a weight loss diet – just as all the experts recommended – and dutifully following it well, you find you don't know how to get off the train. And as you flounder, the experts turn on you and say you are mentally unsound. And in this starving, depressed state, you believe it.

Anorexia is a lethal phase with the highest mortality rate of any disorder.[16] Although it is often undiagnosed, this pattern of behavior occurs (to a greater or lesser degree) in many new dieters but is only labeled as anorexia in the small percentage who sustain these behaviors until they are dangerously lean. Those who start at a higher weight may exhibit equally unhealthy and restrictive eating patterns, yet the behaviors may be unacknowledged – or even celebrated.

Some individuals remain trapped in this stalemate for a long time. The length of time someone is prepared to endure extreme deprivation varies depending upon the surrounding circumstances. For example, a model who is constantly in the critical public eye and whose job requires maintaining a lean physique may endure the discomfort of hunger for an extended period. There are numerous factors influencing the length of time someone is prepared to endure a particular discomfort, but the longer the restriction is pursued, the stronger the desire to eat becomes.

In most cases, this hunger eventually becomes intolerable, and the individual enters the next phase and begins to oscillate wildly between the two competing survival drives.

Binge Eating, Bulimia, and Yo-yo Dieting

At last, in the face of desperate hunger, the floodgates open. In the aftermath of these extravagant binge episodes, more dramatic compensation tactics are often considered. With a painful and distended stomach, the individual may discover that vomiting provides fast and immediate relief – eliminating the excess calories and the pain in the stomach. This purging tactic takes the replication of sham eating experiments to a whole new level. Of course, vomiting severely weakens flavor-nutrition relationships, exacerbates hunger, depletes nutrient levels, and, if continued, can end in death.

As with anorexia, *bulimia nervosa* is considered to be a complex mental disorder with numerous intertwined psychological roots. However, if weight loss is the goal, minimizing the effect of seemingly out-of-control binges can be seen as a logical response.

Those who are unable or unwilling to vomit may instead initiate punishing exercise regimes or undertake fasting. Regardless of the chosen approach, a new diet is almost certain to resume, along with the vow to increase willpower and try harder tomorrow.

This endless treadmill (researching, finding a diet, testing it, discarding it, and then starting the process all over again) can feel like a kind of entrenched madness, but it is *logical hypothesis testing:* the desperate hunt for the dietary rule that corrects the problem.

Unless someone wishes to endure a life of hunger or a life of fatness, the only viable solution in this scenario is to find *a way of eating that allows both survival needs to be met.* Each new diet is a way of splitting and examining food-related stimuli in the hope that doing so delivers a *reliable behavioral rule.* Each diet attends to a particular set of food-related cues in the hope of unearthing where the danger hides. Perhaps fat is bad. Perhaps gluten is bad. Perhaps sugar is bad. Perhaps fructose is bad. Perhaps meat is bad. Perhaps carbohydrates are bad. Perhaps plant foods are bad. And on and on.

Hypotheses are tested and discarded one by one. Sometimes, it takes time to realize a hypothesis is incorrect. Common diets are popular *precisely because they deliver short-term benefits* (resulting in an influx of fans who spread the diet to new hosts). Vegan diets, for example, flood the system with vitamins, nutrients, and numerous other beneficial plant compounds that are lacking in the standard American diet, often delivering dramatic health improvements in the short-term. Doctors and influencers become convinced they have found the solution (as well as a marketing opportunity) and leap onto the bandwagon. With long-term adherence, however, plant-based dieters may begin to suffer from poor teeth, skin issues, bone weakness, joint pain, fatigue, and depression. (Searching YouTube for "why I'm no longer vegan" delivers many sobering anecdotal tales.)

Similarly, ketogenic diets – including the most extreme form, carnivorism – initially seem to offer the holy grail. The body is flooded with nourishing fats and proteins – a particular benefit for those who have previously been on plant-based diets. Some may find that blood pressure stabilizes, skin clears, muscles strengthen, energy resumes, and depression lifts. With a greater length of time spent in ketosis (a metabolic state in which the body primarily burns fat for energy instead of carbohydrates), these diets also provide many of the benefits of fasting – while continuing to deliver a valuable stream of nourishment – and can hence facilitate amazing health transformations. In delight, another set of doctors and influencers leap onto the bandwagon. However, behind the scenes, the negative consequences of ongoing adherence can begin to mount.

Although long-term research into the ketogenic diet for weight loss is limited, a much more extensive body of research exists regarding the use of a ketogenic diet to treat health conditions. Of 28 children placed on the ketogenic diet for over six years as a treatment for epilepsy, for example, 82% ended up below the 10th centile for height.[17] This growth restriction occurred after, but not before, the initiation of the ketogenic diet.[18]

These and other studies identify potential complications associated with long-term adherence to a ketogenic diet, including hyperlipidemia, cardiac disease, gastrointestinal disorders, vitamin and mineral deficiencies, bone fractures, and kidney stones.[19 20]

After consuming a low-carbohydrate diet for an extended period, any attempt to broaden the diet may result in digestive issues, even when consuming previously tolerated foods (this is likely due to temporary alterations in gut bacteria, as described in chapter 7: *Disruption of the Microbiome*). It can thus seem as though the individual is now intolerant to a wide array of foods.

Insulin sensitivity can also deteriorate despite initial improvements – causing further issues if carbohydrates are suddenly reintroduced. Thyroid function may also decline,[21] accompanied by hair loss, cold hands, and cold feet. It is also interesting that Dr. Paul Saladino, author of *The Carnivore Code* (2020) – one of the most popular carnivore diet books currently for sale on Amazon – has revised his thoughts following publication and now believes that carbohydrates do indeed play an important dietary role.[22]

Between these two extremes lies the full gamut of dietary options, each supported by enthusiastic doctors, nutritionists, and fans. The experts are at open war with one another, and the public is led in endless, desperate circles.

Although popular diets often inadvertently exclude many deceptive foods, they rarely provide the complete spectrum of nutrition required for optimal health. In other words, although these popular diets sometimes correctly isolate the offender, they draw the line in the wrong place, losing many genuine survival rewards in the process. As such, these diets often initially seem to work, and may be recycled and tried repeatedly in the hope of emulating the conditions that led to initial 'success' without realizing that the diet itself is flawed. Each attempt is shorter-lived, and hopelessness grows.

As time passes, the diets become more obscure, restrictive,

and desperate, eliminating whole food groups or types of food. Such strategies are appealing, as they require less willpower. A rule to never eat wheat or to only consume animal products is far simpler to follow than weighing food at every meal, counting calories, or tallying points. Furthermore, when a diet is restricted to only a few items, hunger for these flavors quickly satiates, and it thus seems as though appetite is 'under control.' Of course, when veering from the diet, appetite returns in full force.

Hypothesis testing can take time. Cognitive psychologist Claude G. Čech from The University of Louisiana at Lafayette explains that the length of time it takes to discriminate between two items depends upon how similar they are. Čech notes that if animals are asked to select between two items that are almost identical, they may acquire a state of "experimental neurosis." For example, Pavlov's dogs became "extraordinarily agitated and snappish"[23] when asked to discriminate between two very similar ovals.

Like Pavlov's dogs, attempting to solve this endless dieting fiasco can leave you irritable and snappish. You may wonder how you can be so smart yet fail at this supposedly simple thing.

As the pool of plausible hypotheses diminishes and the failures mount, the gaps between each new diet widen, and binge eating may extend for days, weeks, or years. The situation begins to feel hopeless, and the effort required to initiate each new diet grows.

If someone fails repeatedly – sliding further from the goal at every turn – summoning the enthusiasm to try again is hard.

This back-and-forth debacle can last for decades. As the lack of nutrition, gorging, and purging take their toll, the need to restore health grows in priority, while the necessity to maintain an attractive physique may wane.

Although having an appealing figure is a valuable asset at

any age, it is most critical in those who are young and single – about to enter the mating pool. Thus, the older one becomes, the harder it can feel to initiate another taxing dietary regime – particularly when all prior attempts have failed.

Eventually, it may dawn on you that the endless restriction might be part of the problem. You may recall a time – long ago – when you *just didn't think about this stuff* all the time.

And with this insight, you finally attempt to *stop dieting.*

Intuitive Eating

First, you waste years of your life trying to diet. Then you waste years of your life trying to stop.

When moving away from restrictive diets, another group of professionals emerge. These experts encourage 'mindful' or 'conscious' eating, chewing each mouthful slowly, and avoiding distraction during mealtimes (just in case it has escaped your attention that you inhale the contents of your pantry in one sitting). You are encouraged to exchange food rules for *intuition*, and vow never to weigh yourself or restrict food intake, endeavoring to attend to 'genuine' hunger cues, whatever these might be. You may attempt to rate hunger using charts and scales, stopping while 80% full or 'comfortably full' (in case the problem is a slight volume miscalculation). You are encouraged to condemn anything that might contribute to body-image issues and focus on health alone, making efforts to embrace a voluptuous physique at any size.

There are many valuable lessons to be gleaned from the intuitive eating movement – such as the importance of listening to the body and noticing how food makes you feel – just as there are many valuable lessons to be learned about nutrition during the dieting phase. But without understanding how flavor deception distorts and manipulates appetite, this approach is often futile.

Despite the admirable goal, intuitive eating typically results in steady weight gain. As long as flavor-nutrition relationships are unreliable, hunger remains high. Reassured that this process can take years, you press onwards, consuming deceptive food whenever the desire arises, making sure never to restrict yourself. You may stock the house with previously forbidden items, eating these in liberal quantities as part of ongoing 'recovery.'

Just like the earlier phases – intuitive eating often begins with a glorious feeling of hope – joy at finally allowing hunger to be filled. Stomach-bursting binges may subside, leaving in their wake large flavor-enhanced meals and frequent grazing, punctuated by 'final feasts' whenever dieting is reconsidered.

If sustained attempts to 'eat when hungry' lead only to weight gain, you may eventually resort to time-based approaches, trying intermittent fasting, one meal a day (OMAD), three meals a day, and so on, in case the issue is lack of structure.

You may idolize your childhood, cursing your first diet, and wishing with all your heart that you could go back to the way you used to be. It may escape your attention that most children do not have free access to junk food, a ready supply of money, or a car to drive to the shops whenever they wish. If you had access to these things as a child, who knows how 'normally' you would have eaten.

Post-starvation hunger does *not* explain why someone who abandoned restrictive dieting years ago should *still* struggle to maintain a healthy weight. Nor does it explain why some children are overweight from a very young age, long before dieting or body-image issues take hold. Nor does it explain why some people develop 'binge eating disorder' *without ever having dieted at all.*

You see, the dieting is almost an anomaly – a smokescreen. It conceals what is really happening and distracts you from seeing the truth. Dieting increases the likelihood of being conned by deceptive food...but *it is not what conned you.*

If deceptive food did not exist, you might *still* have attempted a crazy diet as a youngster...but when hunger became too much, and you gave up on that ludicrous idea, after a short period of compensatory overeating, you would have settled back at a normal, healthy weight.

In fact, if deceptive food did not exist, you would almost certainly *never have dieted in the first place.* This is because not only would you have already been a healthy weight, but there would be *no obesity crisis,* and society would not have developed a pervasive fear of fatness.

After testing intuitive eating for some time, it one day sinks in that even though you stopped restricting long ago, the overeating remains. It is with this realization that the true horror of your predicament emerges.

'Compulsive' Eating

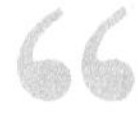

> ...he drinks in the morning before he allows himself to see anyone; he drinks again in the car on the way to work; and he nips at the bottle in his desk until it is time to go to lunch where he throws down a few more.
>
> — JAMES ROBERT MILAM AND KATHERINE KETCHAM, *UNDER THE INFLUENCE* (1984)

After years of resistance, seesawing between plump and thin, obesity finally begins to get the upper hand. You may resort to hiding wrappers, concealing the evidence as if it were a fine art, even though the evidence is right there, on the torso and limbs.

If supply gets low, you may find yourself concocting bizarre mixtures from household ingredients, attempting to recreate the intense flavor profiles you crave.

Comments from loved ones may become tinged with frustration: thinly veiled critiques and biting, angry barbs. You may wonder if a lack of support is the problem and may move house, change jobs, separate from spouses, any wretched thing in an effort to spur positive change.

In a last bid of desperation, you may employ public 'willpower hacks' (group weigh-ins or public weight loss challenges), hoping that the shame of it might force good eating patterns to remain on track – locking in good behavior and protecting against subsequent 'willpower lapses.'

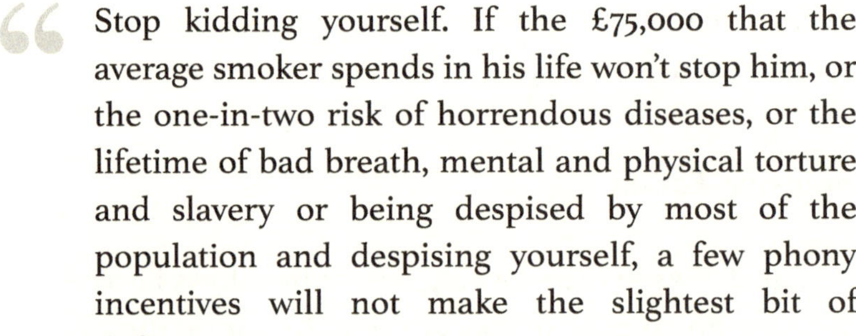

> Stop kidding yourself. If the £75,000 that the average smoker spends in his life won't stop him, or the one-in-two risk of horrendous diseases, or the lifetime of bad breath, mental and physical torture and slavery or being despised by most of the population and despising yourself, a few phony incentives will not make the slightest bit of difference.
>
> — ALLEN CARR, *THE EASY WAY TO STOP SMOKING* (2010)

At breaking point, you may cry, "Enough is enough!" and throw all deceptive items into the trash, dousing the remainder with vinegar or ketchup to prevent yourself from later retrieving it.

There is no escape from the fact that *something is terribly wrong*. You may fear you are closing the gap between normality and those who occupy concrete reinforced beds in documentaries about the morbidly obese.

At some point, despair sets in. A quiet sorrow edges into your soul. When you've battled with deceptive food for an extended period, a sludgy, brain-thick misery envelops you, and you cannot tell if it is the result of weight gain or if the misery was there all along.

Even if you excel in other areas, failing at this one thing can somehow seem to invalidate all else.

To make matters worse, it can feel that turning the situation around would now require such an enormous undertaking that it may very well be impossible – requiring years of effort, not to mention the *deprivation.* But even though fixing this thing seems as though it might take forever, you still *really want to do it* – because surely anything is better than this.

The problem is it feels like you have lost all motivation and self-control. Perhaps you *could* change if you really put your mind to it, but there is always a reason why the time to do so is never now.

As hopelessness grows, diagnoses like *binge eating disorder* and *compulsive eating disorder* come to mind. You may wonder if you are irreparably screwed up, ruined, incapable of change.

This awful, repetitive Groundhog Day – in which you procure deceptive items, smuggle them home, guzzle them down, hide the evidence, vow to change, and then wake up and do it all over again ad nauseam – feels inescapably like *addiction.*

Not everyone travels through these behavioral phases in the order described, nor enters the journey at the same point. Someone raised in poverty, for example, does not need to undergo a restrictive diet to experience extreme hunger. Similarly, a child whose caregivers stock the pantry with an unlimited supply of deceptive fodder may launch into sham eating from a very early age without any preceding diet necessary.[24]

Some people may find themselves snared at different stages along the journey due to individual life circumstances. Others may cycle back and forth through the stages like a hellish, eternal merry-go-round. And, after 'compulsively' eating for years, you may finally summon the strength to throw yourself back to stage one, ready to embrace the whole filthy cycle again.

At some point, however, you reach a stage that can only be described as *desperation.*

The Dark Before the Dawn

> "Food was my guru, my lover, my sage. It seduced and defined me. And, ultimately, it deceived me.
>
> — JASMIN SINGER, *ALWAYS TOO MUCH AND NEVER ENOUGH: A MEMOIR* (2016)

Eventually, no amount of flavor molecules surpasses the predicted nutritional need, and engaging with a deceptive item – even in extreme amounts – barely lifts you from the trough of misery in which you reside.

As obesity climbs, others begin to judge you more overtly. Sometimes, you might even catch glimpses of what could be disgust in people's eyes, or worse, indifference. The larger you become, the more invisible you feel. This change is particularly noticeable when the weight gain is rapid, and you still remember how people *used* to treat you – as though you were a normal, valuable human being. These reactions shine light upon the obvious and unavoidable fact that you have a *problem*, just as the drunk stumbling and slurring down the street has a problem. The evidence is pasted all over the body, on full display for the world, and you and everyone else knows it.

But worse than the condemnation and judgment from others is the self-loathing, the shame and regret at knowing that you somehow brought this on yourself...and the absolute despair that you don't even really understand why.

It can seem that the odds of salvation for those who reach this phase are unimaginably low – that the prospect of turning the situation around is close to hopeless; the behavior so entrenched, so unshakable.

It isn't.

Just as extreme hunger predisposes someone to stumble across a deceptive item, repeatedly engaging with a counterfeit and suffering the harm first-hand *predisposes you to find the way out.*

Do you think it is mere chance that you are reading this book? Do you think you are here out of blind luck? No. You took a punt on this book by an unknown author because you know that somehow, somewhere, *there is a way out.*

You are doing everything right. You are precisely where you should be – seeking the information necessary to escape.

Psychologists William Miller and Janet C'de Baca found that immediate, life-changing insights often arrive as "an unexpected flood of hope in a time of great darkness" or "a great burden having been lifted."[25]

> One thing that comes out in myths [...] is that at the bottom of the abyss comes the voice of salvation. The black moment is the moment when the real message of transformation is going to come.
>
> — JOSEPH CAMPBELL, *THE POWER OF MYTH* (1991)

Addiction is not a mental disorder that 'overtakes' an individual at a certain point. It is not an inherited or acquired behavioral flaw. It is a *predictable and logical pattern of behavior* that arises when engaging with a misleading circumstance that *pretends to deliver what is needed.*

Many diet books contain tips or tricks to help control an unruly appetite, with guidelines that make restriction less taxing on the will. But this is an absurd back-to-front approach. It's like you fell in love with an abusive partner, and they're so irresistible that you must build fences around them so that you are never left alone in the room together, and your paths never cross.

There is a far easier way out. You can *see what the deceiving entity really is* and *fall out of love.*

The moment the wool is pulled from your eyes, behavior changes – not out of compulsion or necessity, but because you *no longer want that deceptive entity anymore.*

It doesn't matter how physically weak or sick something has made you – or how desensitized the internal sensory system has become – because that's not what keeps someone coming back.

Love is like a spell. The flavor spell was first cast at parties and special occasions when you were young. But it was hammered home while you were starving, and deceptive food pretended to save you.

Addiction is a misplaced love.

The good news is that love isn't magic. It is an emotion built on belief. And *beliefs can change* when the right information comes to hand.

10

ERRORS OF PERCEPTION

AT THIS POINT in the book, some readers may wish to test out these ideas (if so, please wait until the final guidance is given). Others may see the logic in the argument and agree that, in many respects, the concept of intermittent reinforcement of flavor makes sense – yet retain a smidgen of doubt. Still others may fear that although they *could* initiate change if they really wanted to, it probably wouldn't endure – that their problem is more intractable, more permanent somehow.

> "...almost every alcoholic or addicted person I've ever known initially believed that they were "the exception to the rule." They allowed that it might all be true for everyone else, but not for them.
>
> — DAVID E. SCHOEN, *WAR OF THE GODS IN ADDICTION* (2009)

Although it is critical to see precisely how and why deceptive flavors mislead bodily sensors and to understand that intermittent reinforcement is at the root of all addiction – oddly, understanding this is only *part* of what is required. The biggest challenge in addiction is *not* the physical recalibration (this is transitory and can be rapidly undone) but the *false beliefs that are acquired while the sensory manipulation is undetected and misunderstood.*

I used to find it bizarre that if I imagined waking up in the body of a heroin addict (with no prior experience of how I got there), I was certain I could escape. No matter how awful the withdrawal symptoms were, I knew I had within me whatever was required to break free. I was absolutely certain that I would never take another dose of heroin because I understood, without any shadow of a doubt, that *continuing to take the drug makes everything worse*, whereas stopping involves a short period of bodily discomfort, after which everything improves.

It seemed absurd that despite being so certain about my capacity to end hard drug addiction (if I woke up in this state), I had no such confidence regarding something with a withdrawal period that was so ridiculously mild by comparison.

Why was I so confident about the former yet hopeless about the prospect of breaking free from deceptive food? Why is it that some individuals can take highly addictive drugs in hospital settings yet return home, withdraw without apparent difficulty, and get on with the rest of their lives? Why is *waking up* in the body of a drug addict different from a lifetime of personal engagement and first-hand experience?

It is different because the difficulty of escaping an addiction is *not* the intermittent reinforcement itself, nor the recalibrated internal systems, but the *incorrect beliefs that are acquired as a consequence.*

There is a famous analogy about baby elephants who are chained to a stake while young. As baby elephants, they tug and pull at the chain but cannot break free. Eventually, they learn that escape is impossible and give up trying. As strong, fully-grown elephants, who could escape in one second, they do not even bother to tug on the chain. What keeps the adult elephant trapped is not the chain but the *incorrect belief it holds about the circumstance.*

If someone repeatedly engages with a deceptive item across many months or years, they are forced to generate several possible explanations for their behavior. Although deceptive sensory signals are the error that sets the whole downfall in motion, another set of errors congregate in the mind *in an effort to explain the first error.*

Flavor mimicry is invisible to the naked eye. It is not immediately obvious how misleading molecular signals distort appetite or reduce taste and smell sensitivity. If something misleads, the truth is concealed. The tendency in this situation is thus to draw *false conclusions* about why overeating occurs.

The more convincing an explanation seems – the more it appears to fit your particular circumstance – the more likely it was to be believed. False beliefs *always appear very plausible.*[1] They must do – or they would never be believed. These misperceptions about addictive behavior are often shared and adopted by others in the same trap and parroted by experts – making it seem as if these explanations are verified by sheer social consensus.

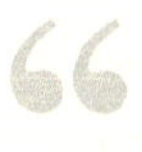

> All addictions are surrounded and supported by a collection of powerful lies, or delusions. Taking control is the process of identifying those lies and discovering the truth.
>
> — GILLIAN RILEY, *HOW TO STOP SMOKING AND STAY STOPPED FOR GOOD* (2007)

Timothy Wilson, professor of psychology from the University of Virginia, makes the somewhat disconcerting observation that others can often predict our behavior better than we can ourselves.[2] On the face of it, this sounds preposterous. How can others better predict our behavior if they don't have access to our thoughts or feelings? It makes more sense, however, when you realize that the way we decipher our own motives is exactly the same way that others do: *by observing our behavior*. Wilson suggests that our stake in the outcome can sometimes be a disadvantage, biasing us toward interpretations that paint our performance in a favorable light.

Shocking experiments have been carried out in patients with severed connections between the left and right brain hemispheres (so that one half of the brain cannot communicate with the other). If an experimenter holds up a message to only one of the patient's eyes (i.e., an instruction asking the patient to stand up and do something), the participant will carry out the instruction. But when asked to explain what they are doing, the left brain hemisphere (responsible for language), which has *not* sighted the instruction, generates a plausible yet incorrect explanation and states it as fact.[3] The implication is that our beliefs about why we do something are merely *logical guesses* – our best estimation of truth – and that these guesses are sometimes formed *before we have all the information to hand.*

If someone leaves a drug treatment center, detoxified and physically strong, only to dive headfirst back into the very same trap, the re-emergence of this behavior is not due to a character flaw or residual differences in bodily sensors...but *faulty beliefs that the individual retains about the situation.*

Allen Carr, who discovered the most successful stop-smoking method of all time, talks about the "little monster" (the body's physical recalibration to nicotine) and the "big monster" (the incorrect beliefs that infiltrate the mind as a consequence –

which he also refers to as the "brainwashing"). Carr explains that the little monster is very easy to overcome – but that debunking the brainwashing is the primary challenge.

Carr's method of escape involves presenting a series of logical, common-sense arguments, each debunking popular explanations for why people *think* they smoke cigarettes. During in-person seminars and one-on-one discussions with smokers, Carr heard the same beliefs about smoking over and over again: *it relaxes me; it helps me cope with stress; it helps me feel calm; the withdrawal period is unbearable; I have no willpower...*and on and on. Carr became an expert in convincing people that these beliefs were faulty and that there was a far more accurate way of viewing the situation. Eventually, it sinks in that there is only one reason why someone smokes: a tiny physical recalibration that has no more power over them than a common cold. As this realization dawns, people find themselves not *dreading* putting down the cigarette but *eager* and *excited* to do so.

Carr's books can seem blindingly obvious and repetitious in places. But what is obvious to one person is not obvious to another, and vice versa. Each individual holds different beliefs about a circumstance due to the differing experiences of their lives. What one person views as self-evident, another may perceive as absurd. Some people never acquire popular viewpoints or experience a particular situation that extinguishes a common belief.

For example, in the case of weight loss, I used to be certain that some form of 'resisting hunger' was necessary. It was not until I followed a whole-food, paleo-type diet that I saw that eating to appetite really was a viable method of losing weight. (Of course, at that time, my definition of which foods were 'acceptable' was far too narrow, but until I had this experience, I simply did not believe that eating to appetite would ever work for me.) In other words, the experiences we have throughout life impact the current beliefs we hold about the situation.

Carr found that it could sometimes be a *single belief* that kept someone in the nicotine trap. Midway through a presentation, he would often be interrupted by someone telling him they suddenly got it – that he needn't say another word – they would never smoke another cigarette again. Crucially, however, the vital information triggering this insight was often different for each individual. This is because every person believes different things about their behavior, and most require the debunking of several beliefs in sequence before the glorious truth sinks in.

Exposing these false beliefs is critical because successfully navigating away from a deceptive item requires not only an accurate model of the misleading entity but an *accurate model of the navigating lifeform* (you).

There is an almost universal tendency among victims of deception to view themselves as a fundamentally flawed human being: deficient, disordered, and *different* from others in some vital way.

It is thus not enough to understand how deceptive flavor distorts appetite if you still believe that overeating can be caused by negative emotions or provides a way to cope with boredom, for example. It is not enough to understand how intermittent reinforcement prompts increased engagement if you still believe that addiction is a confusing powerlessness-type condition from which escape is difficult or rare. In other words, it is not enough to evict a deceiving entity if their lies still infiltrate your castle. To be permanently free of a misleading counterfeit, *all associated misconceptions must be rooted out and cleaved away*.

Ending an addiction is a thought-related challenge. It requires not only changing how you perceive the deceptive item, but changing how you perceive *yourself*. The original Alcoholics

Anonymous book describes this transformation as an enormous emotional rearrangement:

> Ideas, emotions, and attitudes which were once the guiding forces of the lives of these men are suddenly cast to one side, and a completely new set of conceptions and motives begin to dominate them.
>
> — ALCOHOLICS ANONYMOUS, *THE BIG BOOK* (1939)

It was *normal* to start dieting in a society where deceptive food is prevalent and everyone is preoccupied with weight. It was *normal* for conventional diets to fail because these approaches do not accurately identify the culprit. It was *normal* for dieting to increase the likelihood of eating large volumes of deceptive food. It was *normal* for this overeating behavior *not to be understood at first* – because the influence of deceptive flavor signals is not yet widely known. And it was normal, given this circumstance, that you might eventually turn the finger of blame upon yourself.

But to eat like a normal person and maintain a healthy weight across time, you must first see that you *are* a normal person, doing what any competent lifeform would have done in this situation, given the information you had to hand.

To behave accurately, we must have *accurate behavioral rules.* The *right* choices cannot be made if the rules are wrong. Yet (and this is the magic part), the *right* rules can extract you from any deceptive environment (no matter how corrupt the data has become) because the right rules *account for the corruption in the data.*

The moment false beliefs are exposed – and you may

have started this process already – the path to freedom is revealed. The moment you understand fully that overeating in this context was the *normal, expected behavior* – and that *every purported benefit offered by the deceptive item is an illusion built upon sensory error,* walking away from the counterfeit becomes easy. This is because when something is seen to deliver *only a survival loss*, you just don't want that thing anymore.

To understand this more clearly, consider the consequences of losing a 10-cent coin. For most, losing such a small amount of money is inconsequential. But this doesn't mean that you willingly walk around throwing 10-cent coins from your wallet. No matter how slight a downside, *there is no incentive to incur a loss for no reason.* Unless, of course, this loss is *predicted to be offset by another gain*.

Every human being who has been snared by a deceptive circumstance knows the downsides of engagement with painful, personal clarity. The key to escaping an addiction is not to re-examine these awful downsides in the hope that it might spur change but to *turn attention toward the perceived upsides* (the advantages or benefits the deceptive item appears to offer) because it is *these misperceptions that drive the seeking.*

We are now at the part of the book where we begin to defuse common misconceptions about dieting, weight loss, and overeating.

The aim is to reach the point where you can see that *all of this drama* was caused by a simple sensory trick – that the body was duped by a molecular sleight of hand – and that *nothing else is wrong.*

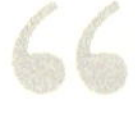

Deduction is like a game of Battleship. You are falsifying each place where the answer does not reside. But it is even more effective in deception,

> because you can pay close attention to where societal pressure forbids you to look...
>
> — ETHICAL SKEPTIC, *X STATUS* (2022)

Fat Genes

> It is of no help to be told that our subject will drink provided he was born under a particular sign of the zodiac which shows a preoccupation with water or provided he is the lean and thirsty type or was, in short, "born thirsty."
>
> — B.F. SKINNER, *SCIENCE AND HUMAN BEHAVIOR* (1965)

A common belief that people hold about weight gain is that the problem is genetic – at least in part. After all, some rare individuals regularly eat deceptive food while remaining lean. Identical twins, separated at birth and raised in different households, often have body weights that are far more similar to each other than they are to their adoptive parents or siblings.[4] Furthermore, some genetic conditions (such as Prader-Willi syndrome) are correlated with obesity. Finally, evidence suggests that epigenetic changes (inherited alterations in the way genes are expressed) may play a role in the propensity to gain weight. For example, children conceived during famine are more likely to be obese,[5] and children of overweight mothers are also more likely to be obese as adults (but interestingly *not* children from those same mothers after they have had obesity surgery).[6]

Collectively, these ideas imply that weight gain might involve an obese-prone genotype. The 'thrifty gene hypothesis' posits that some humans carry a gene that guards against starvation yet fails to protect against overeating. According to this hypothesis, excess food was historically rare (unlike famines) and could not exert evolutionary pressure – leaving people with a tendency to fatten in times of plenty.

Luckily, the thrifty gene hypothesis is not borne out by the evidence. Although starvation was indeed a common threat historically, there were also frequent periods when food was abundant (such as during annual harvests). Even in times of abundance, traditional diets do not lead to widespread obesity. In his book, *The Obesity Code* (2016), Jason Fung describes how the Tokelau tribe from the South Pacific consumed a diet rich in coconut, breadfruit, and fish, which could be readily accessed throughout the year. Yet, the Tokelau had no issues with obesity until industrialization and Westernized dietary influences came into play.[7] In fact, it has long been noted that the obesity epidemic follows introduction of the modern food supply.

> Research published in The Journal of the American Medical Association reveals that within a year of arriving in the United States, 16 percent of new immigrants become obese for the first time in their lives.
>
> — RANDALL FITZGERALD, *THE HUNDRED-YEAR LIE* (2007)

Furthermore, the weight of animals and humans is often vigorously defended in *both directions* around a 'set point,'[8] with biological control mechanisms encouraging a stable weight via adjustments in appetite, energy levels, and metabolism.[9] The hormone leptin, for example, which varies with the amount of body fat, is suspected to play a crucial role in regulating this set point.[10]

Of course, when nutrients are delivered via intermittent reinforcement, with unpredictable flavor-nutrition patterns increasing appetite, maintaining this set point is no longer feasible. As such, experts note that the set point theory does not seem to apply to people consuming a Westernized diet.[11]

If humans were genetically primed to build energy reserves in preparation for an impending famine, the tendency would be to overeat at *every single opportunity*. Yet satiety signals often kick in long before the stomach is at maximum capacity. Those who have fed toddlers know this is true. When toddlers are no longer hungry, they push the food away, sometimes throwing the whole plateful to the floor. This happens well before the stomach is swollen and distended and occurs for the very simple reason that *once nutritional needs are met, there are survival benefits to stopping eating*.

In his book *Decisions, Uncertainty, and the Brain* (2004), neuroeconomist and neuroscientist Paul Glimcher describes elegant game theory models that are applied to how animals hunt and forage for food. Every time a predator pursues a particular food source, it must forgo another activity. For example, a lion cannot chase an antelope while simultaneously pursuing a gazelle. Nor can the lion engage in non-food-related activities at this time. Like all lifeforms, the lion must make complex behavioral decisions – the outcomes of which directly impact its survival. Glimcher notes that a predator's overall aim isn't to consume as much food as physically possible by hunting non-stop...but rather to *minimize the time spent hunting* by being more efficient, leaving it with more time to engage in other essential survival pursuits.[12]

Imagine two men in a tribe. One rests by the fire, gorging non-stop from the food pot. He is sleepy, full-bellied, and slow –

at risk of being attacked from behind. His body is cumbersome and a hindrance to running, leaping, and fighting. His counterpart, on the other hand, prances around the camp, attending to other important survival needs. He uses spare food to barter with others for prize possessions. He socializes with tribe members, cultivating friendships and alliances. With all the extra time spent *not eating*, he conducts daring feats, acquires more food for winter, builds a stronger home for his family, and teaches his offspring how to survive. He engages in productive activities, such as preparing skins for clothing, bones for adornment, and crafting weapons.

One of humanity's great achievements is that we learned to cultivate and cook energy-rich foods, freeing us from the burden of non-stop hunting, foraging, and eating. Those who thrived during the last few thousand years are not those who binge ate all the supplies before anyone else could get their hands on them, but those who carefully stored, preserved, rationed, and bartered food while trading the excess to garner other critical survival assets.

It is important to remember that time spent on one activity is *taken from another*. It is completely unreasonable to expect that we are predisposed to *eat until maximum capacity at every single opportunity.*

The real blow for the thrifty-gene hypothesis, however, came with the advent of genetic screening tools, which enabled large-scale genome-wide association studies to search for links between genes and obesity. Different versions of genes, called alleles, are located at specific sites on chromosomes in every human cell and code for various traits and characteristics. By 2016, more than a hundred alleles were found to correlate with body weight.[13] Experts were surprised to discover that the cumulative effect of these alleles was minimal. Most appeared to influence body weight by less than 150g (about one-third of a pound) per allele.[14] The combined effect was estimated to account for only 1-2% of the variance in BMI.[15] In other words, despite extensive research, no 'thrifty gene' has yet been discovered.

Variations between humans certainly exist. Some people probably *do* store slightly more weight than average, just as some breeds of cats or dogs tend to be slightly plumper or leaner than others. However, these variations are *minor* and do not explain why one man is a sprightly 180 pounds (81kgs), while another of the same height clocks in at 300 pounds (136kgs).

Even in the case of rare genetic mutations linked with extreme feeding abnormalities and early-onset severe obesity, the mechanism by which these mutations contribute to obesity remains unclear.[16] [17] In Prader-Willi syndrome, for example, infants often start life with weak muscle tone and limited movement, leading to a poor suckling reflex and feeding difficulties (sometimes termed *infantile anorexia*),[18] which results in poor growth. Only when the child is older and capable of acquiring food independently does the behavior shift towards ravenous food-seeking (typically between the ages of 4 and 8).

Perhaps these early feeding difficulties cause nutritional deficits that subsequently *increase hunger* (just as might occur with babies conceived during famine). In other words, much like those who engage in restrictive dieting, perhaps this mutation sets up the conditions by which the child is *far more likely to be seduced by deceptive food.*

Not only are genetic mutations linked with severe obesity exceptionally rare (sometimes reported in single cases worldwide)[19] and hence unable to explain why such a large percentage of the population is overweight, but many of those who carry these mutations *are not overweight at all.* For instance, the *MC4R* mutation is present in 1-6% of extremely obese individuals, yet is also present in those who are normal-weight and lean.[20] When a subset of the general population of Germany was screened for MC4R mutations, only six carriers were found – none of whom were obese.[21] In other words, not only is a genetic culprit elusive, but any potential candidates appear to be spread throughout the entire population (both fat and thin) to a greater or lesser degree.

Even without complex genetic analysis, the indisputable conclusion one must reach is that rapid population-wide changes to body weight *can only be environmental in origin*. When sweeping changes occur to a population's health in a very short timeframe, the issue *cannot be genetic* because genetic changes at a population-wide scale take many generations to manifest. Slow-paced genetic adaptation is not sufficient to explain rapid changes in community health.

It is also essential to note that when a survival reward is delivered via intermittent reinforcement, seeking that reward more frequently is not only expected but the optimal response (see chapter 5: *Increased Engagement*). If essential nutrients necessary for growing and healing the body arrive in an unpredictable way, a competent lifeform *must seek those nutrients more often*. Searching for a genetic anomaly to explain the *optimal behavior* is not quite the right approach. Furthermore, if vast numbers of a population exhibit the same behavior, we cannot, by definition, attribute this to a 'rare' genetic issue.

If genetics do not play a role in obesity, why were there a few people who were overweight in the past? Although far less prevalent than today, records dating from medieval times indicate that obesity has been around for a long time.[22] The ancient Greek physician Hippocrates, for example, born around 460 BCE, noted obesity's association with other diseases. There are also well-known examples of people who were fuller-figured one hundred years ago, and many historic paintings depict voluptuous individuals. Doesn't this suggest that a certain percentage of people are naturally predisposed to gain weight in any environment?

It is critical to remember, however, that although intermittent reinforcement within the food supply has exploded in recent decades, deception is not a new tactic (see chapter 4: *Masters of Deception*). The process of refining sugar can be traced back to ancient civilizations. Refined sugar became increasingly widespread in Europe around the 15th century, with the advent of colonial sugar plantations presumably accounting for plump physiques within the upper classes during this period.

But what about weight gain among lower-class citizens? A much older form of deception in the food supply may account for this. Water sources in ancient times were sometimes contaminated with bacteria and other pathogens, making alcoholic beverages safer to drink – and leading to far greater consumption of alcohol than we might suppose. For example, a researcher who attempted to document the diet of 13th-century overweight monks estimated that their daily intake included four pints of watery beer, four pints of ale, and a flagon of wine.[23]

Alcoholic beverages contain ethanol, one of the most ancient deceptive substances utilized by man. Like benzodiazepines, ethanol binds to GABA receptors,[24] strengthening the inhibitory effects of the GABA neurotransmitter, leading to feelings of sedation and relaxation. As with all deceptive substances, long-term usage causes receptors to recalibrate, prompting increased consumption over time. Unlike water, alcoholic beverages also contain calories and may explain the rare cases of obesity in historical situations where the food supply was otherwise absent of deception.

Outside of these rare examples, however, traditional populations who rely predominantly on genuine, flavor-honest fare do not suffer from society-wide weight-related problems.

Any time spent lamenting genetic lottery is time wasted. Food manufacturers *love* it when we blame an internal flaw – because this makes the problem an intrinsic, permanent part of the *individual* – and makes it far less likely that we will lift our eyes and notice the devious little trick they are playing.

Remember, too, that if a mother's gene expression can change during her lifetime to reflect a new food supply (and this adaptation be passed on to the child), logic must insist that the *child's* gene expression can change back in *their* lifetime when a different food environment is perceived.

No one carries a gene that says, 'overconsume to the point of death.' If identical twins are both overweight, while adoptive families are thin,[25] there are numerous other genetic traits that might explain this besides the one that is feared. Perhaps, for example, some people carry a 'high achieving, diligent, follow-rules-closely' trait or some other awesome characteristic that has big pay-offs in ordinary circumstances but backfires spectacularly when following flawed advice like '*lose weight by eating less than you need to survive.*'

In other words, inherited variances may prompt some people to diet more aggressively, setting up the circumstances whereby they inadvertently become more susceptible to being fooled by deceptive food.

There are innumerable inherited reasons why someone might have been more likely to dive headfirst into the deceptive food trap, but *none* of these reasons hinder your ability to leap out.

> ...when the cultured cells you are studying are ailing, you look first to the cell's environment, not to the cell itself, for the cause.
>
> — BRUCE LIPTON, *THE BIOLOGY OF BELIEF* (2016)

Slim Junk Food Eaters

Even so, you may know someone who remains lean without apparent effort despite consuming deceptive foods. Isn't it bitterly unfair that such people get to enjoy a positive perception of deceptive foods their whole lives? Surely these individuals have it best of all?

Before answering this question, let's examine why someone might be in this situation.

Firstly, the person you *assume* regularly consumes deceptive foods might not actually do so. We often encounter others at gatherings and social events where spreads of prepared food are available. Many people eat items on such occasions that they would not ordinarily consume. This can create a false perception of their typical diet.

Secondly, people who appear to 'eat whatever they like' may simply eat freely from butter, cream, cheese, potatoes, rice, and so on, which are often cast as dangerous and fattening yet are flavor-honest. Someone who consumes a plentiful supply of such foods while occasionally ingesting deceptive items is in a far better position than the chronic dieter who limits entire food groups or reduces calorie intake to starvation levels before sham eating large volumes of deceptive food. Those who eat ordinary foods to appetite, without dieting, rarely exacerbate hunger to emergency levels and are far less likely to undergo a deceptive food binge. As such, these individuals are prone to drift into obesity over decades, explaining why many people appear to effortlessly maintain a slim physique while younger, yet find this ability melts away with time.

It is also possible that a slim junk food eater might be snared by another addictive circumstance. Deception of any kind pulls attention and resources away from competing activities, diverting attention from hunger. This is obvious in the case of a heroin addict, but even 'milder' addictions impart this effect. For example, teenagers who regularly play computer games are far more likely to skip meals.[26] You may have also noticed that although many heavy users of energy drinks are overweight, a percentage remain exceptionally lean. This is because the intermittent reinforcement caused by the added stimulants within the drinks prompts greater intake of the deceptive beverage over time. If this drink is low-calorie, the individual may not gain weight despite a deteriorating mood, declining health, weakened enamel, and degrading bone structure due to the high volumes of phosphoric acid that are often added to boost acidity and tanginess. (Of course, many energy drink consumers *are* overweight because these drinks frequently deliver high calories and contain flavor deceptions that distort and manipulate flavor-nutrition relationships.)

Finally, it is important to consider the possibility that a slim person's physique might not be as effortlessly maintained as you imagine. Many of those with dietary struggles hide this from others, even from loved ones. Perhaps the person you *assume* is effortlessly slim implements dietary restriction behind the scenes.

I recall one occasion at university when I decided to have a public 'feast day' with my flatmates. We ordered pizzas, and I baked enormous cookies to have with ice cream for dessert. At this time, I was cycling incessantly between starvation diets and obscene binges. That evening was one of the very few occasions when I let loose in front of others. As I shoveled pizza down, a friend asked in shock, "How do you eat so much without gaining weight?"

Another time, my sister informed a friend that I struggled with dieting and binge eating. Her friend apparently found this unbelievable and told her she thought I was "effortlessly thin." At that time, I was not, in any way, effortlessly thin. I was living an internal nightmare, clinging to that state by the skin of my teeth.

> Before you start envying these people who post pictures of their idyllic lives on social media, remember that the grass is often greener on the other side because it's false.
>
> — WILLIAM PORTER, *ALCOHOL EXPLAINED 2* (2019)

It is also worth noting that a significant number of people who remain outwardly slim have high levels of *visceral fat*. This type of fat hides deep in the abdominal cavity, wrapping around internal organs. Associated with serious health complications,[27] visceral fat cannot be seen with the naked eye and is far more challenging to diagnose. Those who are thin on the outside yet fat on the inside (TOFI) as a result of consuming deceptive food may have very little evidence that anything is wrong.

Remember, too, that weight gain is only *one* of the possible downsides of consuming deceptive food. Slim junk food eaters can still get hypertension, insulin resistance, Type 2 diabetes, non-alcoholic fatty liver disease, and so on. They may not experience weight gain, yet they can still develop metabolic syndrome, feel depressed and fatigued, have terrible skin, chronic inflammation, and suffer the general all-purpose malaise that comes from not feeding the body what it needs.

Every lifeform needs a critical supply of nutrients to move, grow, and regenerate. Slim junk food eaters might not suffer visible damage, but this does not mean the damage isn't occurring out of sight or at a slower rate. Many health issues, especially those related to poor nutrition, can take years or decades to manifest.

It is also worth noting that although genetic changes cannot explain the dramatic onset of the obesity epidemic, genetic variances *may* explain the tiny percentage who remain ultra-lean while eating large volumes of deceptive food. For example, researchers recently analyzed a genetic database of over 47,000 people and found that a mutation in the ALK gene was associated with a very low BMI.[28] Furthermore, deletion of this gene in both fruit flies and mice resulted in thinness, even when consuming an otherwise fattening diet. Unfortunately, malfunctions in the ALK gene are also associated with cancer.

In fact, one of the first lessons you learn when raised around livestock is that animals that don't fatten in the ordinary way often have something wrong with them. Although some breeds of cows are certainly slimmer than others, *all breeds can achieve a healthy weight when conditions are right* – accompanied by sleek, glistening fur and bright eyes. If an animal remains thin, underweight, and scrawny no matter what you do, it almost always indicates a problem.

There are many health conditions that interfere with a person's ability to store fat. For example, lipodystrophy is a condition that can cause someone to store fat in the liver and muscles rather than around the body, leading to a lean and muscular appearance. Lest this sound advantageous, severe complications of this condition include liver failure, heart failure, and sudden death.[29]

Intestinal disorders may also present as a difficulty in gaining weight. These are often hard to diagnose and may remain undetected for many years. Conditions such as Celiac disease, Crohn's disease, and Cystic fibrosis, for example, can hinder the absorption of nutrients, leading to poor growth, fatigue, weakness, infections, and numerous complications related to inflammation and nutrient deficiencies.

However, let's imagine that you know an ordinary, seemingly

healthy individual, without any known hidden dietary issues, who remains lean despite frequently consuming deceptive food. Surely *this* individual is lucky?

To answer this question, let's imagine there is a poison that sickens 75% of those who take it, with some of these people dying. If a population is dosed with this poison, are the 25% who survive without obvious detriment lucky?

Well, of course, they are. Remaining alive and in good health in the face of apparent disaster is a tremendous survival asset.

But if these people *keep on willingly taking the poison* despite witnessing what happens to those around them, are they still lucky? Or might another word perhaps be more appropriate for this behavior?

If a chronic poison-taker escapes the negative consequences while continuing to take the poison, yet their identical twin chooses to avoid the poison entirely, which of the two is in a better position?

After all, even if the poison-taking twin has *zero detectable side effects*, there are almost certainly residual traces of damage within the body. No one *benefits* from taking poison. Who knows what undetected health anomalies are festering inside the chronic poison-taker. Furthermore, because the poison-taking individual holds a belief that makes them prone to *keep taking the poison*, sooner or later, their luck may run out.

Of course, some readers may object to this analogy. No one would *willingly* take poison. But what if that poison was cunningly manipulated so that it *seemed like something good* – so whenever people consumed it, they experienced a small dose of pleasure? In this case, might the poison-taker not think they were fortunate to be able to access this delightful pleasure without the obvious consequences?

As will be discussed shortly (see chapter 10: *Delicious Taste*), there is no free pleasure in this survival game. Whenever pleasure is signaled in error, bodily systems recalibrate accordingly. Prediction errors are always paid for, with interest.

There is a documentary on YouTube titled *Fast Food Baby* (2020),[30] which shows parents feeding young children large volumes of deceptive food. The comment section rips these parents to shreds, just as people vocally condemn those who feed animals poorly. Society evidently has very strong reactions to the idea of feeding children and animals deceptive fodder. Yet, interestingly, it is perceived as normal to feed these same items to ourselves.

If someone believes that those who consume deceptive foods without obvious detriment are *luckier* than others, it means that the individual still perceives the deceptive food eater to be *gaining a benefit*. Perhaps the benefit is simply the ability to relax about diet and eat without concern?

Imagine you had the option of being locked inside a specialist facility while being fed flavor-honest food until you were nourished and healthy. Just prior to departure, the doctors offer to take you to a room and delete all of your diet-related memories: the yo-yo dieting, the overeating, the shame – all gone. For all intents and purposes, you would emerge from this room as a slim, 'normal' eater – and could then approach any food-related situations in a relaxed manner, without worry.

The prospect of erasing dietary memories and returning to 'normal' can seem a marvelous option. However, it is critical to realize that erasing dietary memories would not so much restore a state of normality but a state of *naivety*.

Naivety is certainly pleasant while it lasts (see chapter 9: *The Charm of the First Encounter*), but it is fraught with risk. If you returned to a state of naivety, there would be nothing to stop you from sliding back into the very same trap again.

One day, you might eat a little bit more deceptive food than intended (after all, these foods don't satisfy and increase hunger, prompting the intake of a greater volume to obtain adequate nutrition). Soon enough, you might decide you were ever so slightly plump and would respond in the obvious manner of *eating a bit less*. Then you would get *hungry*, and one day, willpower would run out, and you would gravitate toward deceptive food, and lo and behold, it would taste wonderful because you were *hungry*, and it pretended to offer exactly what you needed.

Enduring this drawn-out tragedy once in one lifetime is bad enough, but do you know what would be worse? Wiping the slate clean and *doing it all over again*.

When someone has no personal experience of the dangers of a particular circumstance, it is easy for them to write off the activity as harmless. In the early phases of engagement with any addictive item, the situation always seems filled with such promise and potential. The honeymoon phase is a time of careless naivety, because it is not yet clear how this particular deception can run life astray.

Someone who avoids a counterfeit has not *lost* something that others still retain; quite the reverse. An individual who encounters deception and walks out the other side has gained something incredibly valuable: *the truth*.

No one is lucky to engage with a counterfeit that systematically takes what it promises to deliver.

Gaining weight after eating deceptive food is certainly unpleasant. But this experience offers a phenomenal silver lining. It offers a clear and unambiguous warning sign that *something is wrong*.

It is *never* beneficial to welcome a traitor into your home and *not know the traitor is there*.

If the torment of weight gain has been at such a level that it has propelled you to seek a solution, then far from condemning you, that torment has saved you.[31]

If an enemy shows you his true face, do you know what an advantage that gives you? Furthermore, as you come to understand what has truly been laid out here – that this trick is replayed in every single addiction – this understanding offers protection not just from deceptive food but from every addictive thing.

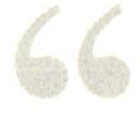

> Contrary to clinical lore, achieving remission does not typically lead to drug substitution, but rather is associated with a lower risk of new SUD [substance use disorder] onset.
>
> — CARLOS BLANCO, MAYUMI OKUDA, SHUAI WANG, SHANG-MIN LIU, AND MARK OLFSON, *TESTING THE DRUG SUBSTITUTION SWITCHING-ADDICTIONS HYPOTHESIS* (2014)

You are not one of the unfortunate ones who must be extra careful around this particular deception. You are one of the lucky ones because when you see deceptive food for what it really is, you're free.

Don't envy the junk food eater. With time, they will notice the change in you, and they will envy you.

Sluggish Metabolism

Another common belief is that extreme dieting might cause durable changes to metabolism or thyroid function. It has long been recognized, for example, that cycling livestock through periods of deprivation is a cost-efficient way to fatten them. When dietary restriction is followed by unlimited access to food, animals often experience a period of accelerated growth, during which food is converted into fat and muscle at a faster rate than before. This phenomenon is known as 'compensatory growth'[32] and is observed in many animal species as well as plants.[33] Farmers have a considerable interest in this strategy because it allows livestock to be fattened for lower feed costs.

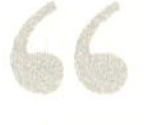

> ...every stockbreeder knows that the most effective way to fatten pigs for market is first to starve them. This knowledge goes back at least 2,500 years.
>
> — GEOFFREY CANNON, *DIETING MAKES YOU FAT* (2019)

The Biggest Loser study, which revealed that most contestants on the popular television show regained the lost weight, played a pivotal role in convincing the public that dieting 'damages' the metabolism. This study found that six years after the grueling episodes ended, contestants were still burning approximately 500 fewer calories per day than expected.[34]

The fear at the heart of these arguments is that caloric deprivation might prime the body to protect against future famines by storing fat more aggressively than before. Those who have experienced post-diet binge eating and the rapid weight gain that follows know how convincing these ideas can feel.

However, a critical detail is often overlooked in discussions about metabolic adaptations: compensatory growth in animals ordinarily *ceases when the deficit is recouped.* In other words, if an animal is fed a restrictive diet and becomes thin and scrawny in the process, it does indeed typically experience accelerated growth once an ample food supply returns. Yet, this accelerated growth *almost always stops once an optimal body weight is achieved.*

This 'optimal weight' varies depending on the species, the animal's age, and the extent and duration of the deprivation. In some cases, animals never achieve the expected size and stature and remain stunted and small their whole lives. Others catch up to controls and then resume normal growth. Still others overshoot, growing slightly larger and more robust than expected. But what *doesn't* happen is that they continue gaining weight until they are morbidly obese. Instead, metabolic adaptations *revert to normal* once an animal's optimal physique is restored.

Interestingly, well-controlled human studies yield the same findings. In one experiment, overweight postmenopausal women were put on a highly restrictive 800-calorie-per-day diet, with all meals provided, until they achieved a normal BMI (this took approximately 2-3 months, with the precise timeframe varying, depending on how long it took each individual to lose weight). During the dieting phase, metabolic rates dropped by an average of 6% and remained at this reduced level throughout the weight loss period. However, when calories were increased to maintenance levels after the diet had ended, metabolic rates *returned to normal within only ten days*. In other words, even with an extreme caloric deprivation, no lasting changes in resting metabolic rate and thyroid hormone levels were observed.[35]

Another study compared the rates of weight loss between women with a history of yo-yo dieting and those without. The study found *no significant differences in weight loss* between these two groups.[36] Another study found that those who had lost weight dieting and then maintained this weight recovered their expected resting metabolic rate, whereas those who *regained* the weight did not.[37]

Why would people who regain weight (including those in The Biggest Loser study) suffer ongoing metabolic disturbances, whereas other individuals – and all animals – do not? The clue may come when you consider that neither animals (nor humans within well-controlled studies) typically *refeed upon deceptive food.*

If deceptive items offer the illusion of nutrition in the post-diet period (hence exposing bodily systems to intermittent reinforcement), a dietary emergency remains. Attempting to quell hunger with deceptive food is akin to putting out a fire with gasoline.

When the body does not have a reliable method for finding the raw materials it needs to build and heal itself, *conserving resources* (precisely the function of a slowed metabolism) makes a lot of sense, just as pinching pennies is wise if one's next source of income is uncertain.

It is also worth noting that prior to taking the final metabolism measurements in The Biggest Loser study, participants were *weighed daily for two weeks*. Although their weight was described as "relatively stable" during this period, the actual trend was for participants to slightly lose weight across these two weeks – indicating that some form of dietary restriction may have been at play. I can only speak to my own reaction in this circumstance, but if I were being weighed daily by scientists scrutinizing my weight, I would not have been able to help subtly normalizing my intake during this period. If any of the participants did indeed modify their diet at this time (intentionally or otherwise), this change in behavior alone would have impacted the final metabolism readings, further complicating the results.

Fortunately, the unavoidable conclusion one reaches after examining both animal and human data is that the metabolic changes that occur as a result of restrictive dieting are *rapidly reversible.*

Large Serving Sizes

Another common belief is that burgeoning portion sizes are to blame for the obesity epidemic. The increase in serving sizes over the past few decades is well documented,[38] with numerous restaurants and fast-food chains opting for bigger dinner plates, wider pizza pans, oversized muffin tins, and so on.[39] The largest single-serve drink from MacDonald's, for instance, now holds over four times the volume it did in 1955.[40] Some suspect that the increased serving sizes in different countries might influence differing obesity rates.

Studies have indeed found that larger serving sizes can lead to increased consumption in the short-term. These studies also indicate that this increase in calories is not offset at the following meal. One study that captured the public's attention was a 'bottomless bowl' experiment, in which soup bowls were surreptitiously refilled while people ate, with the actual portion size concealed. It was found that participants with refilling bowls consumed more soup,[41] implying that reducing plate size (and monitoring portion size) might be an appropriate tactic.

However, a critical eye must be cast over these studies. Brian Wansink, the lead author of the soup bowl paper, was later found to be encouraging his team to engage in 'p-hacking' – the practice of manipulating data to make it seem as if a finding has statistical significance when it does not.[42] Wansink was later removed from his teaching and research roles, and a large number of his papers were subsequently retracted.[43]

There are several reasons to be cautious when interpreting portion size data. Firstly, long-term investigation into the 'portion size effect' is lacking, and a direct causal link between serving size and body weight has yet to be established. Some researchers go as far as to state that the "evidence supporting the proposition that exposure to large portions increases weight is very weak, if not absent altogether."[44]

A major complication when interpreting the results of portion size studies is that a significant percentage of the adult population is actively dieting or attempting to lose weight at any one time (up to 50% by some estimations). Dieters are typically hungrier than others and are more likely to rely on external cues as gauges for how much to eat rather than modulating food intake in response to internal bodily signals. Dieters are particularly vulnerable to consuming more when the amount of food is *concealed or misrepresented in some manner*.

It is also worth considering that a substantial number of participants in scientific studies are university students. Unlike the general population, this cohort is more likely to face financial constraints and may capitalize on the provision of 'free food' within studies by consuming more than they ordinarily would.

The main problem with portion size studies, however, is that scientists typically use manufactured foods because these items are easier to prepare and store in a laboratory setting. Using manufactured foods also makes it straightforward to measure and define portion size, achieving greater control over experimental variables. As such, the majority of portion-size experiments use highly processed snacks, such as flavored crisps – which rarely trigger a full signal at any stage, regardless of whether a small or large portion is eaten. In such scenarios, tweaking cues relating to portion size is far more likely to alter intake.

The use of deceptive food within portion size studies also explains why intake at subsequent meals is not dented. Deceptive foods deliver very little nutrition and thus do not quell appetite; rather, the intermittent signals *increase* appetite.

One of the best studies to put a nail in the coffin of the

portion size argument was a 2018 study in which households were provided with sugar-sweetened cola in 250ml, 500ml, 1000ml, or 1,500ml bottles to see which portion sizes prompted greater intake.[45] Each household received the same volume of cola, but in different-sized bottles, delivered over the course of four weeks. The households with smaller bottles drank the most and reported consuming more than one bottle at a time. The smaller bottles were perceived as being more convenient and portable and were regarded more positively, prompting greater consumption overall.

A similar study tested whether a smaller plate would impede consumption among buffet eaters. It did not. The "small dish size prompted more trips to a buffet bar to obtain more self-served food items."[46]

After all, if portion size was really to blame, why don't people just avoid large serving sizes? Alas, 'portion control' is simply calorie restriction by another name. And like all popular weight loss strategies, it has dismal outcomes long-term.

Elevated hunger leads to larger serving sizes, not vice versa. When deceptive foods are consumed, people are nudged toward eating larger volumes, which manufacturers then compete to deliver. The solution is not to attempt to satiate an elevated appetite with a smaller plate but to *reset hunger back to normal.*

Insufficient Money, Energy, and Time

At my heaviest weight, I spent my days caring for a preschooler and baby while juggling household chores. In the evenings, I stayed up late, growing a fledgling business, before snatching a few hours of sleep and waking up to do it all over again. During this period, life felt relentless and never-ending. The idea of overhauling eating behavior on top of everything else felt as though it might be too much to bear.

While exhausted and overweight, it can feel as if the body is working against success – as if there is no viable way out. In other addictive situations, the genuine item is often a molecule within the body – hence avoiding the counterfeit is all that is required. When it comes to food, however, the genuine item must still be consumed. There is no doubt that preparing a nourishing, home-cooked meal is more laborious than ordering takeout.

Luckily, simple, quick meals are all that is necessary to turn this thing around. Cooking can be surprisingly efficient, particularly when using recipes such as one-pot meals, sheet pan dinners, and slow cooker dishes. Many home-cooked meals take little time to prepare and can be ready in a shorter time than it takes for takeout to arrive.

It takes only a few minutes to throw a hunk of meat in the oven with chopped tubers and vegetables sprinkled with herbs before baking everything until succulent and tender. It takes only a few minutes to boil some eggs and potatoes, open a can of tuna, and throw everything onto a plate alongside chopped vegetables and fruit.

Home-cooked meals do not need to take long nor require culinary expertise. Furthermore, every convenience of modern life can be utilized in this endeavor. In many parts of the world, fruit and vegetable boxes can be ordered online – as well as meat boxes and other produce, such as locally harvested nuts. Some regions even have suppliers who deliver fresh milk or traditionally baked sourdough. Furthermore, it is *exciting* to see a kitchen filled with beautiful, genuine foods.

Part of the problem is that until the situation is clearly understood, the prospect of initiating another dietary change is often accompanied by a feeling of resistance. The real challenge in avoiding deceptive foods is not finding fifteen minutes here and there to prepare a nourishing meal, but in *seeing the situation as it truly is*. It is not *time* that presents a barrier to any particular activity, but the *interpretation of the situation*, which impacts motivation levels and prioritizing of tasks. After all, there are some daily activities that you find time for, regardless of how busy you become.

Another common worry is that eating predominantly flavor-honest food might be too expensive and unjustified in the current economic climate. Many genuine foods are indeed more expensive than their deceptive counterparts. For example, fresh meat is typically more costly than processed meats containing various filler agents, emulsifiers, stabilizers, nitrates, and added flavors. Similarly, freshly squeezed fruit juice is more expensive than reconstituted shelf-stable juices or soft drinks.

When flavored filler substrates replace nourishing ingredients (see chapter 4: *Concealing Flavor*), the resulting product is almost always more affordable. Government subsidies can also favor the inclusion of deceptive ingredients like corn syrup, further reducing the cost of these items. Fresh produce, on the other hand, is typically more expensive to transport and store, with swings in seasonal availability.

Despite this, consuming flavor-honest foods is readily achievable, regardless of budgetary constraints. A wide range of genuine foods remain very affordable in many parts of the world, such as potatoes, fresh milk, frozen vegetables, legumes, apples, and so on. Furthermore, when meals are filling and nutrient-dense, less is eaten overall, resulting in additional cost savings, even once the price of more expensive genuine foods – such as meat, butter, and cheese – are factored in.

When fully home-cooked meals are compared with takeout, a home-cooked meal is almost always the less expensive option. These savings magnify if meals are cooked in bulk and frozen. One study that tracked the cost of food for families with children who converted to a healthier way of eating found that they spent less money on food over time.[47]

If poverty appears to justify the purchase of deceptive fare, it is worth noting that animals fed demineralized diets often perish *faster* than those fed nothing at all.[48] [49] This is because when a low-nourishment diet is eaten, the need for vitamins and minerals to digest, excrete, and transport these compounds around the body can *exceed* the amount of nutrition coming in. In other words, digesting a deficient diet can draw upon the body's reserve of *stored nutrients.* In such circumstances, an animal becomes progressively weaker and malnourished despite eating more food.

Every dollar spent on genuine food is an investment that has a flow-on effect on all other aspects of life. Eating genuine food saves time and money in numerous unexpected ways – improving immune function, reducing inflammation, and contributing to overall well-being and productivity, leading to fewer sick days, boosting energy levels, and making it easier to keep on top of daily tasks. Combined with increasing self-confidence, this can translate into improved job performance and other financial gains.

Health, energy, and time are some of the most valuable assets we have. We only appreciate the value of good health when it is gone – and it then becomes evident that we would pay almost anything to have it back.

How many years have you struggled with dietary matters? How much time and money have you spent researching potential solutions? How much energy have you dedicated toward solving this thing?

Consuming nourishing, genuine food is *never* as expensive nor time-consuming as not eating it. Nutrients are what the body is *built* from, and these building blocks can only be effectively located and utilized if they arrive in reliable flavor-nutrition patterns that the body can read.

Bariatric Surgery

Another belief some people hold is that bariatric surgery might be an easier option than implementing dietary change. Various surgical methods are marketed as a solution for weight loss. For example, gastric bypass artificially reroutes the digestive system, skipping parts of the stomach and small intestine, with the goal of reducing food intake and nutrient absorption. Another procedure, the gastric sleeve, removes part of the stomach, limiting food intake. Adjustable gastric banding involves the upper part of the stomach being encircled with a band to create a smaller pouch. Gastric balloons can also be inserted within the stomach in the hope of artificially inducing fullness. Biliopancreatic diversion alters the normal digestion process by making the stomach smaller and rerouting the small intestine. Finally, aspiration therapy involves placing a tube from the stomach to an external port on the skin – in direct mimicry of sham eating experiments. These ports allow users to empty a portion of their stomach contents into the toilet by connecting the tube to an external device – a strategy that some have termed "medically sanctioned bulimia."[50]

The idea that surgically removing part of one's body or inserting foreign objects into the digestive tract is considered a viable weight loss solution is a testament not only to the lucrative potential of this field but the desperation felt by those who struggle with overeating.

Surgical interventions often come with painful post-operative periods and numerous potential complications, ranging from staple line disruption (the breakage or loosening of surgical staples, which can lead to the leakage of stomach contents), ulcers, stomal stenosis (the narrowing of the opening created between the stomach pouch and the rest of the stomach, restricting the passage of food), band erosion (gradual wearing away of the surgical band, which can lead to infection), excessive bleeding, internal hernias, gastroesophageal reflux (the backflow of stomach acids into the esophagus), and acute gastric distension (sudden and severe swelling of the stomach, often due to trapped air or fluid, which can lead to pressure on surrounding organs and may require emergency treatment).

Many bariatric surgery patients experience deep regret following the procedure, not only due to the physical discomfort, but the realization of what it means to never again be able to sit down and enjoy an ordinary meal with friends and family. Post-surgical dining typically requires following rigid dietary instructions, such as "chew meticulously, never drink with meals, and wait 2 hours before drinking after solid food is consumed."[51]

Although some individuals experience improvement with time, interviews with long-term bariatric patients do not offer reassuring reading.[52] One patient notes that although he no longer appears to be at risk of heart attack and diabetes, he now has blood pressure problems and a high risk of osteoporosis, despite only being 35 years of age, and describes his teeth as "breaking like crackers."[53]

Gastric bypass recipients may develop an imbalance within the microbiome, with an excessive overgrowth of bacteria interfering with nutrient absorption. With the stomach and intestine no longer functioning as intended, patients can come to realize they have signed up for a lifetime of side effects such as chronic nausea, bloating, vomiting, and 'dumping syndrome' (unpredictable diarrhea). These complications add infinite complexity to daily life.

> You have to plan everything. It is not easy to do something spontaneous. If it is a diarrhoea day I cannot go into town, and if it is a constipation day I cannot go either because of the pain, and I need to bring emergency food to avoid blood pressure fall.
>
> — JOHN, BARIATRIC PATIENT, QUOTED BY ANITA BERG, *UNTOLD STORIES OF LIVING WITH A BARIATRIC BODY* (2019)

Although bariatric surgery can deliver impressive weight loss, the combination of rapid weight loss with low nourishment often leads to a higher chance of excessive loose skin. Although aspects of life improve as obesity diminishes, this is often offset by other health complications. Unsurprisingly, interfering with the critically important human digestive system "establishes a vulnerability to unforeseen, unknown, unacknowledged and not yet curable health problems."[54]

These ongoing complications are often due to malnutrition. Bariatric patients are thus typically required to take large volumes of supplements. Deficiencies can arise nonetheless, including protein malnutrition, which may require 2-3 weeks of hospitalization, and iron deficiency.[55] (See chapter 4: *Supplements and Fortification* for an indication as to why supplementation does not appear to reliably solve the problem.)

Approximately one-third of bariatric surgery patients develop gallstones, and 10-15% need surgery to remove the gallbladder.[56] Other complications include metabolic bone disease,[57] short-term memory loss, hair loss, cold intolerance, reduced sex drive, mood swings, and pervasive low energy.

It is also worth noting that the glowing testimonials about weight loss surgery found online often come from those only a few months or years out from the procedures. Less commonly shared are stories from those who regain the lost weight – an outcome that is more prevalent than people might suspect,[58] [59] but far more shameful to talk about because it can feel as though the last resort has failed.

The reason bariatric surgery does not guarantee durable weight loss is not just because these methods compromise the vital functioning of the human digestive system but because they do nothing at all to address the reason why people overeat in the first place. Patients quickly discover that weight loss surgery does not solve 'food problems' nor remove cravings.[60] One paper notes that the common predictors of weight gain following bariatric surgery include increased food urges and "concerns over addictive behaviors."[61] In other words, the very same behaviors that are present in almost all of the target clientele.

> The surgery is on your stomach, not your head. [...] Food addiction doesn't go away overnight just because you're incapable of eating all of the things you want to eat.
>
> — SIERRA MCCONNELL, THE ATLANTA JOURNAL-CONSTITUTION, *9 THINGS NO ONE TELLS YOU ABOUT WEIGHT-LOSS SURGERY* (2018)

Consequently, many patients resort to 'cheating the system' and finding ways to get around surgically-imposed limits, such as constantly sipping molten ice cream through a straw. The artificially reduced stomach capacity can also stretch (known as pouch dilation), and band slippage or staple line disruption can enable greater food intake, with rapid weight gain often following.[62] The 'effectiveness' of weight-loss surgeries thus declines with time.

Unlike a failed diet, however, surgical intervention is often irreversible. Gastric bypass and sleeve gastrectomy cannot be undone as they involve permanently removing a large portion of the stomach. Although adjustable gastric banding is more easily reversed, tissue damage or scarring may remain. Biliopancreatic diversion is also difficult to undo due to the extensive changes it makes to the digestive system. These operations typically leave the recipient with severe, lifelong alterations to the functioning of the body, which cannot be reversed.

It is also worth noting that those who successfully maintain weight loss in the years following surgery often report using traditional weight loss strategies such as exercise and counting calories. Even when weight loss is successfully maintained, individuals often face ongoing stigma,[63] due to the perception that they have taken the easy road out.

Eight years after surgery, one patient notes:

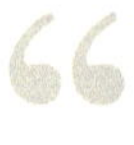

> Bariatric surgery is like playing with nature. The body is as it is for a reason. It is created in a certain way... it is not meant to be redesigned.
>
> — ROGER, BARIATRIC PATIENT, QUOTED BY ANITA BERG, *UNTOLD STORIES OF LIVING WITH A BARIATRIC BODY* (2019)

Marketers of these techniques prey on the desperation experienced by people when nothing else appears to work. These interventions not only fail to deliver an optimal health outcome but reinforce the notion that the individual is *so broken and flawed that cutting out part of the body is the only solution.*

Rest assured, there is a far easier way out – a way that restores the body to its original factory settings and leaves the amazing digestive apparatus fully functioning and intact.

Weight Loss Drugs

While weight loss drugs have experienced much controversy over the years, many still hope that a pharmaceutical treatment might offer the solution. Unlike obesity surgery, popping a pill certainly seems rather effortless.

Since the mid-20th century, various weight loss drugs have been introduced, each promising effective results with minimal effort. In the 1990s, Fen-Phen, a combination of fenfluramine and phentermine, became a popular weight loss solution but was withdrawn after it was linked to heart valve disease.[64] Another drug, sibutramine, was approved in the late 1990s but was later pulled from shelves in multiple countries due to the risk of high blood pressure, irregular heart rhythms, heart attack, and stroke.[65] Other weight loss drugs, such as rimonabant, were suspended mid-trial due to the gravity of side effects.[66]

Despite these setbacks, the quest for a pharmaceutical weight loss solution continues. The latest drug to surge in popularity is semaglutide, marketed as Ozempic. Ozempic mimics a chemical that naturally occurs within the body called glucagon-like peptide-1 (GLP-1). This gut hormone plays a crucial role in regulating blood sugar levels, slowing down gastric emptying, and reducing appetite. Due to GLP-1's role in stimulating insulin release,[67] drugs targeting this hormone were originally developed as a treatment for Type 2 diabetes. However, it was subsequently observed that GLP-1-mimicking drugs induced weight loss, making patients feel full sooner and less interested in food.

The natural version of GLP-1 is created predominantly within the gut and is released by the body in specific quantities at specific times, rising after meals, reflecting the volume of glucose consumed.[68] Between meals, GLP-1 levels fall (and become very low during periods of extended fasting). GLP-1 also has a circadian element[69] and varies according to the time of day.

Whereas the natural version of GLP-1 within the body is carefully tailored to the precise nutritional circumstance, a weekly injection of Ozempic creates higher levels of GLP-1 at all times, including between meals. This is marketed as helpful because those who are overweight or obese often appear to secrete less GLP-1 after meals than others.[70] However, between meals, obese people typically have *elevated* baseline secretion of GLP-1. In other words, the highs and lows of natural GLP-1 secretion are blunted in many overweight and obese patients.[71] The implication is that these individuals might have malfunctioning hormones, requiring pharmaceutical intervention.

As a consequence of artificially elevating GLP-1 levels, patients often experience disinterest in food, as if they had just eaten a large, satiating meal. Furthermore, when they *do* eat, Ozempic patients reach satiety faster and typically consume less food overall. Ozempic users are often shocked at how different life is when one actually feels full after eating – and describe how it feels to be able to go about their day without being distracted by constant thoughts of food.[72] Many patients wonder, in astonishment, if this is how normal people feel.[73]

As a result of taking Ozempic, however, there are now two versions of GLP-1 within the body – the naturally occurring hormone and the counterfeit.

Although the naturally occurring GLP-1 hormone is primarily degraded within the gut,[74] the full blast of Ozempic enters the bloodstream, where it does not break down for a very long time. You see, although GLP-1 and Ozempic are similar, they are not quite the same. Ozempic contains deliberate structural modifications to prolong its half-life (the time it takes for blood concentrations to reduce by half) and shares only 94% of its amino acid sequence with GLP-1. This means the counterfeit is similar enough to slot into the same receptors but is cleared far more slowly by the body. Whereas natural GLP-1 has a half-life of only a few minutes, Ozempic has a half-life of approximately *one week*. This allows Ozempic to be administered by weekly injection rather than requiring doses at every meal.[75]

Of course, as you might suspect, adjusting the rate at which the body processes a vital chemical signal can have several unintended consequences. One of these consequences appears to be a delay in stomach transit time (the time it takes for food to move through the stomach), explaining the common side effects of nausea, diarrhea, and vomiting.[76] One study found that five weeks after taking liraglutide (a drug in the same class as Ozempic, which also mimics GLP-1), food movement through the stomach was significantly delayed, taking 70 minutes for the stomach to empty on average, rather than four minutes in those who did not take the drug.[77] Another study found that after taking Ozempic for twelve weeks, patients still had 37% of food solids sitting in the stomach four hours after eating, whereas those in the control group had none.[78]

Delayed gastric emptying might explain case reports in which long-term Ozempic users develop 'cyclic vomiting syndrome' (whereby vomiting is so frequent that it prohibits ordinary employment) and 'stomach paralysis' (in which stomach function is severely slowed).[79]

After taking Ozempic for two years, one woman had difficulty swallowing and began vomiting. Doctors discovered that her stomach was packed full of undigested food. Another Ozempic user found she was throwing up food she had consumed several days prior, indicating an extremely delayed stomach transit time.[80]

The process by which the body disassembles food into its molecular parts and transports these elements around the body is critical for survival and is hence controlled with extreme precision. If a drug interferes with this process, the body cannot ignore this change. When food begins to move through the stomach too slowly, the body dials the GLP-1 signal down. One way this appears to be achieved is by decreasing sensitivity of the vagal nerve (which transfers signals from the gut to the brain) so less of the GLP-1 signal gets through.

This recalibration process begins from the very first counterfeit dose. One study found that the delay in stomach emptying time was reduced even between the first and second meals after administration of a GLP-1-mimicking drug.[81]

In addition to the tolerance that develops in response to delayed gastric emptying, other forms of recalibration also occur. A 2020 study, for example, found that mice acquire tolerance to the glucose-lowering effect of GLP-1 drugs after chronic exposure.[82] A 2021 paper discusses the decreasing efficacy of GLP-1 mimicking drugs and notes how continuous stimulation of GLP-1 receptors leads to desensitization.[83] Another study speculates that tolerance to the stomach-emptying effects "could lead to the recurrence of overeating and deterioration of glycemic control."[84] A Japanese paper discusses how the long-term use of GLP-1 mimicking drugs can result in 'rebound' high blood sugar levels due to acquired tolerance to GLP-1[85] and notes that this weakens the effect on appetite. Another study noted that semaglutide patients experience an increased pulse rate compared to placebo.[86] Rodent studies have also found an increased risk of thyroid cancer.[87]

There are many unknowns about the impact of Ozempic usage. Long-lasting GLP-1 mimicking drugs "target multiple nuclei within the brain"[88] [89] (including regions implicated in stress response and emotions).[90] One Ozempic user noted that after taking the drug for a year, their zest for life was missing. Another defined emotions as "flatter,"[91] while another described "living in a fog."[92]

Jens Juul Holst, a biomedical science professor from the University of Copenhagen, explains that there is a "price to be paid" for taking these GLP-1-mimicking drugs and notes that people rarely stay on them long-term.[93]

Any effort to artificially reduce appetite is doomed to fail. Many drugs have a weight loss effect – as the heroin user might attest. In fact, GLP-1-mimicking drugs initially create what is described as an "acute anorexic response."[94] Yet, while new users rave enthusiastically about this phenomenon and the subsequent reduction in food-related 'noise,' others offer quiet warnings about the re-emergence of cravings one year down the track. Long-term Ozempic users begin to report that dosages no longer seem to be working.[95] [96] Another study concluded that when the drug is stopped, the weight returns.[97]

This rebound effect was described by an Ozempic user who could not afford the drug anymore. Despite believing they had established good eating patterns, ten days after ceasing the drug, they found that a voracious appetite returned, hitting them with an "insane vengeance" and culminating in "the worst binge" of their life. Another user explained how they became a "raging bull" around food after ceasing the drug.[98]

In short, like all counterfeits, Ozempic cultivates the opposite of what it pretends to cure – leaving the individual with an even wilder hunger.

First, food manufacturers make money selling products spiked with isolated chemicals that communicate a false nutritional signal. Then pharmaceutical companies make money selling isolated chemicals that pretend to offer a solution while escalating the very same problem. In other words, corporations clip the ticket at both ends, while the consumer remains suffering in the middle.

Weight loss drugs are "littered with false starts, failures in clinical development, and withdrawals due to adverse effects"[99] and have historically delivered "insufficient efficacy and dubious safety."[100]

Even a basic understanding of intermittent reinforcement makes it clear that all pharmaceutical weight-loss methods must fail. Obesity cannot be fixed with a pill because it is neither a disease nor a malfunction of the body. As Calley Means accurately notes, "Obesity is not an Ozempic deficiency."[101]

An elevated appetite is the *correct response* to intermittent reinforcement within the food supply. All efforts to modify this response will be resisted and counterbalanced by the body.

Hunger signals are carefully calibrated to optimize survival. When a drug interferes with these vital signals, the body must counter the error.

What is missing in the discussion about GLP-1 levels is that gut hormones are *influenced by diet* (see chapter 7: *Insulin Resistance*).[102] Foods rich in protein and fiber appear to increase post-meal GLP-1 secretion, as does weight loss (also implicating a change in diet). On the other hand, habitual refined sugar intake is associated with blunted GLP-1 secretion following meals, and those with higher BMIs *and* the highest amount of added sugar have the weakest meal-stimulated GLP-1 secretion of all.[103] Furthermore, disruptions in daytime GLP-1 levels worsen as body fat increases.[104]

In fact, GLP-1 is not just expressed within the gut but also in the *oral cavity* in response to *sweet flavor signals*. It turns out that GLP-1 is produced *directly within the taste bud cells* of the mouth and is implicated in taste perception[105] – playing "an important role in modulating taste sensitivity."[106]

Every single piece of this puzzle fits together. In light of the hypothesis presented within this book, blunted GLP-1 expression is not a sign of malfunction but is the *expected response to intermittent reinforcement of sweet flavors.*

When manufacturers interfere with flavor signals, the body rightfully perceives this as a critical error. GLP-1 levels in obese patients are not evidence that something is wrong with the body but a sign that the body is competently responding to *something wrong with the food.*

One good thing has come from people's experience with Ozempic: The drug reveals *how easy weight loss really is when you are not constantly plagued by hunger.*

Of course, there is a far easier and risk-free way of achieving this outcome. You can remove the reason the hunger was elevated in the first place.

Poor Body Image

Many of those who have struggled with dieting and weight gain develop a negative perception of their bodies. Societal pressures and the stigma associated with obesity can lead to low self-esteem and feelings of inadequacy. This is particularly the case when the weight gain is rapid and noticeable. Consequently, eating disorder specialists often advocate for Health at Every Size (HAES), focusing on improvements in health alone, without emphasizing weight loss as a primary goal. Some even go so far as to recommend completely setting aside weight loss ambitions and learning to love the body as it is. The hope is that a positive self-image might break the cycle of problematic eating behaviors. Openly celebrating diverse body shapes is also believed to help discourage youngsters from leaping upon the dieting treadmill.

Many of the intentions behind this movement are well-founded. Just as humans have unique fingerprints, we have individual body shapes. (This is lucky – imagine how boring it would be if we all looked the same.)

Yet, part of the dilemma is that while the influence of deceptive food is misunderstood, the increase in appetite seems illogical, and it hence feels as though the body has malfunctioned. Displeasure toward the body is thus not merely an aesthetic issue but reflects the deep sense that the body cannot be trusted – that it has *betrayed the individual* in some manner and is not operating in the proper way.

It helps enormously to see that the body is not broken or disordered – that it has been behaving exactly as was expected in this circumstance. It helps, too, to understand that ending overeating does not involve punishing the body further but finally responding to its needs in a reliable and predictable way.

However, this does not mean anyone must accept obesity or love how deceptive foods weaken and sicken the human form. In fact, displeasure at this scenario is very useful. After all, if you truly viewed obesity as wonderful, there would be little incentive to change. *Recognizing that something is wrong* is a necessary precursor to escape.

Attempting to love one's physique in the hope that this might spur change is a flawed approach. Poor body image arises as the *result* of pursuing deceptive food – not vice versa. The solution is to expose and avoid the deception at the heart of this situation – so that the body naturally gravitates toward health of its own accord. When this occurs, it quickly becomes evident that the body *works as intended*, and an improved body image is the natural result.

Food Rules

Another common belief is that food rules are part of the problem and contribute toward overeating. Framing foods as 'bad' is believed to invoke a sense of guilt or shame around eating and is feared to promote 'all or nothing' thinking, increasing feelings of restriction and subsequent binge eating.

These concerns can feel particularly valid, especially when overeating emerges following the implementation of a strict diet. Furthermore, because 'forbidden' items are often prioritized during binge sessions, and these restrictions appear to precipitate the binge, it can seem entirely plausible that overeating is itself exacerbated by a rigid and unforgiving dietary approach.

A wariness of food rules is very understandable in the chronic dieter because conventional diets almost always get these rules wrong. As such, these guidelines often restrict access to genuine foods, creating a deprivation of calories or nutrients that increases with time. After subjecting oneself to such misery for an extended period, it is no surprise at all that an aversion to dietary rules may develop.

No one likes following incorrect rules. It is *sensible* to discard an approach that leaves one irritable and hungry while limiting access to nutrients. But it is equally foolish to believe that all food rules are wrong.

In fact, the *right* rules are an essential part of life. Toddlers learn food rules from a very young age. For example, most youngsters learn not to eat random insects or inedible plants. These lessons are vital because many substances are toxic and wholly unsuitable for human consumption.

All humans abide by numerous food rules on a daily basis, often without even consciously thinking about it. For example, people commonly follow the rule: *don't eat raw potatoes* (these contain solanine and chaconine, which can be toxic in high amounts). Without the raw potato rule in place, some might suspect that crunching on a raw potato would be convenient – just like eating a raw carrot. Yet, we follow this rule without issue, despite often not knowing anyone who has fallen sick eating raw potatoes. We follow this rule with ease because we attribute a *survival loss* to this action – and, rightly or wrongly, we *believe it*. As a consequence of this belief, we have no desire to eat raw potatoes.

Of course, this decision is aided immensely by the fact that raw potatoes *don't taste very nice*. Indeed, the slightly bitter, cool, damp interior of an uncooked potato *accurately reflects its survival value*, making it far easier to follow this rule.

You may have also noticed that people typically don't object to allergy-based rules. Although some people certainly wish a food allergy did not exist, no one considers these guidelines *unwise*. Being 'allergic' to something means that an item is known to deliver a survival risk for that individual. If something is known to be harmful, avoiding that item is considered a sane and sensible approach.

Much of the fear around dietary rules centers upon the notion that restriction *itself* might provoke a rebellious response. However, it is critical to see that food rules only risk rebellion when someone is forbidden from accessing something they want. If a child is forbidden from eating dirt or raw chicken, they will likely follow such rules with ease. If a child one day eats some dirt on the back of a lettuce leaf, it is highly improbable that they will run to the garden and begin shoveling dirt down their gullet at top speed, knowing the rule is now broken.

Rules only feel like restriction when they *invoke a sense of loss*. It is not the presence of a 'rule' that causes a problem but whether or not an individual *wants to follow it*. If someone believes that an item delivers a benefit, a rule prohibiting access to that item is met with resistance and discomfort because it appears to compromise access to a survival reward.

The solution is not to abandon *all* food rules and start

scoffing down dirt, raw potatoes, and raw chicken – but to find the *right* rules.

The *right* rules immediately leapfrog you out of this trap – rapidly resetting the sensory apparatus, rebooting appetite, restoring health, and cultivating a sense of confidence that spills over into every arena of life.

Even better, the correct rules are soon revealed to be effortless and *enjoyable* to follow because they accurately isolate the threat on one side while leaving all of the reward freely available on the other.

With the right rules, there is zero sense of loss or restriction. This is because when a hoax is abandoned, nothing genuine is lost...because the reward was never there.

Boredom Eating

Many people believe that boredom drives overeating. It has even been suggested that there is such a thing as 'boredom hunger,' as differentiated from 'genuine hunger.'

Boredom is the restless state that arises when there are no obvious survival needs to address. During periods of boredom, people scan the environment, sifting through priorities, attempting to decipher precisely what to do. Some believe that eating provides a distraction from this state, just as some smokers believe that cigarettes offer an activity to keep their hands busy.

To remedy 'boredom eating,' therapists often recommend compiling a list of alternative activities, such as calling a friend, partaking in a hobby, listening to music, reading a book, going for a walk, and so on. Here is another suggestion to add to the list: The next time boredom strikes, why not trim a patch of lawn with scissors and carefully count the blades of grass? If a deep craving strikes, you could measure the blades of grass and sort them according to height.

No doubt, you reject this 'boredom solution' as pointless and absurd – despite the fact that it would keep your hands busy and occupy the brain. Such actions (of which there is an almost infinite supply) are very unlikely to enter consciousness as a possibility, regardless of how bored one gets. This is because, unless you are a botanist conducting an experiment, trimming grass with scissors is predicted to have *zero impact upon survival* (remember the third rule of the game). Hence, it is very difficult to summon an interest in such activities.

In fact, many actions *never* enter contemplation as a boredom solution. For example, if you became exceptionally bored tonight, would you snort cocaine? (If you would, replace this activity with something you would never do.) The point is that boredom alone is not enough to make you do something that you do not want to do.

Of course, many people *do* eat while bored. One study found that people were more likely to overeat in a bored state than in any other.[107] Another study gave participants a dull and interesting task, along with access to wheat crackers. Both obese and normal-weight participants ate more crackers during the dull task.[108]

It is critical to note, however, that although eating while bored can and does occur, boredom is never the *proximal cause* of the overeating. To understand this, consider another bodily urge: the need to visit the bathroom. While engaged in work tasks, you can often ignore the pressure gradually building upon the bladder. But as soon as you have downtime, you are far more likely to visit the bathroom than you were a moment prior. Although boredom *coincides* with the bathroom visit, the ultimate cause of the bathroom trip is the *increasing pressure upon the bladder*. You can ignore bladder sensations until a more convenient time, just as you can temporarily ignore hunger until you have a spare moment. However, in a state of boredom, *unattended bodily signals are far more likely to be 'heard' and acted upon*. While bored, there is nothing left to distract from the nagging sensation of hunger.

Repeatedly overeating during periods of boredom does not indicate a boredom problem – it indicates *an elevated appetite problem*. When appetite is restored to ordinary levels, the presence of boredom or otherwise becomes irrelevant.

The role of hunger in overeating is revealed when people take drugs that impact appetite (see chapter 10: *Weight Loss Drugs*). Although artificially modifying appetite has numerous unintended consequences and is not recommended for many reasons, the fact that weight loss can and does occur in this circumstance supports the notion that it is *hunger*, rather than boredom, that drives overeating.

This is also revealed when someone is sick and loses their appetite. A sick person may feel miserable and lethargic, lying around with nothing to do. Yet, the propensity to overeat at such times is low – despite often being incredibly bored.

In short, addressing boredom without fixing the elevated appetite is like mopping the floor while having a leak in the roof. It is a temporary solution that delays rather than remedies the problem. This is obvious when caring for a toddler who is hungry and cranky. Reading a story or doing a silly dance may temporarily pacify the child, but the moment the distraction is over, the irritable behavior returns. The optimal solution is not for the caregiver to run themselves ragged, generating an endless stream of entertaining activities, but to *feed the child the nutrition it needs*. The moment hunger abates, the toddler transforms back into their ordinary self, and the unending stream of distractions is no longer required.

It may have also come to your attention that eating itself is not particularly riveting. Although a novel dish may captivate attention for a moment or two, most people eat while busying the mind with *other* things: chatting with loved ones, reading a book, watching television, or surfing the internet. It is rare for people to sit alone in a room doing *nothing else but eating*, contemplating how intellectually stimulating the activity is.

Isn't it curious that with the enormous plethora of potentially interesting activities available in the modern world, a repetitive hand-to-mouth action with severe negative social and health consequences is chosen as a boredom solution?

Of course, this is *not* why eating is chosen. Eating is selected during periods of boredom to *quell the aggravation of hunger*. When appetite is exaggerated by deceptive foods, hunger becomes an almost permanent background companion – and in times of boredom, these sensations are much harder to ignore.

Even if it were possible to cram every day full of entertaining activities from dawn until dusk, an elevated appetite would soon find opportunities to be heard, regardless. It may have come to your attention that many people lead perfectly busy lives yet still manage to overeat. In fact, such people often fear that an *excess* of activities is to blame. This is why people sometimes recommend *avoiding* distractions while eating (such as not eating in front of the television) to allow full focus to be placed on the meal. According to this hypothesis, eating while bored should be *advantageous* because it allows full attention to be placed on the food.

In other words, while some believe distraction *impedes* good food choices, others see the *absence of distraction* (boredom) as the cause. Two completely opposite states are blamed for the same problem.

Understanding that boredom is not the cause of overeating is critical because if someone still believes that an uneventful life is part of the problem, the situation can feel much harder to resolve.

On the other hand, when you see how *deceptive food causes an elevated appetite* and that this elevated appetite drives all forms of overeating (whether bored or not), you can address the issue with laser focus.

You might also be pleased to know that fixing an elevated appetite not only eliminates so-called 'boredom eating' but naturally leads to a *reduction in boredom*. When healthy and energetic, you are far more inclined to take part in interesting activities. In other words, as appetite and weight normalizes, life becomes a lot less boring of its own accord.

> As an ex-chain smoker I can assure you that there are no more boring activities in life than lighting up one filthy cigarette after another, day in day out, year in year out.
>
> — ALLEN CARR, *ALLEN CARR'S EASY WAY TO STOP SMOKING: REVISED EDITION* (2015)

Do you know what's really boring? Never going out with friends because you think you're too fat.

Do you know what's really boring? Not partaking in outdoor activities because you're unfit and ashamed.

Do you know what's really boring? Not swimming in the ocean because you hate how you look in a swimsuit.

Do you know what's really boring? Spending year after year researching how to escape this insane trap.

Boredom is the result of overeating, not the cause.

Stress and Emotional Eating

One of the most popular explanations for overeating – in fact, for addictive behavior of all kinds – is that it is a coping mechanism for unpleasant emotions or stress. The idea is that certain foods (not broccoli, for example) induce a pleasant and soothing sensation that helps to take the edge off uncomfortable feelings.

Numerous potential psychological reasons for overeating are offered, such as feelings of loneliness, sorrow, depression, worthlessness, inadequacy, hopelessness, shame, resentment, and anger. Emotional eating is believed to be an attempt to manage, numb, or silence intolerable moods that may stem from poor relationships, unsatisfying careers, childhood neglect, abuse, trauma, and other sources of distress. Eating in this context is viewed as a kind of self-medication and is considered to be disconnected from genuine hunger signals.

Emotions can undoubtedly impact physical conditions. For example, it is well-known that stress can modify the functioning of the immune system, and tension headaches sometimes arise in response to stressful circumstances. Many people believe that eating disorders and addictions fall under the same kind of 'mind-body' umbrella.

The idea that addictive behavior might arise as a coping mechanism for stress appears to align with evidence from the famous 'Rat Park' experiments conducted by Bruce K. Alexander.[109] In these experiments, Alexander explored the effect of the environment on morphine-addicted rats. Rats isolated within small, barren cages will readily consume morphine when given the chance. Alexander discovered that when these same rats are released into large enclosures with climbing platforms, exercise wheels, and numerous rats of the opposite sex, they reduce their intake of morphine, begin having fun, and get on with the business of making babies.

In light of these findings, it can seem plausible that humans might overeat to 'fill an emotional void' or to disengage from the stresses of life, and that addressing an unpleasant surrounding environment might solve an overeating problem. Unlike rats in experiments, however, humans cannot instantly migrate to an idyllic paradise. Furthermore, even if such a transformation were possible, it has long been noted that many rich and famous individuals with seemingly perfect lives succumb to addiction. Although the emergence of an exciting external environment can certainly distract for a time (as the rats might attest), even quite dramatic lifestyle changes – moving to a new city, taking on a new job, or starting a new relationship – often do not impart durable behavioral change. Consequently, addictive behaviors can seem to follow an individual from circumstance to circumstance, like a stench they cannot outrun.

After years of futile attempts to modify the external environment, people may eventually conclude that the problem is not so much an external issue but a flaw that resides within. They begin to suspect that, somewhere along the way, they developed a maladaptive coping strategy – a tendency to initiate unhealthy behaviors in response to stressful situations or unpleasant emotions.

Numerous self-help books, cognitive behavioral therapists, support groups, and emotional eating treatment programs build upon this idea, offering strategies to help people 'stop using food as a crutch' and 'heal emotional hunger.' These tactics include implementing mood-boosting replacement activities such as talking with loved ones, meditating, exercising in the fresh air and sunshine, and learning to accept one's feelings as they really are. So-called 'emotional eaters' are encouraged to keep mood logs, identifying 'emotional triggers' and establishing times at which overeating might be prone to occur. Throughout these endeavors, experts recommend avoiding judgment and practicing self-compassion if the overeating behavior continues.

If you have tried such approaches and found them lacking, it is because the concept of emotional eating is built on a false premise. Although emotions certainly appear to play a role, it is not in the way commonly assumed. Difficult as it can be to believe, *chronic overeating is always driven by genuine hunger*.

This prospect can feel exceptionally implausible, particularly if overeating occurs while the stomach is full. Eating while full is believed to be a tell-tale sign of emotional eating – because if the stomach is full, an individual surely cannot possibly be genuinely hungry. On the other hand, if eating occurs out of loneliness, for example, this might explain why the eating would continue, if the unpleasant emotion persists.

When the role of intermittent reinforcement in the food supply is undetected and misunderstood, an elevated appetite appears illogical, making it far more likely that blame will be cast where it does not belong. Moreover, because the hunger arising in response to intermittent reinforcement often feels markedly different from ordinary hunger (as it does not involve a lack of calories), it can seem plausible that this is a separate type of hunger – perhaps one arising for emotional reasons.

Ordinarily, hunger includes several recognizable symptoms, such as food cravings, a feeling of emptiness in the stomach, and, in severe cases, weakness or light-headedness due to low blood sugar levels. However, exposure to intermittent reinforcement of flavor escalates the *need for nutrients* while simultaneously delivering an excess of calories. This leads to a unique type of *sensory-specific* hunger, which is absent of many of the commonly recognized hunger symptoms. For example, with a ready supply of calories, 'empty stomach' sensations or feelings of faintness and dizziness are rare. Instead, the predominant symptoms are *cravings directed toward the flavors predicted to supply the missing nutrients* (see chapter 3: *Hunger and Satiety*). Because sensory-specific hunger does not always feel like ordinary hunger, it can seem that something else is to blame.

Another reason sensory-specific hunger is often misinterpreted as emotional in origin is that all forms of stress, including hunger, create what is known as a *nonspecific stress response*[110] – a generic set of bodily symptoms that occur across all states of stress, regardless of the cause.[111] A nonspecific stress response is experienced as a restless, irritable, anxious feeling – the general sense of unease that something isn't right. When multiple stressors are present, the nonspecific stress response grows – it is cumulative. In other words, if an individual has more than one stressful situation, an additional load of nonspecific stress is experienced.

When I was new to dieting, a primary motivation for subjecting myself to various modes of self-starvation was to improve my physical appearance and boost dating endeavors. If something went sour in a particular romance, I would often simultaneously abort the diet and begin to eat. For example, at age 20, I wrote the following diary entry after discovering that a boy I loved had kissed someone else:

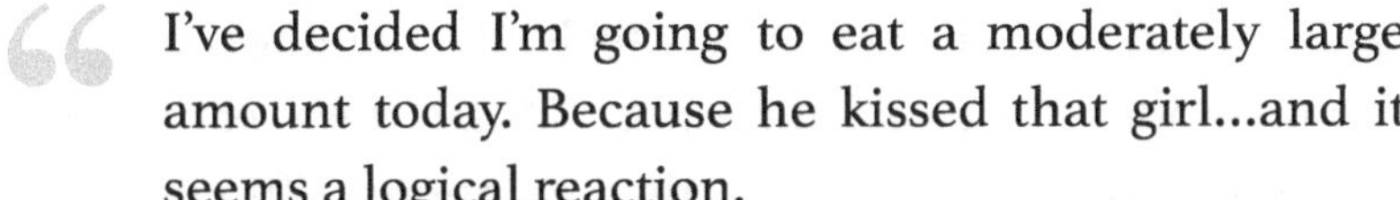

> I've decided I'm going to eat a moderately large amount today. Because he kissed that girl...and it seems a logical reaction.

In a very literal way, the doomed romance appeared to act as an 'emotional catalyst,' directly prompting overeating (behaviors that subsequently spiraled). I truly felt in this circumstance that I was eating for 'comfort,' and in many respects, I *was*. But the comfort received was the *alleviation of hunger*.

You see, at that time, I was constantly trying to hold down a ravenous appetite as a result of extreme dieting. While heartbroken, it was that much harder to endure the added misery of food restriction. If life is deteriorating in some manner, the prospect of voluntarily embracing *another* stressor can feel that much more challenging.

> " People with eating problems may or may not have enough love in their lives, but one thing is certain: they do not have enough good food when they need it.
>
> — JEAN ANTONELLO, *BREAKING OUT OF FOOD JAIL* (1996)

Dieting is a stressor and eating lifts the burden of that stress. Deceptive food is *also* a stressor because intermittent reinforcement increases hunger. In this way, both dieting and deceptive food cultivate the same stress.

Someone who alternates between restrictive dieting and periods during which deceptive foods are consumed thus remains in an almost constant state of stress. After struggling with dietary issues for years, people often become so acclimatized to the nonspecific stress response whirring away in the background of their lives that it feels like the new normal – and may evade conscious detection. What does *not* escape conscious detection, however, is the temporary lifting of this state whenever deceptive food is consumed.

As flavor molecules lock into taste and smell receptors, it appears that the solution to the nutritional emergency has been found. A portion of the hunger-related nonspecific stress response immediately abates, reducing agitation and delivering a greater sense of calm. For a brief, fleeting moment, a sense of semi-normality returns.

Of course, it doesn't restore complete normality. Although eating deceptive food temporarily reduces a portion of the hunger-related stress, it doesn't take away the damage caused to the body (it increases it), nor does it eliminate the knowledge that, by taking this action, the situation is getting worse. Eating deceptive food slightly dampens down the misery; it doesn't deliver *joy*. It doesn't restore the sense of peace and tranquility that you would have had all along if you had never encountered the deceptive item in the first place. Deceptive food delivers only a small and fleeting measure of relief (a temporary lightening of the load) by *pretending to solve the very problem it creates.*

This is why eating deceptive food always appears to provide some form of emotional support, regardless of the situation, and why many people find themselves overeating in both happy *and* sad situations – because the nonspecific stress response of hunger is present at all times. When hunger is elevated, it is harder to cope with the bad times *and* harder to enjoy the good times – like walking around with a thorn in your foot.

Unfortunately, as the consequences of overeating climb, the cumulative stress response grows, and life feels increasingly unmanageable.

> Once the fish are hooked, you can reel them in again and again, for years—you are filling a positive role, giving them what they cannot get on their own. They may never suspect that you are turning them like a thumbscrew...
>
> — ROBERT GREENE, *THE 48 LAWS OF POWER* (2000)

Deceptive foods temporarily alleviate the very hunger they create. After each engagement, the individual is left fatter, weaker, and sicker – with an added dose of hopelessness, despair, and shame thrown into the mix. In this scenario, there appears to be only two options: succumb to the cravings or undertake a conventional diet to undo the damage. Unfortunately, both of these options *elevate hunger* and hence perpetuate the constant, ongoing stress.

With an elevated appetite, even returning to a *normal* intake can feel impossible and akin to initiating a restrictive diet because an ordinary volume of flavor molecules is not predicted to deliver the optimal volume of nutrition (see chapter 6: *Tolerance and Escalation*). When the role of intermittent reinforcement is not understood, *all options seem unworkable*, and the situation appears increasingly unresolvable.

This lose/lose/lose situation is why many of those snared by deceptive foods come to feel that they must have some kind of emotional issue. And when a caring counselor suggests the problem might be emotional in origin, it often feels undeniably true. Of course, the prospect that one is suffering from an emotional 'problem' further diverts attention from what is really going on and promotes the inaccurate and unhelpful notion that something in the individual is fundamentally flawed.

> Long-term therapy aimed at understanding how one eats to "fill an inner emptiness" as if it is an individual quirk is dubious in an environment when two-thirds are overweight and almost everyone will overeat if dining on supernormal stimuli.
>
> — DEIRDRE BARRETT, *SUPERNORMAL STIMULI* (2010)

Do you want to know the hilarious truth? The natural human response to stress is a *lack* of hunger. As a teenager, before I ever went on a diet and before 'food problems' emerged, I often participated in high school drama productions performed before large crowds. This induced considerable anxiety before opening night. On such occasions, my stomach would seem to close completely, with hunger vanishing. Similarly, when I began dating, the nervous anticipation prior to each outing made it almost impossible for me to eat.

A reduction in appetite during stressful situations is the normal human response because withdrawing resources away from digestion leaves the body alert and prepared for 'fight or flight.' The natural human tendency in stressful circumstances is thus to *empty* the digestive tract – resulting in nervous bathroom trips and the sense that one's stomach contains 'butterflies' or is 'tied in a knot.' In fact, food avoidance is the natural human response to all forms of stress...except one: *hunger*.

If you overeat in response to a stressful or emotional circumstance, it is not because you have developed a maladaptive coping mechanism but because *one of your stressors is hunger*.

Stress only dissipates when we *remove the cause of that stress*. To illustrate this, imagine you need to visit the bathroom; yet, due to unforeseen circumstances, you cannot leave the premises, no bathrooms are available, and you are in public view. In this scenario, you are likely to feel restless, nervous, and agitated. As time progresses, you might even feel panicky. Although listening to music or chatting with friends might provide a temporary distraction, such strategies are doomed long-term because *they do not resolve the problem*. As the hours pass, the desire to visit the bathroom increases, and the corresponding urges grow in severity and frequency, dominating your thoughts, regardless of the effort put into 'coping strategies.' The only way to restore a sense of peace and calm in this scenario is to *remove the source of stress* by emptying the bladder. No other activities suffice.

Even if there *were* a way to switch off the stress of any particular circumstance by engaging in an unrelated activity (which there isn't), it would never be advisable to do so. The body's stress response communicates vital information and acts as an alarm bell. Without an alarm bell, a lifeform has no incentive to escape a survival threat. In fact, they may not even know the threat is there.

Some infants are born incapable of experiencing physical pain. Sadly, this condition is life-threatening because, without these bodily signals, it is far more challenging to understand when things are going wrong. Like pain, a stress response provides a *vital signal protecting you from emergent survival threats.*

Although stressful situations are certainly unpleasant, there is something far worse: misleading items that quietly pretend to remedy a crisis while making that same crisis worse.

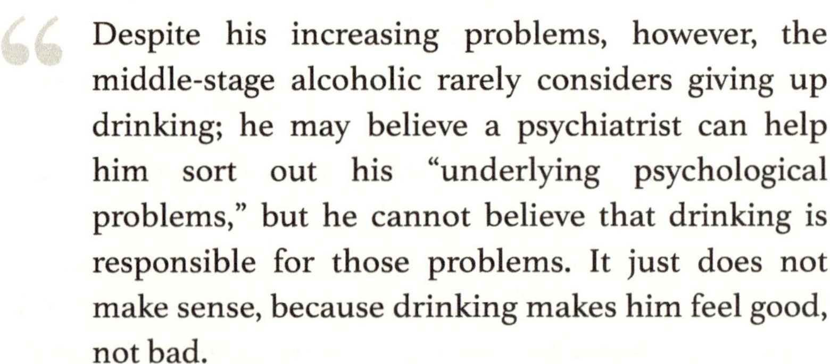

> Despite his increasing problems, however, the middle-stage alcoholic rarely considers giving up drinking; he may believe a psychiatrist can help him sort out his "underlying psychological problems," but he cannot believe that drinking is responsible for those problems. It just does not make sense, because drinking makes him feel good, not bad.
>
> — JAMES ROBERT MILAM AND KATHERINE KETCHAM, *UNDER THE INFLUENCE* (2011)

One of the great strengths of Kathryn Hansen's book, *Brain Over Binge* (2014), is that it spells out that there is no need to resolve any stressful circumstance or emotional 'side issues' in order to end an overeating problem. Just as it is futile for the heroin addict to 'work on their emotions' while continuing to dose themselves with a substance that dysregulates emotions and increases stress, it is pointless to attempt to improve emotional responses while escalating hunger at every turn.

Overeating is not a mental health problem – it is a *deceptive food problem*. It is the predictable and logical pattern of behavior that arises in response to deception within the food supply. Molecular mimicry *deceives the very sensory apparatus tasked with moderating food intake*; no amount of 'emotional work' can ever solve this problem.

Turn attention away from the emotions and focus instead on the purported 'medicine.'

Deceptive food does not heal emotional issues or dull negative emotions; it exacerbates them. It provokes a self-perpetuating cycle of misery that goes on and on and on until you stop it.

Self-sabotage

Another common explanation is that addictive behaviors might be a form of self-sabotage, driven by past experiences of abuse, trauma, or low self-esteem. It has been proposed that self-hatred or self-loathing might manifest as overeating, with obesity providing a form of self-punishment. Tragically, it appears humans are capable of inflicting great harm upon themselves in certain circumstances – with suicide being the most extreme example. In a similar vein, some believe that obesity can become a deliberate means of sabotaging ambitions or goals – offering a convenient cover story for not confronting life's challenges or advancing a career – with these behaviors potentially adopted due to a fear of failure or a sense of unworthiness.

Others believe that obesity might be embraced as a means of

deterring unwelcome or inappropriate sexual advances, with weight gain acting as a "defense mechanism."[112] In this case, obesity is seen as a way to "desexualize"[113] the body and avoid unwanted attention – perhaps as the result of childhood abuse or as a strategy to avoid temptation and minimize the odds of straying from a marriage.

While these explanations may seem to make sense on the surface, it is essential to examine the situation closely. Remember that all addictive circumstances are accompanied by a great deal of confusion about why the individual is acting in this way. If someone can point to a traumatic event in their past, it is very easy to assume that this might be to blame. It is worth noting, however, that many people who have experienced trauma do *not* go on to develop disordered eating habits, and many of those *without* a history of trauma still struggle with overeating.

After all, if discouraging unsolicited advances was the goal, there are numerous simpler and faster ways to achieve this outcome without risking the health consequences associated with obesity. Similarly, if someone feels unworthy of success and wishes to compromise career progression, you might be aware that there are many ways to underachieve and procrastinate without resorting to weight gain. Finally, if overeating is sought as a form of self-punishment, why is the activity not made a little more punishing? For example, someone could seek out foul and revolting things to eat – or escalate weight gain by glugging down glasses of sugar and oil.

Has it struck you as odd that this form of 'self-punishment' involves eating delicious things? Is it slightly curious that this so-called method of 'self-destruction' makes people feel temporarily *better?*

There are no doubt a few rare individuals who really do wish to become obese for various reasons and deliberately set out to do so. However, if you are reading a book about how to stop overeating, we can safely conclude that you are not one of them.

Of course, some might fear that self-sabotage is a *subconscious* goal – that the individual is acting against their own interests despite consciously knowing that doing so is unwise. After all, if someone chooses to overeat, and overeating leads to destruction, it appears evident that, at some level, the individual is *choosing* self-destruction. What is forgotten in this line of argument is that the negative consequences of a particular behavior are *never why that behavior is chosen.*

If you buy an item of clothing and hand over money to the cashier, you certainly lose money. But the *reason* for engaging in the transaction is not to lose money but to *gain a new item of clothing*. The self-sabotage hypothesis mistakes the *price* people are prepared to pay *for their reason for doing it.*

Turn attention away from the detrimental consequences and focus instead on what deceptive food *appears to give*. Ask a better question: *why are you prepared to pay that price?*

No lifeform ever embraces a survival threat unless doing so appears to be *offset by a greater survival reward.*

As an example, the mating rituals in some species of praying mantis result in death for the male, who is eaten by the female during or post-copulation. The male makes the ultimate sacrifice in exchange for the chance of transferring his genes into the next round of the game.

Similarly, humans are often willing to enter life-threatening battles if doing so helps their relatives or offspring survive. In other words, self-sacrifice can be a logical strategy in this survival game.

Devastating as it is to contemplate, even suicide can be understood in this light. If an individual's use of resources appears to compromise the success of close relatives, removing oneself from the game can tragically be perceived as reducing the "burdensomeness toward kin."[114] Similarly, if someone perceives their own situation as hopeless, or feels that their existence disgraces the family, self-extermination can sadly seem a rational option. In other words, suicide is predicted to emerge whenever an individual (correctly or otherwise) deems that their genes would be better off without them.

This lens also explains non-suicidal self-injury, such as cutting. Self-harm behavior immediately alerts others that something is wrong, acting as a public alarm system, often eliciting care responses and resources from others. A large study analyzing responses from those with a history of self-harm found that the behavior was perceived to serve a beneficial purpose. Many viewed self-harm as a way to "seek help from someone" or a strategy of "letting others know the extent of my physical pain."[115]

Even ordinarily unpleasant actions can be experienced positively when linked with a greater survival reward. For example, if electric shocks are connected to a lever that delivers food, the shock itself can become a signal of reward.[116] In this way, those who engage in self-harm can find these behaviors enjoyable if the action is followed by a benefit.[117] In fact, some people report that self-harm can even feel *addictive* – presumably because the response to such shocking acts is often *variable and intermittent.*

What this means is that 'self-sabotage' is only ever undertaken (whether consciously understood or not) with the hope of improving the survival odds of one's genes. Every act of 'self-punishment' is a desperate move undertaken by an individual in an effort to acquire a better outcome for their genes.

No lifeform willingly sets out to destroy its own prospects. *Avoidance of known survival threats* is an unbreakable, foundational rule in the game.

Overeating is not an extermination method. Those with suicidal ideation typically implement the fastest and most painless method available. Nor is overeating a cry for help. Unlike the response to self-inflicted wounds, the typical response to weight gain – as you may be well aware – is not an immediate outpouring of love, kindness, and support.

Whereas self-inflicted wounds are painful openings through which the life force visibly flows out, eating is the action by which life-sustaining nutrients *flow in*. It is the action by which we obtain the essential raw materials necessary to *live*. Overeating is not self-harm; it reflects the *desperate urge to live.*

The only problem in this situation is that the molecular patterns ordinarily associated with nutritional rewards have been intermittently *paired with threats*, creating unpredictable flavor-nutrition relationships.

Overeating is not self-flagellation; it is the expected outcome of intermittent reinforcement of flavor. And all of these problematic eating behaviors return to normal as soon as a reliable stream of sensory signals is restored.

Entrenched Habits

Another popular notion is that overeating is a deeply rooted habit. This idea centers around the understanding that repeating an action creates connections between synapses in the brain. As actions are repeated, these connections strengthen, allowing neurons to activate more quickly. This concept is encapsulated by Donald Hebb's famous rule: "Cells that fire together wire together."[118]

Although it is widely acknowledged that it often takes longer than 21 days to 'automate' a new habit, the general consensus is that, with enough patience and repetition, a new behavior will eventually 'stick' and become ingrained, with unused neuronal pathways weakening and withering away.

The process of habit formation occurs across all areas of life. For example, when learning to walk, we initially toddle around, tripping and falling, before this action becomes effortless, carried out without conscious contemplation of each muscle movement or balancing technique. A similar process of habit formation occurs when learning to ride a bike or drive a car. These activities require concentration at the start but become increasingly effortless as time passes.

There is a clear survival advantage in being able to learn and repeat common behavioral sequences. Habit formation saves time and frees the brain for other tasks. Consequently, an experienced driver can often maneuver a vehicle, hold a conversation, attend to traffic cues, and abide by road rules all at once. Habits are well-oiled behaviors, and every human successfully forms and breaks habits throughout their lifetime.

Why is it, then, that a habit that brings shame and destroys health can feel so entrenched and difficult to change? The key insight missing from discussions of habit formation is that *habits are about efficiency; they are not about choice.*

To understand this, imagine you are a cave dweller living partway up a cliff above a river. Each day, you follow a precarious path hewn into the cliff face, traveling down to the riverbed below. After following this narrow path for years, you, like other members of the tribe, can skip nimbly along it, knowing where every foothold and handhold is. As there is no other way to access your cave, this habit is repeated several times a day.

Now imagine that another member of the tribe discovers that there are, in fact, *two* paths leading up the cliff face, both of equal distance and difficulty. After trying the new path out of curiosity, you decide to stick with the existing path because familiarity makes the journey safer and faster. In this case, the existence of the habit *does* influence the decision because the advantage of *already knowing the path* counts in the original path's favor.

However, imagine that a group of tribe members decide to construct a new, safer path. They hew out a wider track from the cliff face and add safety barriers so careless children do not tumble into the water below. Once completed, it is evident that the new track is both shorter *and* safer than the original. It also has the added advantage that you can easily carry things up to the cave because two hands are no longer needed to aid the climb.

In this scenario, the benefit of 'already knowing the path' is revealed to be infinitely small in comparison to the benefits of using the new track. Even if you have used the original path your entire life and have the most 'ingrained,' 'wired in,' 'deeply entrenched' track habits, should it take 21+ days of intense, focused effort to ensure that you remain on the new track? Do you imagine it would be difficult to override existing 'brain wiring'? Do you expect to constantly fight unpleasant 'urges' tugging you back to the old path?

Perhaps, on autopilot, you might sometimes leap onto the old path by mistake before realizing you had taken a wrong turn. In this circumstance, do you expect to be overwrought with sorrow at having *destroyed the habit of walking on the new track?* Or would you simply drop from the old path onto the new one and continue prancing along it, delighting in how safe and wonderful it was?

If you saw that 30% of the tribe persistently chose the old, narrow path while 70% obtained the benefits of the new, safe track, would you suspect that the 30% had an ingrained habit problem? Perhaps you might feel that, with any improvement in technology, a significant portion always refuses to adapt. But is this refusal due to ingrained habits? Do these people *try* to take the new track but find the old habit too difficult to overcome?

Isn't it more likely that rather than suffering from an ingrained habit, 30% of the cave dwellers simply hold a different belief? Perhaps they feel that the old path offers fitness advantages. Perhaps they built the old path in their youth and feel resentful that it has been usurped. Perhaps they doubt the excavation capabilities of the tribe and consider the new track a landslide waiting to happen. There are numerous reasons why someone might choose the old path, but none of these involve something called a 'stubborn habit.'

What would happen if an old-path user saw a lion blocking the way ahead? Now, the old path is not only narrow and precarious but leads to almost certain death. The new track, by comparison, waits, unblocked, offering a safe route home.

Does it seem reasonable that *any* part of the individual's mind would argue for staying on the old path? Can you envision the cave-dweller inching miserably toward the lion, wishing they could go on the new track but feeling as though their habit had condemned them to the old path? Would they suffer the urge to move along the old path, *just one more time*, promising themselves that they would evade the impending danger soon?

When a familiar path is revealed to be a dangerous one, with the cons outweighing the benefits, *we change course*. The brain *always* takes the best course of action given the information it has to hand. There is no such thing as an 'autopilot mode' that traps a lifeform into repeating an action it *knows is the wrong choice*. The human brain is never designed to get programmed into a rut and stay there until it dies.

Changing to the new track *does* require concentration for a day or two, just as any new behavior requires a few days of attention and focus. When traversing the new track, you need to learn where the steps are, where to turn, how to move along at speed, and so on. Every new action requires conscious attention for a short time. But what it *doesn't* require is an *ongoing battle of desire.*

Should I do this? Will I? Won't I? I mustn't, but I want to!

It is this back-and-forth argument that makes some behaviors seem harder to change than others. This internal argument arises whenever a circumstance is *not yet fully understood.* This internal argument is particularly prevalent when *deception muddles the data* and the truth is not yet seen.

The difficulty in changing an addictive behavior is not the automation process, nor the complexity of the behavior itself, but *the conflicting data that guides the choice.*

Eating behaviors, like all behaviors, contain a habitual element. But this habitual element is *not what makes the behavior feel difficult to change.*

If someone feels as though they are battling against an entrenched habit, it is because *an argument rages within*, causing them to flip-flop between paths. They see a threat in one direction, but they also see a reward.

Imagine the difficulty the cave dwellers would have if the two tracks were so similar they could not readily distinguish between them or if an enemy kept sneaking in and digging perilous holes on the safe track so that what *appeared* to be safe was not.

It is the *muddling of the data* that makes addictive behaviors initially feel difficult to change because it takes time for the truth of the situation to become clear.

But surely it is clear? Isn't it obvious that consuming less deceptive food would be beneficial?

Well, for a start, most people are unaware of what deceptive food even *is* – or how to define it. Secondly, although consuming *less* is certainly advisable, how much less? In what circumstances is it appropriate to engage with something that deceives the sensors? Should one *never* consume, or moderate carefully? How does one approach this misleading entity, given the extreme level of infiltration in the modern world? If it *were* clear, you wouldn't be reading this book.

We will get to these questions soon. For now, please rest assured that ingrained habits are not part of the problem.

Delicious Taste

People offer endless reasons for why they overeat. But perhaps the simplest and most honest explanation is that deceptive foods *taste nice*. The whole point of manipulating flavor and adding misleading ingredients to the food supply is to drive sales and maximize profits. This ploy only works if these strategies make foods taste *better*.

When people crave a food, they mentally simulate chewing and swallowing that item, imagining the flavor and texture as it moves around the mouth, slides down the gullet, and enters the body. What is craved in this circumstance is the pleasant feeling as flavor molecules lock into taste and smell receptors, signaling that a nutritional reward is forthcoming.

Gillian Riley, author of *How to Stop Smoking and Stay Stopped for Good* (2007), describes a fascinating study in which smokers receive an injection containing nicotine along with another injection that does not. Despite only one of the injections delivering a hit of nicotine to the bloodstream, smokers could not distinguish between the two. As a consequence, they experienced no difference in cravings. A similar study concealed alcohol within intensely flavored vitamin drinks and gave these to alcoholics. These alcoholics reported no increase in cravings after consuming the alcoholic beverage because the presence of alcohol was *not detected by the sensors*. In contrast, when the alcoholics consumed a non-alcoholic drink that they thought *did* have alcohol in it, cravings spiked.[119]

These studies appear to provide evidence that responses to addictive substances are 'all in the mind,' but it is far more accurate to say that our perception of *anything* is all in the mind and that we can only respond to something *if we first know that thing is there.*

Imagine someone transferred a million dollars into your bank account. If the money sits there without your knowledge, you would experience no shock, pleasure, or surprise. This does not mean that money has no survival value or that the presence or absence of money is inconsequential. It simply means that you cannot respond to something without first being alerted that the thing is there.

Pleasure attaches to a cue that *indicates the acquisition of a survival reward.* Throughout history, the only way that nutrition ever entered the human body was through the gateway of the mouth. In other words, the way the body *recognizes that nutrition is arriving* is by detecting the preceding flavor cues.

It is the *pleasure experienced while eating a particular flavor* that provides the primary motivation for returning to it – because it is this pleasure that predicts the incoming nutritional reward.

In *The Cure for Alcoholism* (2012), Roy Eskapa describes a treatment known as the Sinclair Method, which exposes the crucial role of pleasure in addiction. Alcoholics undergoing this treatment take naltrexone one hour before they drink. Naltrexone is a drug that blocks the brain from experiencing pleasure. Thus, when alcohol is consumed, the negative side effects of drinking remain (the loss of control, the stumbling, the hangover), but no pleasure is experienced. Over time, the association between drinking alcohol and pleasure weakens, resulting in a reduction in the desire to drink.

There are four difficulties with the Sinclair Method. Firstly, it relies on people voluntarily choosing to remove the pleasure of an activity they enjoy. As you can imagine, some drinkers simply stop taking naltrexone. Secondly, it requires ingesting a drug (which sets up intermittent reinforcement and side effects of its own). Thirdly, it can take a long time for the extinction process to kick in, during which alcohol continues to be consumed, resulting in ongoing damage to the body. Finally, because the brain cannot experience *any* pleasure while under the influence of naltrexone, pleasure is simultaneously removed from *all other activities that occur at the same time as drinking* – such as socializing, sexual interactions, and so on.

The Sinclair Method thus has many serious pitfalls. Still, the fact that it *does* curb drinking in those who continue to take the drug at the appropriate time illuminates something vitally important: *that the desire to drink is maintained only by the pleasure experienced while doing so.*

You may think this sounds logical. After all, who would drink alcohol if the experience wasn't pleasant? However, recall that this is not why most alcoholics think they *do* drink. Like all other addictions, alcoholism is blamed on many different factors – emotional challenges, genetics, boredom, stress, traumatic childhood, and so on. The documentary *Drinkers Like Me* (2018) by Adrian Chiles provides a captivating look at the explanations commonly offered by heavy drinkers (this is a great watch for overeaters because seeing the same excuses fall from the mouths of others is highly valuable). Yet, despite drinkers believing numerous reasons are to blame, when they take naltrexone as prescribed, they find the desire for alcohol fades away, even though *every other aspect of their life remains the same.* Their career is just as stressful or mundane, their home life just as dull or problematic, and their genes and life history exactly the same. The only difference in this circumstance is that they *no longer enjoy drinking* and, consequently, no longer want the drink.

It is essential to note, however, that it is not *the loss of pleasure*, per se, that cements this change. You see, these individuals still know that, at any time, they could stop taking naltrexone and access that 'pleasure' again. These are people who previously struggled to stop drinking at any cost. Yet, despite knowing they *could* return to the pleasure of drinking, they choose to stop drinking entirely. Why?

The answer is that *turning off the pleasure* allows people to *see the truth* about alcohol without the deceptive label attached. Karen Dion, who documented her experience of taking naltrexone on YouTube,[120] recalls that once the pleasure of drinking was gone, she realized that alcohol *only brought her down* – that it delivered *nothing beneficial*. In other words, removing the pleasure forces the individual to acknowledge that the reasons they *thought* they were pursuing the deceptive item were false and that all they were doing was chasing a fleeting dose of pleasure.

Kathryn Hansen, author of *Brain over Binge* (2014), reached a similar conclusion when she tried the drug Topamax as a treatment for bulimia. Although she did not take Topamax for long due to the unpleasant side effects, the experience had a profound impact on how she perceived the problem. Because Topamax reduced her binge eating while all other aspects of her life remained the same, it made it clear that the issues she *suspected* were contributing to the problem could not be to blame.

This is a very important distinction because it means that people really only pursue a deceptive item for one reason: *the pleasure of doing so.*

Think about this carefully: If a food tasted *unpleasant*, would you overeat it?

Imagine that you are home alone, with three large buckets on the table. One bucket is filled with oil, one with refined sugar, and the other with plain cooked white rice. In other words, you have at your disposal a liberal supply of fat, sugar, and refined carbohydrates – the three commonly blamed culprits. Imagine, too, that you are well-fed and have just eaten a large, satisfying meal containing all food groups.

Would you eat from the three buckets?

Perhaps you might take a few spoonfuls of rice. Maybe you would pick up a handful of sugar and chew on it curiously for a bit. But would you sit down and get really stuck in and binge eat until you felt sick? Would you haul the buckets in front of the television so that you could enjoy an evening consuming these things to your heart's content?

If someone came into your house and saw you lapping from the bucket of oil and asked why you were doing it, would, "I felt bored," or "I felt stressed," or "I just have a habit of overeating," or "I didn't have time to prepare anything more healthy," or "the serving size of oil was just so large, I couldn't resist," or "I have thrifty genes and thus feel compelled to take advantage of all caloric opportunities" provide an adequate answer?

When the pleasure is gone, *every excuse collapses.*

Some readers may think this argument is unfair. Of course we only overeat things that taste nice. So, now, let's imagine replacing the items in the buckets with three delicious *flavor-honest* foods – those you find pleasurable in their natural form – perhaps a bucket of fresh peaches, a bucket of apples, and a bucket of freshly seared salmon (or any other genuine, flavor-honest food that you like). Again, assume that you have just eaten a full, satiating meal.

Would you eat from the buckets?

Of course, you probably would try *some.* After all, the nutrition found in fresh peaches, apples, and salmon may not have been present in the prior meal, so it makes sense to have a little. But would you continue eating until you felt bloated and sick? Would you feel compelled to throw the excess in the trash to prevent yourself from gorging on these items tomorrow?

No matter how delicious a flavor-honest food is, the more you eat of it, the more satiated you become. This is because genuine foods *deliver the nutrition they promise*, and as the item is consumed, hunger is steadily replaced with satisfaction and contentment.

Deceptive items, on the other hand, do *not* deliver what they promise. Consequently, fullness signals from the gut are delayed or non-existent, and the desire for *more* remains firmly switched on.

In *The Freedom Model for Addictions* (2017), authors Steven Slate, Mark Scheeren, and Michelle Dunbar explain that every choice we make is made in the pursuit of happiness. In other words, at every moment, we act in the way that is expected to make us feel *better.*

Of course, this doesn't mean that our actions always result in this outcome or that every decision is *correct*, but that the *intention* is always to move away from pain and toward happiness. This is how the survival game works.

To understand this, consider studying for an exam. Sitting in a room and cramming boring information into the brain is seldom enjoyable. In fact, for many people, virtually any other activity – including tidying a bedroom from top to bottom – is preferable. The common belief is that, in situations like this, we must embrace something unpleasant for future gain. The idea is that we *willingly choose to suffer* in order to acquire a future benefit. However, careful analysis implies that this is not quite what happens. You see, for many people, there is, in fact, *one thing worse* than the tedious monotony of studying: *failing the exam.* If you fall into this category, as the exam draws nearer, the anxiety about *not studying* grows. This anxiety is driven by the knowledge that if you don't get your act together soon, there will not be enough time to learn the material, and you risk failing the exam. At some point, this anxiety overwhelms the desire not to study, and you go into your room, open your books, and begin.

Even if studying is perceived as painfully boring, at some point, *it eventually becomes the most enjoyable option.* It is not that studying becomes '*fun*,' and you certainly wouldn't say it makes you 'happy,' but as the exam looms, studying becomes more enjoyable than putting up with the anxiety of not studying.

Emotions in the present are modulated by future expectations. In other words, what we *believe* about a situation – and how we predict it will unfold – *directly influences how we act in the present.* This is why learning the truth about a deceptive circumstance can *alter behavior.*

Some readers may believe they now have a good understanding of the tricks used by the food industry to seduce the tongue – yet, for some reason, this hasn't eliminated all of the desire. Such individuals may feel that, *unlike the foolish naltrexone drinkers*, they already know that all they get out of this transaction is a temporary dose of pleasure. The problem is that they *like* this pleasure, and the prospect of minimizing access to these deceptive delicacies can seem too much to bear.

Surely, there is nothing wrong with a little pleasure, now and again? Isn't there an advantage to artificially boosting one's mood, even if this is not directly linked to a tangible survival reward? Isn't feeling better *itself* a benefit (the advantage of a positive mood, for example)?

After all, most experts agree that meals are not *just* about nutrition. Sitting around a table with loved ones imparts numerous survival benefits. Surely there are occasions when consuming these misleading items *simply for the deceptive pleasure of it* is justified? Isn't it reasonable to sometimes eat for *pleasure* rather than the cold, hard, analytical pursuit of nutritional gain?

Get this absolutely clear in your mind: pleasure is not a trivial sensation that can be thrown about willy-nilly. Pleasure is a vital signal in this survival game. *No one* experiences pleasure for the 'fun' of it – pleasure *is* inherently fun because it *reliably coincides with the acquisition of a survival reward.*

If an individual wants fun, irrespective of the consequences, heroin would fit this bill. Yet, the reason heroin doesn't appeal to most people is that any documentary about heroin use quickly makes it clear that *something about the pleasure is acting as a decoy* – that rather than signing up for a lifetime of pleasure, the heroin user is really signing up for a lifetime of pain.

You see, the crucial yet commonly overlooked aspect of the pleasure argument is that although pleasure plays a fundamental role in addiction, the pursuit of pleasure is not the entire story. After all, no matter how flavorsome a deceptive item tastes, it doesn't seem feasible that for a mere pleasant mouth sensation, you would ever sacrifice so much.

When you first tasted deceptive food as a young child, did you think, "Wow, this thing tastes so fantastic that I am going to sacrifice my whole life just to consume it?"

In the aftermath of binge eating, with a painful, distended belly, do people ever think, "Wow, I'm on such a high. This is so awesome. I'll be sure to do this again, several times a day, for the rest of my life."

The notion that people pursue deceptive items *only for the pleasure of it* is very close to the truth. But it misses one fundamental piece of information. The defining characteristic of every addictive item is *not* that it offers pleasure but that it *offers pleasure in error.*

Consequently, when the sophisticated survival machine that

is your body detects this error (which it always does), internal bodily systems recalibrate, and *less pleasure is experienced with the next engagement.*

Misleading molecular signals dupe the body about the nutritional reward coming in. When this reward does not arrive as anticipated, taste and smell receptors recalibrate, reducing sensitivity, so that both deceptive and genuine flavors taste worse going forward (see chapter 7: *Downregulation of Taste and Smell*). In other words, the need for nutrition grows *while the pleasure experienced per unit of flavor falls.*

Deceptive foods lure consumers with a pleasurable eating experience yet systematically degrade the ability to experience flavor so that every meal becomes progressively less enjoyable, until even ten junk food binges deliver far less pleasure than would have been available from a single nourishing meal. Like all addictive items, they steal the very thing they promise to deliver.

If your friends played a trick on you and told you that you had won a million dollars, you might leap and jump with joy. But if this was revealed to be a joke, your excitement would certainly deflate. Would you then request the trick be played on you again, so that you could delight in the thrill of false news once more?

Situations that induce pleasure by masquerading as a reward while elevating one's need for that same reward and surreptitiously delivering a threat are not trivial forms of entertainment. Deceptive foods fool the sensory apparatus, allowing a trojan horse to enter the gates. It is as if you order steel, timber, and bricks to repair your castle, and the enemy sells you sludge, sticks, and silt.

Do you know what happened when scientists worked out how to directly stimulate the pleasure centers in the brain? In the 1950s, James Olds and Peter Milner implanted electrodes in the brains of rats, allowing them to self-stimulate these regions by pressing a lever.[121] Did the rats benefit from a delightful increase in mood? No, they pressed the lever repeatedly, forgoing all other activities until the researchers had to urgently intervene to prevent their death.

It is *never* advantageous to be relaxed, calm, and blissful while another lifeform steals your eggs from the nest.

Deceptive food doesn't deliver pleasure; it thieves it. It doesn't cure boredom; it cultivates it. It doesn't heal negative emotions; it makes one progressively more anxious and depressed. Deceptive food saps productivity, degrades health, and ruins every aspect of life.

You have been duped by a sensory trick set in motion by food manufacturers who profit from this precise deception.

This trick has been played by one organism against another since the dawn of time.

This is the snare of addiction.

A Mild Problem

There is a growing consensus that *something* about the modern food supply is addictive.[122] Some blame food addiction on *sugar* or *fructose*, although these molecules in fruits and whole foods do not appear to create the same effect despite being chemically identical. Others blame food addiction on the *insulin rush* caused by high-carbohydrate foods, despite many traditional populations eating a liberal supply of grains, tubers, and honey without apparent difficulty. Others blame food addiction on the specific combination of *salt, fat, and sugar*, even though it is almost impossible to mix up a solution of salt, oil, and sucrose that is remotely appealing. Others blame *energy density*, even though people rarely binge upon plain glasses of oil or sticks of butter. Others suggest *palatability* might be to blame, despite there being many delicious, easily digestible, flavor-honest foods that are *not* regularly binged upon.

In other words, although many agree that *something* in the modern food supply is addictive, there is no consensus about what that addictive thing is. This book lays out the evidence that *molecular deception* is the culprit, illustrating how intermittent reinforcement of flavor leads to a recalibration of taste and smell receptors while escalating appetite.

When it becomes apparent that forms of molecular mimicry within the food supply echo strategies involved in drug addiction, the tendency is to use this as evidence to justify why overeating can seem so resistant to change without really considering that the situation might be *on par* with other forms of addiction.

After all, the overeater doesn't stagger home drunk, slur words, crash the car, or commit crimes to sustain the 'habit.' An overeater can still be a good parent, even if fatigued and less energetic than most. An overeater can still be a good employee or business owner, even if they might delay career advancements or put off opportunities for professional development. An overeater can still be a good friend, even if avoiding social engagements and hiding behind a screen. In other words, overeating is surely a whole lot milder than 'real' addictions.

Some might accept that the same mechanisms are at play but retain the belief that the issue is tamer, involving more trivial aspects of body image and suchlike. Even at the point of morbid obesity, with serious health complications, it seems evident that overeating is not at all in the same league as other addictions – not as deserving of the same horror or fear.

Imagine two murderers who escape from prison. One runs around the streets, firing off a gun and yelling obscenities. He is noisy and vocal, and a few people die.

The other murderer moves quietly from town to town, releasing poison into the water supply, killing inhabitants slowly and imperceptibly over decades. The death toll is in the billions, but because the symptoms are so slight and build up so gradually, no one really notices what is happening, and when they finally do, it is unclear where to point the finger of blame.

Everyone is terrified of the first criminal, but the latter kills far more people.

One reason why overeating can seem so hard to change is that the side effects of each engagement are so slight, and there is no sense of urgency to escape. Like cigarettes, there is a lag between the onset of the behavior and the appearance of severe health complications.[123]

When punishment *rapidly* follows a behavior, the odds of repeating that behavior diminish[124] because the connection between the action and outcome is clear. However, when punishment unfolds gradually, it can take a very long time to notice that a seemingly innocent delicacy is robbing you of almost everything you own.

The most lucrative drugs are not those that kill the victim outright but those that offer a small squirt of deceptive pleasure while imparting an imperceptible threat that slowly degrades the user's life until the drug appears to be the only positive thing they have left. These items have a downfall that is gradual and insidious, crippling the victim incrementally over decades, so the counterfeit merely seems a harmless little vice.

With a gradual decline, the deceptive item is not overtly implicated, and the sufferer believes themselves complicit. After all, they can clearly point to all of those earlier in the process who appear to be happily engaging without apparent consequence, suggesting the substance is not really to blame. Yes, the best kind of customer is one you can fool for life.

Nicotine is considered one of the hardest drugs to quit –

even by those who have discarded far more 'serious' and deadly drugs. It is not really harder to quit, of course, but it is *harder to see what needs to be done*, because the consequences of smoking are far more subtle.

Deceptive foods, like cigarettes, leave the consumer in a slightly miserable, low-grade life, and that kind of existence is far more tolerable than a pastime that can kill you within the hour.

Deceptive food has a *higher death toll than all other deceptive substances,* with poor diet believed to be "responsible for more deaths than any other risks globally."[125]

Awful as it is, hard drugs have a saving grace. Although they are lethal and can kill with a single dose, the gravity of the situation sinks in much sooner. If you find yourself intoxicated, behaving erratically, and stealing from friends, you are far more likely to *wake up to the danger you are in.*

Imagine that the effects of consuming deceptive food happened at high speed – that after just one month, you were morbidly obese, diabetic, and exhausted. As your friends succumbed to this condition around you, you watch them morphing from normal and healthy to bloated and sick before your eyes. Even if they told you how delicious these items were, how they helped them cope, how they felt like the only source of pleasure they had left...you would reel from these items in horror.

Imagine your own life playing at top speed before your eyes – the diets, the researching, the binge eating, the weight gain, over and over again. Play not just your story but that of your family and loved ones in the same trap, and see how the pattern repeats. Notice how consumers end up desperately wanting change, flogging themselves mentally, searching for a way out that allows freedom from the horrid consequences *while retaining the precious source of pleasure*. Notice how people come to hate the cumulative side effects of deceptive food...but they still love *it.*

> "It has been often and truly observed that the addict in many ways resembles a lover with a fatal attraction to an injurious, possibly even a deadly love object.
>
> — FLOYD P. GARRETT, BEHAVIORAL MEDICINE ASSOCIATES, *THE ADDICT'S DILEMMA* (2012)

It is interesting that a single remark from a hypnotherapist allowed Allen Carr to break free from cigarettes. The remark was that smoking is nicotine addiction and that *he was addicted just like a heroin addict.*

One day, there is no escape from the fact that the heroin user, the alcoholic, the smoker, and the overeater are all caught in the same trap.

We call this thing *addiction.*

Powerlessness

Addiction is commonly believed to be a chronic, relapsing 'brain disorder' characterized by 'compulsive' seeking of the addictive item. The condition is believed to involve alterations to the frontal cortical regions of the brain, particularly in areas related to reward and motivation – purportedly predisposing the individual to act impulsively and recklessly. According to this interpretation, whether due to genetics or one's unfortunate life, the addict is cursed with a malfunctioning brain from which there is no easy escape. In short, the popular belief is that there is something fundamentally different about the addict: that they have an intrinsic weakness, a deficiency, an abnormality that results in a "loss of behavioral control."[126]

A common explanation for this purported loss of control is that downregulated dopamine receptors might compromise decision-making (as noted in chapter 5: *Obsession*, dopamine plays a key role in attention, motivation, and the monitoring of prediction errors). Studies have indeed found that obese people, like cocaine and heroin users, have reduced dopamine activity in the brain. It is suggested that these differences might indicate a dopamine signaling 'dysfunction.'[127]

It is interesting to note, however, that even in the depths of an addiction, individuals typically exhibit an *exaggerated* dopamine response when contemplating the addictive item in question.[128] In other words, the issue does not seem to be an *incapacity to produce dopamine*, but rather that the brain strategically directs this response toward the activity that appears best able to *solve the problem*.

Imagine you had a bullet wound leaking blood onto the floor. If a scientist flashes a cheery image at your face, should the brain's pleasure centers joyfully light up as they ordinarily might? Is it appropriate to enthusiastically contemplate romantic involvement, cute pets, or goals for the future while blood pools about the feet?

Summoning enthusiasm for less-critical activities in the face of a life-threatening disaster is not an optimal response. In fact, behaving in such a way would be a serious design flaw. If someone detects that their life is being systematically run into the ground by a deceptive circumstance, a dampened dopamine response to less critical side issues is *wise*.

Addictive behaviors involve a misleading item that appears to offer a vital survival reward while simultaneously imparting a threat – increasing the need for the very reward it pretends to deliver. This presents a highly confusing and risky situation, demanding focus and attention (see chapter 5: *Obsession*). This tuning of attention toward the deceptive item is a crucial short-term adaptation that *aids escape*. In other words, the observed dopaminergic changes in the brain of an addict are not impairment nor the *cause* of the addiction but the *logical and optimal response*.

In *The Hypothesis Testing Brain* (2010),[129] Jakob Hohwy makes a compelling comparison between the common perception of addiction and delusional beliefs that sometimes arise when people face an unusual circumstance that they do not yet understand. Hohwy argues that delusions are a logical attempt to explain unexpected anomalies or errors in sensory data – with the delusion appearing to be the best way to make sense of evidence that doesn't fit prior expectations about the world.

Hohwy gives the example of rubber arm experiments, in which a fake rubber arm is placed on a table in front of a person seated at a chair, positioned as if it was their own arm resting on the table (their real arm is concealed out of sight, motionless, under the table). If the experimenter taps the fake arm at the same time as tapping the real arm, participants quickly come to perceive the tapping sensation as *coming from the fake arm on the table*, despite knowing it is not.

Hohwy argues that in this scenario, the brain is forced to make sense of conflicting streams of data. Visual information from the eyes suggests that the tapping occurs on the table; sensory data from the skin indicates the arm is *under* the table. In this case, the visual information (which comprises two separate pieces of evidence – seeing both the arm *and* the tapping) wins out over the skin sensations. Thus, an incorrect perception – the feeling that one's arm *really is on the table* – is experienced as true.

Hohwy gives another example of stroke or dementia patients who come to believe their body is under alien or demonic control. These patients often appear completely rational and reasonable in all other areas of life yet become convinced that an external power influences their bodily movements. Hohwy explains that if muscles no longer move the body in a predictable way (as might occur after a stroke), the brain has difficulty making sense of bodily movements. It can thus seem as if the individual is no longer the one in control.[130]

If someone doesn't set out intending to overeat to the point of becoming overweight or sick, yet repeatedly does so, suffering relentless cravings no matter which dieting or 'non-dieting' approach is followed, it is easy to see how they might conclude that hunger is *out of control.*

Bessel van der Kolk, author of *The Body Keeps the Score* (2015), presents fascinating ideas about the aftermath of trauma. He proposes that when unpleasant bodily sensations are not *reliably eliminated by one's actions*, the natural tendency is to *distrust what the body is saying* – because listening to these signals doesn't appear to help. For example, if a child grows up with an abusive parent whose behavior is unpredictably volatile, irrespective of how the child acts, the child may learn to distrust their own behavioral cues. Van der Kolk points out that this mistrust leaves people feeling stuck and immobile because, without this internal guidance, it is never clear how to act.

To understand this, let's reconsider the urge to urinate. It may seem that the urge to visit the bathroom emerges from the subconscious at unpredictable times without direct behavioral control. Yet, this is not the case. People have tremendous influence over whether or not they experience the urge to go to the bathroom at any given moment. For example, we quickly learn that this urge disappears when the bladder is emptied and is unlikely to return for some time unless there are other confounding factors involved, such as infection. We also learn that if we pre-emptively go to the bathroom before a long trip, we can avoid this particular discomfort for some time. We understand, too, that drinking an enormous volume of water brings the sensation back faster. In other words, whether or not we experience the urge to go to the bathroom is *reliably influenced by our actions* – and is hence very much under behavioral control.

The problem with addictive circumstances is that they *mislead the body*, so the resulting bodily sensations *do not appear to make sense*. The more deceptive food is consumed, the louder appetite squalls until intake appears wholly absurd and unreasonable. Even after consuming enormous volumes of deceptive food, hunger may remain switched on – when logic dictates that it should not.

These anomalies in outcome alert the brain that *something in its map of the world is wrong*. To uncover the error, the brain begins testing hypotheses, trialing different ways of modifying food intake in an effort to restore predictable and reliable hunger sensations. However, because these dietary approaches are implemented without a full understanding of the situation, the solutions do not endure. As health deteriorates and the pool of potential solutions dwindles, the situation feels progressively dire.

Those who study complex systems – such as insect colonies, the internet, the global economy, and the human body – have discovered that these systems share universal characteristics.[131] One of these characteristics is a vulnerability to *cascading failure*.

Melanie Mitchell, professor of computer science at Portland State University, explains that although complex systems are often resilient to minor mishaps, a critical error can set in motion a rolling failure across the entire network.[132] When something vital malfunctions, another part of the system must carry the load, increasing the odds that this part, too, will break under the strain.

Mitchell describes how the failure of an important hub in an electricity network can cause its load to be rerouted to another, causing the next hub to fail, and so on, like dominoes, until the whole network is brought down. When this happens, failure can spread through surrounding networks that rely on electricity, such as healthcare systems, financial systems, defense systems, and so on. If a tipping point is reached, the entire system may collapse. Catastrophic failure of this type can sometimes be traced back to a single error.

Addiction is a form of biological cascading failure, driven by a sensory error. Because the error is not obvious at the outset and because testing behavioral hypotheses does not immediately reveal the solution, a rolling collapse begins. One by one, ancillary systems start to fall: energy, mood, friendships, relationships, productivity, income, health.

As the failures mount, the brain becomes increasingly challenged to explain what is going on. Eventually, only one hypothesis may remain standing: *hunger is out of control.*

Failing at diets over and over again drums a false belief into the brain: *appetite has run amok* and you are *powerless to stop it.*

Acceptance of this belief marks the devastating moment at which the powerlessness delusion takes root. It is the moment at which the individual decides they have acquired a baffling and mystical condition known as *addiction.*

At first, the notion that one might be suffering from a 'relapsing brain disorder' can provide relief. After all, the addiction narrative is far more forgiving than the 'lazy, zero-willpower' narrative. The prospect that part of the brain – through no fault of one's own – might be unable to resist or relinquish the allure of certain addictive substances really does appear to align with the evidence. It can truly feel as though a mysterious power – something separate from conscious desire –

tugs the individual indiscriminately back toward the very thing that destroys them.

But, soon, comfort lapses into despair.

After reading addiction literature or attending treatment programs, a sense of hopelessness may arise. If there were initially two arguments raging within the skull (one arguing to consume and one arguing to stop), the addiction narrative adds fuel to the wrong side of the fire.

What is the point of fighting this thing if relapse will occur anyway? Who wants to spend a lifetime battling willpower? How is that even possible? It is no surprise that after the onset of the powerlessness delusion, intake often increases.[133]

Like other popular beliefs, the powerlessness delusion is contagious, which is one reason why addiction appears to run in families and between groups of friends. The delusion jumps from mind to mind, appearing to offer a viable explanation for what is going on.

If others insist this type of powerlessness does not exist, it is easy to argue that this is because they haven't experienced addiction themselves and thus cannot understand. In fact, the powerlessness delusion appears so good that the circular logic fuels itself.

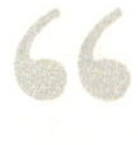

> The label of addiction is attached to the behavior because the person is assumed to have lost control of the substance use; when asked why the person has lost control, the answer is that he is addicted. In other words, addiction causes addiction.
>
> — DON ROSS, CARLA SHARP, RUDY E. VUCHINICH, AND DAVID SPURRETT, *MIDBRAIN MUTINY* (2008)

Powerlessness is a deadly hypothesis. It initiates a self-perpetuating prophecy because it implies that permanent escape is impossible. It implies that even 'success' might involve ongoing struggle and lack, fighting against an intrinsic deficiency, overcoming cravings one day at a time. This outlook can make it feel like hope is lost even before the escape begins.

If someone believes they have an inherent weakness, the capacity to take the necessary action is severely curtailed. Like the elephant chained to the stake, they haven't yet realized they could *immediately stand up and walk free.*

Of course, deep down, most people admit that no one *truly* loses control over their actions. The problem is that it just doesn't feel that way.

To understand this, imagine you are desperately thirsty in a desert, and someone sits beside you with a bucket of water and only lets you have one teaspoonful. In this situation, you would almost certainly experience unbearable cravings for water. You would probably find it easier to not even *see* the bucket than to taunt yourself with a single teaspoonful. Even knowing the bucket was nearby might be enough to initiate tortuous water cravings.

When appetite is elevated to extreme levels, having none is easier than having one, and restricting intake to a small serving can feel impossible. An elevated appetite can make it seem as if an individual lacks the ordinary level of control – because the *logical explanation* for the elevated need is not understood.

Increased engagement is the *normal response* of any healthy lifeform to intermittent reinforcement (see chapter 6: *Tolerance and Escalation*). Addictive behaviors are no different from any other type of behavior. The only difference is that the sensory data informing the choices is *misleading* and communicates a false picture of what is going on.

There is no powerlessness in addiction. There is no

mysterious affliction. There is only the *belief* in all of these things.

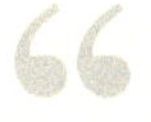

> ..."addiction" does not actually exist as a state of loss of control or hopelessness but only as a state of belief in loss of control and hopelessness.
>
> — MICHELLE DUNBAR, STEVEN SLATE, AND MARK SCHEEREN, *THE FREEDOM MODEL FOR THE FAMILY* (2018)

Imagine you could travel back in time and care for your younger self. Watch that wonderful, innocent child grow up and begin to struggle with deceptive food. Watch as your younger self goes to war with hunger. Watch as they flounder and struggle. As a young adult, filled with potential, imagine they come to you with tears in their eyes because they can't *fix* this thing. Something must be terribly wrong; they must be *broken*...

Take your younger self by the shoulders and *shake* them. Make them see that they're in the same trap as everybody else and that the problem is not *them* – it's the things that are *pretending to be the food.*

Society has been misled by a molecular sleight of hand that recalibrates sensory systems without conscious awareness, escalating hunger in a way that seemed irrational *but was not.*

Addiction isn't powerlessness. It's deception.

It is an interpretation error invoked by a sensory error. It is a predictable pattern of behavior that arises and is sustained when a misleading circumstance provokes *inaccurate beliefs.*

Do you know what the lucky thing is? If addiction is sustained by inaccurate beliefs, it means this isn't a genetic problem, a brain wiring problem, a dopamine receptor problem, an entrenched habit problem, an emotional problem, or any other type of problem. It is an ordinary behavior sustained by faulty beliefs...and beliefs can *change* when refuting evidence comes to hand.

The moment a participant in a rubber arm experiment *moves their arm*, the illusion shatters. The additional stream of sensory data *immediately exposes the truth*, and a more accurate interpretation is revealed.

Without any conscious effort or *will* required on the part of the participant, the brain reassembles the pieces, weighs up the data (just as your brain has been doing while reading this book), and forms a more accurate picture of the world.

After all, if addiction were truly a sign of powerlessness, no one would ever escape. Yet, they do. Despite what is commonly believed, *almost all addicts quit*[134] – often without assistance or fanfare. According to the National Epidemiologic Survey on Alcohol and Related Conditions, the lifetime probability that someone will end problematic substance use is over 90% for alcoholics, 96% for opioid users, and over 99% for cocaine users.[135] A study of individuals with a history of dependence upon sedatives, tranquilizers, opioids, and stimulants found that the lifetime probability of remission was "above 96% for all substances assessed."[136]

Gene Heyman and Verna Mims provide cumulative percentages of those in remission from various addictions, graphed as years after the initial onset of the behavior. Remission rates increase in a smooth curve as more and more people end the addictive behavior over time.[137] According to this data, cocaine is quit the fastest, followed by alcohol and then cigarettes.[138] This order is expected because, as noted previously, the severity of the consequences influences the speed of escape. To put this another way, the time it takes for a deceptive item to be discarded depends upon *the length of time it takes for the individual to see the truth.*

Allen Carr makes a brilliant distinction: he says people think that addicts have no willpower, but what they really have is a "conflict of will."[139] This conflict is driven by the confusing and unreliable data that emerges in the face of intermittent reinforcement.

Many famous, capable, and highly accomplished individuals struggle with their weight. When beta readers volunteered for this book, a flood of requests came in from engineers, doctors, PhD students, and so on. This is *not* a low-willpower cohort.

You are not powerless. In fact, you probably have more willpower than most people you know. It may have even been your extreme willpower that threw you headfirst into this mess – via the implementation of a strict diet that increased hunger and thus increased the likelihood of consuming large volumes of deceptive food.

How many years have you spent trying to remedy this problem? How many books have you read, videos watched, diets tested?

And yet, after all of this, have you thrown in the towel?

No, here you are, reading another book – hunting for clues, fitting together the pieces, and absorbing the truth.

You have willpower in spades. All you needed was *the right information.*

After years of struggling with diets, I feared that I might never solve this thing – that overeating might be something I was stuck with for life – that I would be perpetually trying and failing, never cured.

It wasn't true. Trying and failing is a predictable precursor to escape. Variation after variation is tested until, at last, *the right understanding is found.*

11

THE RIGHT MINDSET

DECEPTIVE FOODS FOOL the sensory apparatus, enticing the consumer to eat to the point of obesity, sickness, and death. Food manufacturers lace products with chemicals that mislead taste and smell receptors, manipulating eating behavior and lining their own pockets in the process. As in nature, these counterfeits arise at the hands of a competing lifeform who stands to benefit from the deception.

Whether the deception is deliberate, malevolent, or malicious does not matter because the outcome is the same: the perpetrator boosts their survival odds at the expense of your own.

Lifeforms will always take advantage of loopholes that allow their genes to prosper. This isn't personal. Deception is as old as life itself. It is the oldest trick in the book.

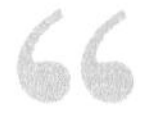

> When he lies, he speaks his native language, for he is a liar and the father of lies.
>
> — JOHN 8:44, *THE HOLY BIBLE* (NIV)

Deception is a problem of living. It is a universal problem. And this is wonderful because universal problems have universal solutions.

In each case, escape requires unveiling the deceit; exposing the trickery; understanding the ruse that has been played (see chapter 6: *Recognition*). When a counterfeit's true nature is revealed, its illusory reign of power ends. When a genuine and counterfeit item are finally recognized as *not being the same*, the brain *corrects the faulty rule*, splitting the cue-set in two. With this distinction, the genuine and counterfeit item are at last *treated differently*.

We are nearly there. Soon, this book will set out the elegant and straightforward practical method of escape that rapidly reverses sensory recalibration and returns the body's hunger and satiety systems to its factory settings – just as you were born to be.

Before we get there, there is one final thing to discuss. You see, unlike other addictive substances, which can be readily identified and isolated, you may have noticed that deceptive ingredients infiltrate the food supply in a rather pervasive manner. This means we must discuss issues relating to *occasional ingestion*.

Moderation

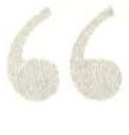

> Give us certain wise rules about this thing, but for the sake of respectable and dignified humanity do not sweep it away from the earth.
>
> — CHANCELLOR CROSBY, *MODERATION VS. TOTAL ABSTINENCE* (1881)

In chapter 6: *Tolerance and Escalation*, simple calculations illustrated how the undetected emergence of a counterfeit cue prompts progressively higher engagement. But what if the counterfeit is *known?* In this case, might careful and rare ingestion be possible?

When consumption of deceptive items is infrequent, in low volume, and offset by ample quantities of nourishing, genuine food, the effect upon appetite is correspondingly small. It makes sense that this would be the case. Minor variations in environmental stimuli are part of the 'noise' of everyday life. The method the brain uses to track and predict survival outcomes cannot be so fragile that one tiny unexpected anomaly should immediately throw behavior off-course. In other words, it *is* possible to reset the sensory apparatus and occasionally consume deceptive foods without detectable changes to appetite. This explains why many individuals may recall a time early in life when they ate deceptive foods occasionally in a seemingly 'normal' manner without apparent issue.

When the sensory apparatus is reset back to normal, occasional engagement with a counterfeit feels far more manageable because these items are not met with a ravenous appetite. Many people move on from bulimia (which, among other things, involves repeatedly binge-eating deceptive foods), returning to an 'ordinary' diet that includes some deceptive items. Similarly, many prior overeaters stop binge eating and lose weight without eliminating every single deceptive ingredient. There are also case studies in which prior alcoholics go on to moderate intake.

After all, if moderation were *impossible* for a certain subset of the population, the implication must be that addiction really does involve some deficit in self-control.

Knowing that it is *possible* to moderate doesn't quite address the real question, however. Are there any *benefits* to doing so? Is moderation the optimal approach?

One benefit of occasionally eating deceptive food is that it provides tangible, first-hand evidence that you are *not* powerless or broken. Of course, if a loved one announced that they were occasionally smoking cigarettes just to prove they could moderate, I'm not sure I would agree this was an entirely valid justification.

And if someone *does* choose to moderate deceptive food, where, precisely, should they draw the line? For the sake of argument, let's assume they wish to operate via an 80/20 rule, consuming a diet that is 80% genuine and nourishing. How will they know when they have exceeded the 20% margin? The whole issue is that taste and smell receptors cannot reliably differentiate between deceptive flavors and their genuine counterparts, so how should someone monitor the intake of these molecules – particularly when quantities and volumes are rarely specified on labels? Should they attempt to measure the deceptive item as a whole – or the tiny chemical ingredients that mislead the sensors? How can they gauge a suitable quantity when these molecules deceive the very sensors tasked with regulating intake?

Remember, genuine foods do not cause these problems. Moderation of carrots is not an issue because when you are hungry for carrots and then eat them, you soon get full and no longer want carrots. Likewise, the appetite for carrots does not subtly grow tomorrow as a result of carrot consumption today. When eating genuine foods, the amount consumed is beautifully regulated by the act itself.

Deceptive foods, on the other hand, do not induce satiation as expected, because the promised nutrition does not arrive (see chapter 3: *Sham Eating*). Even with a well-calibrated sensory system, people still find themselves polishing off bags of crisps or declining a second serving while wishing they could have more. Similarly, parents of young children quickly learn to store cookies and other deceptive items high on pantry shelves to stop youngsters from gobbling these down.

Unlike carrot consumption, the intake of deceptive food is never a stable state. Each engagement subtly adjusts bodily systems, increasing the likelihood that the same flavor will be sought out again. People *can* limit their intake of deceptive items – and this is certainly much easier when appetite is restored to ordinary levels. Yet, the natural tendency is for engagement to climb, which is why such a large portion of the population is overweight or obese, despite not setting out with this goal in mind.

Moderation is possible. However, it requires working against natural hunger and satiety systems, necessitating ongoing conscious decision-making. And if conscious decision-making is required, what are these decisions based *upon?* On what occasions is it suitable to eat deceptive food? Upon what logic should one decide?

Perhaps someone might choose to follow the conventional dietary patterns set out by society, adhering to societal norms. For example, if everyone else has one slice of birthday cake, they, too, take one slice. Operating by such strategies eases the burden of decision-making and, assuming celebratory functions are not attended every day, can indeed work.

However, if someone's social circles regularly consume deceptive items, how can they be sure that abiding by these societal norms is appropriate?

Following societal norms also reinforces the notion that these substances are the ultimate delicacy to be brought out on special occasions. If reducing the intake of deceptive food is good for both the individual and society, how does it make sense to celebrate by consuming these things? What message does this send to others, as well as young children who may soon be ushered into the trap? How does someone get from believing that deceptive food has derailed their life – stolen health, energy, confidence, and time – to believing that it is a harmless, innocent substance to be celebrated?

Almost all of those snared by a deceptive circumstance first desperately wish to return to their prior life of moderation – yearning for the time when they engaged innocently, like a normal person.

But you *are* a normal person. And here you are, joined by an ever-growing cast of other normal people, all playing out the same internal tragedy.

You didn't choose this. You didn't set out intending to overeat, gain weight and acquire negative social and health consequences. But when something lies to the bodily sensors – when flawed data is fed into the navigation system – people end up where they don't want to go.

It *is* possible to reboot hunger and satiety mechanisms, restore taste and smell receptors, and return to occasional consumption; it's true. You, like any other person, could do it.

But is it the best or most enjoyable approach?

If someone concludes that they want to keep eating a deceptive item, but it's dangerous, so they must only have it sometimes, they will always wonder when that time is, and how much they should have. Moderation requires constant effort and vigilance.

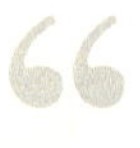

> ...endless tiny decisions that eat away at sanity and attention, constantly testing your will. Should I tonight? What about tomorrow? Does this count?
>
> — EDITH ZIMMERMAN, BODY + SOUL, *HOW TO CHANGE WITHOUT WILLPOWER* (2019)

Of course, you may remember a time when moderation did not seem to take up so much headspace. Surely there is a way to moderate, without obsessing over every little detail? Why was moderation much more effortless early in life?

The answer is simple. Early in life, you were naïve to the danger; now you are not. When a charming mask *slips*, the truth is revealed.

The time of engaging innocently with a con artist has passed. The prospect of casually inviting a counterfeit through the doorway becomes that much more complicated when you know the harm it can bring.

Should you take cocaine on birthdays?

Should the Greylag goose hatch a doorknob just for fun?

Your survival rests upon the ability to sort environmental stimuli into three categories: things that harm, things that benefit, and things that do neither and thus can be ignored.

What should you do with that pesky fourth category – things that mimic survival benefits while systematically destroying your life? Do you really want an approach that allows you to moderate such things?

If someone wishes to moderate, it implies they still believe that deceptive food offers something good – something so wonderful that it might offset all of that bad. Something that, if they are careful, they might find a way to access, while limiting the damage to an imperceptible degree.

What benefit could be worth all of this harm? What *good* does deceptive food bring?

Well, it doesn't deliver the promised nutrition.

It certainly doesn't heal negative emotions, fight anxiety, or alleviate boredom. No – it exacerbates all of these things while weakening and sickening the body to boot.

The vicious joke is that it doesn't even deliver a great flavor experience – it systematically steals the ability to experience flavor, downregulating taste and smell receptors so that each mouthful tastes progressively worse.

Deceptive food escalates hunger, prompts obscene levels of engagement, and provokes ongoing dietary obsession. With each encounter, it pretends to offer the nutritional reward that is so desperately needed while increasing the need for that same nutrition. In doing so, deceptive food offers fleeting relief from the very aggravation it creates.

You know, there's a better way to have relief from that aggravation. A way that gives you relief from the very first moment you wake up until the moment you go to sleep. This is the magic of the Allen Carr method: that what you are seeking is the sense of relaxation and peace that you would have had all along if you had never encountered the deceptive item in the first place.

Some people spend their whole lives rotating on and off diets. Restricting one thing and then another. Always watching the final ten pounds. Wildly ballooning up and then punishing themselves down. Endlessly fighting appetite, never feeling like it is done.

Do you know what is far less painful?

Seeing the culprit and walking away. Being free of it, once and for all.

Does that mean never?

Never

There are lots of wonderful things about *never*.

Consuming a completely flavor-honest diet is the fastest way to reset the sensory apparatus and dial down hunger. It is also the healthiest option: every system in the body is better off for it. Furthermore, this approach sends a coherent message to others (such as children who have yet to fall victim to the trap) and encourages food manufacturers to change their ways. Best of all, it resolves the uncertainty – the endless decisions.

Abstinence is also a popular approach when it comes to other deceptive substances. Although it may seem that most people drink alcohol without issue – it is worth remembering that many so-called 'normal drinkers' wake up with hangovers, embarrassing experiences, and regrets. Alcohol is the third leading cause of preventable death in America,[1] with *one in eight* adults meeting the diagnostic criteria for 'alcohol use disorder.'[2] What is most eye-opening, however, is the number of people who don't drink at all.

According to the 2018 National Survey on Drug Use and Health,[3] *thirty percent* of the US adult population consumed zero alcohol in the past year (with 45% drinking no alcohol in the past month). In older age brackets, these percentages are even higher. In other words, an enormous percentage of the population has realized that the easiest way to be free of the problems of alcohol is *not to drink it.*

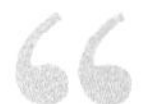

> Focus on the obvious.
>
> If you're doing something harmful to yourself, wouldn't it be good to stop it?
>
> — JACK TRIMPEY, *THE INTERNET CRASH COURSE ON AVRT*, RATIONAL RECOVERY (2014)

Eating flavor-honest food is far easier than any other dietary approach you have tried. It does not limit animal products or fats. It does not limit potatoes, rice, or grains. It does not limit naturally sweet foods, such as fruit, berries, fresh juices, or honey. In fact, *it limits no genuine food at all.*

But what about birthdays and other celebrations? Doesn't *never* make life altogether not worth living?

Well, how fun are special occasions now? How fun are events when you are ashamed of your appearance, overeating in secret, and enduring inner torment and insatiable hunger? Might not special occasions at which you are healthy, satiated, energetic, and confident be a whole lot more enjoyable? Might it not, in fact, be phenomenally awesome to have solved this thing?

If you see someone at a party who is fit, healthy, and strong, selecting only nourishing foods to eat, do you think, "Oh, that poor sod, they're missing out on all the fun in life?"

Imagine you attend a party at your optimal weight – healthy and vibrant – surrounded by your favorite people – including those you haven't seen in some time. The table is spread with delicious, genuine foods: sweet fruits, berries, meats, salads, cheeses – every natural delicacy you can think of. Everyone is laughing and having fun.

Now imagine an identical celebration, except that in the place of the genuine food, there are mass-produced counterparts. The table contains a colorful and gaudy display, mimicking the flavors, textures, and appearance of genuine foods...a little brighter, a little more intense.

Which party is missing something?

Which party has a *lack?*

Make no mistake: It is the deceptive food that conceals the lack. These items are chemical decoys, duping society for monetary gain...but *no longer duping you.*

Never is a wonderful approach. You, like anyone else, could do it. The world needs as many people as possible to stand up and help steer the human food supply back in the right direction.

But it may have come to your attention that there are quite a few potential difficulties with never.

For example, how is it practically feasible, given the extreme level of infiltration? Unlike cigarettes and alcohol, deceptive flavor molecules come in thousands of guises and are wound through an almost infinite array of foods. Over 2,500 chemicals are currently used to manipulate various characteristics of food (not to mention the 12,000 chemicals that may inadvertently find their way into the food supply).[4]

How does one ensure that every meal is 100% genuine and flavor-honest? Will you prepare food from scratch *every single day of your life,* no matter what? Will you purchase 100% additive-free ingredients from vendors you know and trust, regardless of the cost, every single time, without fail (perhaps moving to an organic farm for good measure)? Will you never eat out with others, not once?

It takes an enormous amount of time, money, and effort to ensure that deceptive food is *never, ever* consumed.

And if one *does* attempt never, what happens if a deceptive ingredient is consumed accidentally (an outcome that is quite plausible given the current levels of infiltration)? Does this mean the plan is ruined? Will it induce a sense of failure or hopelessness? The pursuit of never can invoke a kind of neurotic terror of its own.

Never is undoubtedly best. If deceptive foods did not exist, this would be the best outcome for everyone. The problem is they *do* exist, and they are so prevalent that even if someone decided, with the best of intentions, to abstain, the odds that they would succeed, *every meal of their lives,* is so low as to be almost impossible. Complete abstinence is very difficult from a practical perspective.

Never is optimal, but unrealistic. Moderation is exhausting. Where does this leave us? Are there any options left?

Luckily, there is.

An option that delivers the best of both worlds.

Avoidance

What is avoidance? This is the approach you use for all other known survival threats.

Consider the prospect of walking across a busy street in front of a speeding car. You probably don't struggle with the desire to walk across dangerous roads on special occasions, nor feel compelled to vow that you will *never* do so. What keeps you safe from speeding cars is not a vow but rather a clear and unequivocal understanding of the situation.

Despite knowing the threat posed by oncoming traffic, you also understand that there are certain circumstances in which exposure to this risk may be justified – such as when rescuing a child who has wandered onto the road. In addition, you know that streets vary in danger level, with conditions fluctuating (contrast a quiet street with occasional bicycles versus a freeway teeming with speeding trucks). Despite this complexity, you probably don't spend hours fretting about your brain's capacity to evaluate just how dangerous a particular street is, nor require a complicated rule book setting out precisely when you should or should not cross a particular street.

What makes addictive circumstances feel that much harder to navigate is not the complexity of the decision or the number of variables involved but *the difficulty in correctly understanding the situation in the first place.*

Imagine the complication if certain streets were disguised in such a way that they appeared to be peaceful walkways. If you noticed that some individuals kept injuring themselves on this type of street and it was proposed, as a solution, that people should avoid that area of town or only approach in carefully defined circumstances, this might sound particularly risky and problematic in comparison to the far safer idea of *never* approaching. But it is critical to see that the added fear provoked by this circumstance comes not from the inherent danger of the street, per se, but the confusing concealment, which misrepresents what is really going on, making it difficult to discern where the danger hides.

Deception turns an ordinary survival threat into a confusing nightmare because it is unclear how to act around a situation that is misunderstood.

Addiction is caused by a threat disguised as a survival win. Such scenarios threaten not only because they fail to deliver the anticipated reward and instead introduce harm, but because the unexpected outcome causes the sensory apparatus to recalibrate to account for the error. Consequently, each engagement has a *flow-on effect upon the next.*

In the case of deceptive food, this flow-on effect is caused by the decrease in taste and smell sensitivity, coupled with the increase in hunger. This increased hunger prompts higher intake, in much the same way as the pressure on a tightening bladder prompts another trip to the toilet. These sensations don't *remove* choice – the choice remains yours, as it always did – but the data guiding these choices is manipulated across time.

The danger of deceptive food, therefore, is not just the scarcity of nutrition, unwanted additives, and excessive caloric intake consumed during a single eating episode but the *incremental distortion of hunger and satiety across time.* Each mouthful subtly adjusts the learned relationships between flavor and nutrition, *impacting future responses.*

A deceptive item thus presents a far more devious threat than it might first appear. In the case of nicotine addiction, it hence makes sense that *never smoking a cigarette* is the best option. But this evaluation does not, in and of itself, imply that inhaling a single breath of second-hand cigarette smoke (which contains trace amounts of nicotine)[5] is so dire a survival risk that it should *never* happen. In fact, there might be numerous occasions when inhaling second-hand cigarette smoke could be considered a tolerable loss – such as when a non-smoker chooses to sit in a smoky bar to catch up with old friends.

Those who are so afraid of second-hand nicotine that they only venture outdoors while wearing an oxygen mask, or refuse to enter populated areas, are far more likely to incur several other survival losses that greatly outweigh the tiny threat that comes from rare and infrequent exposure to second-hand nicotine.

It *is* possible to never smoke another cigarette. But it is immensely difficult to guarantee that you will never inhale second-hand cigarette smoke again (and thus be 100% nicotine-free your entire life). Never smoking a cigarette is a viable option, but eliminating exposure to every speck of second-hand cigarette smoke in every single circumstance is not.

The issue when it comes to deceptive food is that rather than a few isolated products akin to 'smoking a cigarette,' there is an almost infinite array of deceptive items with differing levels of deception. In other words, there is a sliding scale of severity with numerous shades of grey.

Consider the difference between a manufactured raspberry chocolate product containing fake berry flavors, refined sweeteners, coloring agents, caffeine, theobromine, etc., as well as a handful of freeze-dried raspberries thrown in to cement the deception, versus a homemade sandwich containing eggs, tomatoes, lettuce, cheese, and bread made from organic flour, yeast, sugar, and water. Whereas the former is almost wholly deceptive, the latter is packed with nourishing, genuine ingredients and contains only the tiny addition of refined sugar in the bread. Although the former is far more misleading than the latter, there is no clear dividing line between what is tolerable and what is not.

In attempting to escape the effects of deceptive food,

therefore, we need a simple, effective strategy that allows us to navigate this complexity while minimizing exposure to deception. We need an approach that can accommodate not only accidental consumption but circumstances in which one might *voluntarily choose it* – just as someone might choose to enter a dangerous road to rescue a child.

The strategy we need is *avoidance.*

At first glance, avoidance can seem to be a wishy-washy kind of moderation with vaguer, imprecise guidelines. It is critical to see, however, that avoidance is *not* moderation. You do not moderate crossing a dangerous street; you avoid it.

Moderation implies a kind of *seeking* (albeit with careful rules). Avoidance, on the other hand, is predicated upon the notion that something *delivers a survival loss* – and a survival loss is only ever tolerated if this action is predicted to be offset by a greater survival gain.

Rather than moderation, avoidance is much closer to *never.* It combines the desire of never with the realistic acceptance that sometimes this just isn't possible. Avoidance embodies the *mindset* of never, but is absent the neuroticism. It sidesteps the exhausting demands of 100% abstinence yet retains the freedom and clarity of thought that comes from *never wanting it.*

Soon, we will discuss how avoidance might play out in practical situations. For now, let's examine the process of withdrawal.

Withdrawal

When a lifeform enters a new environment, different data feeds into bodily sensors, and internal systems recalibrate to perform optimally under the new conditions. In some cases, internal systems recalibrate slowly – such as when responding to gradual seasonal change. However, an abrupt environmental change often invokes a correspondingly rapid bodily response, even when adjustments of astounding magnitude are required. For example, when fully-sighted humans are blindfolded day and night while undergoing intensive lessons in braille, the part of the brain usually dedicated to vision (the visual cortex) switches over to respond to *touch* within only five days.[6] Likewise, when traveling to high-altitude areas, the body adapts to reduced oxygen levels by modifying breathing, heart rate, and red blood cell production over several days. Similarly, when moving to a new time zone or initiating a new sleep schedule, the body adjusts sleep-wake cycles, hormone release, and temperature regulation, shifting circadian rhythm by about an hour per day.[7]

Prompt recalibration in the face of environmental change is essential because lifeforms that adapt too slowly – or not at all – risk adverse health outcomes and are more likely to be outcompeted by those who adjust more efficiently. However, this adjustment process must not occur *too* quickly. After all, if recalibration occurred *instantly*, the body would become at the mercy of every fleeting, irrelevant change (imagine the chaos if the visual cortex dramatically rerouted to cater to touch every time you blinked your eyes).

For many human bodily functions, a 3-5 day recalibration period – during which the bulk of the adjustment takes place – strikes an optimal balance. This timescale is slow enough to discount noise and transitory change yet fast enough to minimize serious disadvantage if a significant environmental change occurs.

This is why many addictive substances, despite their vast differences, induce a common 3-5 day 'acute withdrawal phase' during which the body rapidly adapts to the removal of the intermittent reinforcement environment.

Just as moving to a new time zone can result in a few days of 'jetlag,' and entering high altitudes can lead to a few days of 'acute mountain sickness,'[8] discarding a deceptive item may result in a few days of physical symptoms which tail away to undetectable levels over the following few weeks.

Although some addictive substances can trigger quite severe recalibration symptoms, such as 'delirium tremens' during alcohol withdrawal, the good news is that deceptive food withdrawal is incredibly mild. In fact, the symptoms are so mild that many people pass through this phase without even recognizing it as a withdrawal process at all.

There are no tremors, convulsions, or seizures. There are no hallucinations or night terrors. Deceptive food withdrawal involves only a restless, fatigued, out-of-sorts feeling – and, in very rare cases, a headache.

Although these symptoms are incredibly mild, they can trigger the sense that something isn't right.

Perhaps the diet is wrong. Perhaps the timing is off. Perhaps today isn't the right day for change. Perhaps, when all is said and done, it would be better to abort the escape attempt and try again tomorrow.

You see, although the discomfort of withdrawal is incredibly slight, it is *added* to any discomfort that is already present. And when someone has engaged with deceptive food for quite some time, the general state of discomfort is often quite high. Life is not much fun for those who chronically overeat, gain weight, and feel ashamed.

But no matter how uncomfortable things feel – no matter how unpleasant life becomes – it always seems slightly worse whenever deceptive food is set down. It is only *marginally* worse, but if life is unpleasant already, a tiny extra dose of discomfort can feel like the straw that breaks the camel's back.

Stopping is always less comfortable than staying, and that is the trap, in a nutshell.

Of course, if the escape attempt is sustained, the discomfort rapidly alleviates within a few days, and the situation improves in leaps and bounds, such that you soon feel far better than you might ever have imagined possible.

Unfortunately, there is a faster way to remove the tiny added discomfort of withdrawal. Returning to deceptive food immediately restores the flow of misleading flavor molecules and creates the illusion that a high volume of nutrition has been found. This quells the elevated hunger, dampens the aggravation of withdrawal, and temporarily restores the ordinary, slightly more tolerable state of misery.

This relief is only ever partial. It doesn't deliver happiness nor remedy the situation. It temporarily dials down the discomfort and makes life seem slightly more bearable for a fleeting moment while ensuring the same discomfort grows.

And, as the body's physical condition atrophies and the situation deteriorates, hopelessness climbs.

But no matter how hopeless things feel, at least returning to deceptive food temporarily quietens the mild background aggravation.

Because this additional discomfort is present whenever someone *stops* eating deceptive food yet disappears when they return, it can seem that no matter how bad life gets, things are always *slightly better* with deceptive food – and, without it, things are always *incrementally worse*. Consequently, people find themselves miserable eating it and even more miserable without – strengthening the perception that deceptive food helps with all manner of unrelated things (see chapter 10: *Stress and Emotional Eating*).

Deceptive items sting with their tail. They entice with a sensory illusion, exposing bodily systems to gradually escalating intermittent reinforcement. Yet, the most insidious aspect is that whenever an escape attempt is made, everything feels momentarily worse.

Although the illusory flavors are the lure that baits the trap, it is the mild discomfort of withdrawal that swings the trap door closed. In fact, it can prompt someone to reach out and willingly bolt the door to the cage.

You see, once someone believes that life without deceptive food is the less happy option, continuing to eat it is the logical choice. What is the point having health and fitness, if the behaviors required to achieve this create less happiness than before? What is the point having an appealing body if the process required to maintain this delivers less happiness overall?

The great travesty is that deceptive food not only destroys physical health but systematically runs happiness into the ground. It cons people into staying by always making leaving seem to be the less attractive option.

The reason smokers find the first cigarette of the day the most 'enjoyable' one is that it partially relieves the withdrawal that has built up overnight. In other words, withdrawal is not a phenomenon that emerges exclusively at the *end* of an addiction – but a familiar discomfort that re-emerges throughout (see chapter 6: *The Downfall*) – a discomfort that returns, again and again, until you stop it.

All myths and religions speak of the hero's journey. There is a price to be paid, and the hero must pay it.

Three to five days of slightly increased discomfort is the price of freedom.

It is a tiny price, and you can pay it. Like the fully grown elephant who can stand up and triumphantly yank itself free from the chain – you can break free *the moment you realize it.*

But what if withdrawal *isn't* mild? What if, against all odds, you are struck down with a splitting headache and are so fatigued that you can barely rise from the couch? To really round things off, let's imagine that you have explosive diarrhea and aching bowels, and are so restless that you cannot focus on complex tasks as normal.

Could you bear that discomfort for five days?

What if some of these physical symptoms drag on, and you find yourself occasionally restless for three whole weeks?

Could you take that?

Could you do it?

Escape comes when you can say yes to these questions. When you realize, in fact, that you could endure *any physical discomfort* this situation might throw at you – that, no matter what happens, *you could bear it* – you suddenly see the doorway out.

Deceptive food withdrawal is ridiculously mild. Symptoms may only emerge into consciousness now and again during the first few days, if at all, and you may not experience any physical symptoms whatsoever.

If symptoms *do* arise, they cannot be eliminated. But you can change how you view them. Rather than seeing these bodily sensations as a sign that you are on the wrong path, you can see that these sensations indicate that you are on *precisely the correct path.*

Withdrawal symptoms are the feeling of the body righting itself, restoring the factory settings, putting things back to how they used to be.

Allen Carr reconstrued withdrawal sensations as the death throes of a little monster dying, encouraging the individual to relish and revel in each physical twinge. Those who escape nicotine following Carr's method describe the process using words such as "victory" and "triumph."

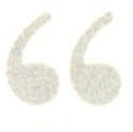

I suffered anxiety and a lack of concentration. I had night sweats; I think that was my body ridding itself of the toxins I had consumed. Some describe the

> experience like a mild flu. I didn't mind my symptoms because they spelled victory.
>
> — ANNIE GRACE, *THIS NAKED MIND* (2018)

There is no need to distract yourself in this scenario, because nothing bad is happening. Recalibration is necessary to escape, and thus the sensations are *desired* and *good*. Withdrawal symptoms are a sign that the deceptive flavor environment has departed; the honest flavor signals are flowing back through. In response, the brain and body are getting to work, steadily correcting things, returning them to how they used to be.

And, as the new flavor data comes in, meal by meal, the cells in the mouth and nose regenerate anew. Like the metaphorical phoenix rising from the ashes, the sensory apparatus is reborn. Within approximately ten short days, *every single taste receptor in the mouth regenerates.*[9] [10] Unlike the sensitive hairs in the ears or the photoreceptors in the eyes, taste cells are unbelievably regenerative.[11] This is because *locating the raw materials necessary to build and heal the body is such a fundamental requirement of life* that the flavor-sensing apparatus is protected at all costs. Even if the tongue is burnt and the cells literally scorched right off, they grow anew.

> “...the entire taste bud and the taste organ, the gustatory epithelium, can be removed or destroyed and will fully regenerate, making one of the very few organs in humans capable of total regeneration.
>
> — PAUL A.S. BRESLIN, *AN EVOLUTIONARY PERSPECTIVE ON FOOD AND HUMAN TASTE* (2013)

Thus, you can be tired, but still happy. Restless, but free.

Because here's the thing: you're not walking *into* hell; you're paying the tiny price to walk out the doorway.

With this approach, you don't fear the withdrawal sensations, you embrace them. Instead of fearing the discomfort, you turn, at last, and face it. You walk toward it with a kind of stubborn confidence – almost excitement – like a marathon runner with aching limbs might feel elation while crossing the finish line.

You don't set out in trepidation to see if you can bear it – you invite in the worst, knowing that whatever comes, you can take it. You carry any withdrawal sensations with a kind of honor – a crazy kind of glory – because in this act you take back your life.

> “...he understood at last what Dumbledore had been trying to tell him. It was, he thought, the difference between being dragged into the arena to face a battle to the death and walking into the arena with your head held high.
>
> — J.K. ROWLING, *HARRY POTTER AND THE HALF-BLOOD PRINCE* (2013)

When you suddenly realize that not only *could* you do it, but that *you can and you will*, it's like a shaft of sunlight streams down upon you, because you realize you can see the pathway out.

Paradoxically, once you reach this point – once you realize that no matter how uncomfortable it might be, *you will do it anyway* – withdrawal becomes easy.

In an odd way, that's the free ticket.

Dissolving Cravings

But what about the cravings? Doesn't intermittent reinforcement of flavor elevate hunger and trigger unbearable cravings for deceptive food?

Luckily, this is the awesome part. With the right mindset, cravings for deceptive items are switched off at their root and redirected to where the genuine reward is found.

Understanding how cravings work is crucial because the aspect of withdrawal that people usually dread is not the few days of mild physical symptoms, but what is known as *psychological withdrawal* – the cravings, irritability, mood swings, and so on.

After all, if ending a lifetime's addiction required only enduring a few days of feeling slightly under the weather, people would escape the influence of a counterfeit easily.

In fact, it *is* easy to escape a counterfeit when the situation is viewed in the right way because, as you will soon see, the correct mindset *switches off psychological withdrawal.*

Psychological withdrawal is best understood as the frustration that arises when someone is prevented from accessing what they want.

Individuals who struggle with cravings months or even years after abandoning a deceptive item do not suffer from a protracted withdrawal syndrome but are haunted by the memory of something they believe offers a benefit. Like pining for a long-lost lover, the torment is kept alive by the idea that they are separated from something good – leaving them moping for a benefit seemingly lost.

This psychological response can create further physical symptoms of its own. Allen Carr gives the example of a child who tantrums for a toy the parents refuse to buy.[12] The child's frustration can lead to tears, a red face, heavy breathing, screams of rage, accelerated heart rate, and many other physical symptoms in addition to the negative emotions. In other words, a changed *perception* can greatly improve the physical symptoms also.

One of the difficulties with addictive circumstances is that although repeated engagement provides first-hand evidence of the awful, accumulating downsides, the illusory upsides appear to magnify in tandem. The more deceptive food one consumes, the greater and more urgent the need for nutrition. As hunger rises, the reinforcing value of flavor thus climbs,[13] and the illusory reward promised by the counterfeit seems increasingly essential. As the 'punishments' rise in severity, so too does the illusion of reward – and with every engagement, the deceptive item appears to play the role of savior.

As downsides accumulate, the decision to pursue the deceptive item becomes plagued with more and more uncertainty, and the hypothesis testing may become frantic. The individual urgently needs a way to access the reward which seems to reside within the counterfeit while avoiding the pain. But because the pain is exacerbated by consumption, and the reward is not where it promises to be found, this is impossible.

A war begins to rage inside the individual's skull, each side of the argument pitted against the other, desperately trying to ascertain what to do. One side of the argument simulates how delicious these deceptive items might be, imagining the flavor molecules sliding over the tongue. In this simulation, the action appears to result in the individual *feeling better* – predicting the arrival of a genuine nutritional reward – and a craving is born. The opposing side of the argument rears up, recalling vows to change and issuing reminders that *this action is ruining everything.*

This internal battle may become so frequent and prolonged that the individual is perpetually distracted by an incessant barrage of food-related noise. It can feel impossible to resolve because engaging with the counterfeit promises to deliver the very nutritional reward that is needed.

When intermittent reinforcement interferes with access to a critical survival reward, a real and escalating emergency unfolds. The only method the body has for resolving a nutritional crisis is *seeking flavors associated with the necessary nutrition.*

Both sides of the argument thus unfold with urgency, knowing survival is at stake. Both sides of the argument are initiated with the individual's best interests in mind, but one set of arguments is *running on faulty data.* An error has entered the system, and this error can bring the whole network down.

A single pivotal insight is often experienced by those who escape addiction. It is the realization that *every argument supporting pursuit of the counterfeit rests upon an error.*

Jack Trimpey, author of Rational Recovery (1996), frames all thoughts promoting substance use as originating from a primitive part of the brain that has mistakenly associated the behavior with survival. Extending Trimpey's ideas, Kathryn Hansen writes:

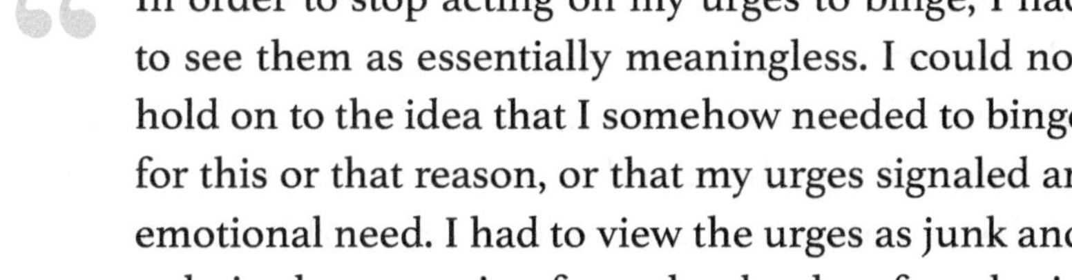

> In order to stop acting on my urges to binge, I had to see them as essentially meaningless. I could not hold on to the idea that I somehow needed to binge for this or that reason, or that my urges signaled an emotional need. I had to view the urges as junk and only junk, emanating from the depths of my brain and not worth any further consideration whatsoever.
>
> — KATHRYN HANSEN, *BRAIN OVER BINGE* (2014)

Glenn Livingston, author of *Never Binge Again* (2015), conceptualizes such urges as a "survival drive gone wrong."

Each of these approaches is a tactic for categorizing bodily signals that might suggest pursuit of a deceptive item as *originating in error* – and thus able to be *ignored by the rational decision-making brain.*

Deceptive foods mislead bodily sensors. The taste and smell receptors – the faithful sentries standing guard at the entrance to the body – have been deceived. The sensory system is fooled and cannot detect it. But *you* can.

You, the one reading this book, are the leader of your multicellular organism. You collate evidence from multiple sources, integrating data from a wide range of inputs, in order to better ascertain truth.

While the mouth and nose faithfully transcribe flavor signals and send this data to the brain, other sensory teams transmit different information, just as the eyes are relaying the information coded within the little black marks on this page.

You are the decision-maker: the truth-seeker. One of your most important roles is to establish truth, because truth (which we might define as *information that is reliable across time*) is the foundation of all accurate behavioral rules.

By culminating data from multiple sources, the brain provides a defense against deception. After all, if individual sensory teams could be relied upon to always get it right, the brain could just kick back and let the body do its job. But that would be a dangerous approach in a world riddled with deception. When deception is at play, individual sensory teams are fallible and require a mechanism to save them.

You are that mechanism. You are the escape hatch. You are the one who *saves the lifeform* whenever an individual sensory team has been led astray.

In *The Biology of Belief* (2016), Bruce Lipton describes how all cells within the body "follow instructions from the head honcho nervous system, even if those signals are in conflict with local stimuli." This means that you can *immediately* extract yourself from any deceptive circumstance – *the moment you are certain that doing so is the right thing to do.*

You see, in order to take command and right the ship, you must be convinced this action is *right*. Ordinarily, bodily systems are *superb* at doing their job – they must be, or your genes would not have made it through so many rounds of this game. Ignoring bodily signals thus *cannot be taken lightly* because doing so without sufficient evidence can lead to peril. If doubt remains – if taste and smell receptors are *right* in this matter and a survival reward really is left on the table – the argument must rage on.

However, the moment it becomes obvious that every purported benefit associated with deceptive food is an *illusion founded on sensory error* – the argument is over. As the truth is revealed, the inner torment dissipates, and the addiction is gone.

To be clear, taking command and righting the ship does *not* involve 'manually overpowering' cravings (such an approach would be nonsensical because the brain supposedly tasked with the overpowering is the same brain that generates any cravings). Manually overpowering cravings is akin to *continuing the argument*, whereas the only way out of this dilemma is to *resolve the argument* (which is what we have been doing throughout this book).

Some experts believe that to be free of cravings, an individual must minimize exposure to so-called 'triggering' circumstances. For example, alcoholics are often advised to stay away from the bar where they used to drink. But even the original Alcoholics Anonymous book notes the futility of such approaches:

> His only chance for sobriety would be some place like Greenland Ice Cap, and even there an Eskimo might turn up with a bottle of scotch and ruin everything!
>
> — ALCOHOLICS ANONYMOUS, *THE BIG BOOK* (1939)

The issue with minimizing exposure to 'triggers' is not merely the practical impossibility but that it doesn't address the real issue. No circumstance can ever directly *cause* a craving. All it can do is provide a reminder of a particular action or suggest that a particular item might be available. Whether this item is then *desired* depends on what the individual believes that action would deliver.[14]

No external environment or internal bodily condition can ever cause someone to crave something they do not want.

You can be starving and have *no desire for deceptive food*, just as you can be miserable and have *no desire for heroin*. It is not the presence or absence of a particular state that determines whether a craving is experienced. Cravings only occur if an item or behavior is predicted to *deliver something good.*

I spent years trying to come up with a method that quietened all cravings for deceptive food without ever noticing it was the final step in every chain of events that needed dissecting. Rather than attempting to minimize exposure to numerous preceding 'triggers,' I needed to direct laser focus upon the *misled wanting* that lay at the heart of it.

A craving is not a bizarre, unexplainable sensation that bubbles up from the ether. It is an expression of *wanting,* and wanting *only arises when a benefit is perceived to be associated with a particular action.*

Allen Carr discovered that the psychological withdrawal (the wanting) can be eliminated *even before you discard the substance.* In fact, when the situation is viewed in the right way, it is possible to pass through the withdrawal period *without any cravings at all.*

Even if a craving occasionally arises, unbidden – perhaps at a rare moment when the truth slips one's mind – the solution is never to fight or battle the craving...but to *recall the truth;* to remember that a *false signal* has been transmitted and an *error* received.

In recognizing the truth, no 'overpowering' is necessary because the brain *turns the craving off.*

The Pathway Out

> Then you will know the truth, and the truth will set you free.
>
> — JOHN 8:32, *THE HOLY BIBLE* (NIV)

Deception is an age-old trick. But escape requires only *one thing:* to see it.

There is a lag in deceptive circumstances between the first encounter and knowing the truth. At the outset, it isn't obvious that deceptive foods deliver only a survival loss. Because these items mimic sensory cues that ordinarily lead to nutritional gain, they are first perceived as *good.*

Because the downsides of each engagement are so insidiously mild, this viewpoint can persist for a very long time. If overeating occurs, it can be hard to believe that the substance is really to blame. It seems much more plausible that the individual might be the problematic one. This notion can feel particularly hard to shake when vast tracts of society thrash around under the same illusion, reassuring each other that these delicacies are not to blame.

But no matter how much deceptive food is swallowed, it never seems enough. No matter how hard one tries, it never seems possible to find a recognizable boundary between the purported 'innocent pleasure zone' and the 'gluttonous danger zone.' Navigating such murky waters requires endless arbitrary rules, following guidance from others – in the hope that *they* have worked it out.

The problem is not that anyone is missing the perfect moderation strategy, but that the good-bad interpretation at the heart of it is wrong. No one can simultaneously move toward *and* away. No one can pursue *and* flee. If something is perceived as both good *and* bad, it is never clear how to act.

As long as a deceptive item is perceived as harmful yet wonderful – enticing yet forbidden – there is no easy way to proceed. There are only tortuous methods requiring willpower in varying degrees.

Even *never* is often tainted with the idea that the individual is *making a sacrifice* – that they are giving up something for their own gain. People thus feel coerced into change – obliged to ride cravings, initiate self-discipline measures, pray for divine intervention, and reaffirm the vow of never, one day at a time.

It *is* possible to restrain desire. People can establish arbitrary guidelines and boundaries, initiating mental handbrakes, granting themselves permission to eat certain deceptive items in predefined circumstances, minimizing usage to what they hope is a reasonable degree. It is certainly possible to constrain desire within limits and regulations...but while one does so, the individual continues to experience the ongoing frustration of *restricting what they want.*

Alternatively, one can give in and let appetite run wild. You can release the handbrake, eating deceptive foods on special occasions, ordinary occasions, in the evenings, during breaks, at meals, between meals, while driving, while working, while relaxing, during stressful times, during boring times, and every time in between.

And you can oscillate endlessly between these two states: succumbing to desire and then curtailing it, pursuing and then resisting – never happy, in either condition.

This nightmare goes on and on and on and on until the day it finally becomes clear that deceptive food isn't good *and* bad; it's only bad. No matter how tiny and imperceptible the consequences of each engagement are, it *always delivers a loss*.

Prior to this shift in understanding, the drama continues: on the one hand, it is wanted; on the other hand, it is not. An endless war that rides on without any solutions or rules to make the pain go away.

Some people spend a lifetime oscillating between desire and restriction...but you can take, in Allen Carr's words, the "*easy way.*"

You see, there exists an unexpected and shockingly easy way out of addiction. It involves seeing that the deceptive item delivers *no benefits at all* – that it is a wolf in sheep's clothing, killing you with each imperceptible blow.

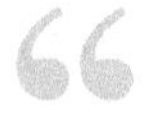

> So I believed both that I loved drinking, and that it was ruining my life.
>
> For me, it changed the day — the morning, the hour — that I realised, finally, that I no longer loved alcohol. That it wasn't making me happy and ruining my life, it was just ruining my life.
>
> — EDITH ZIMMERMAN, BODY + SOUL, *HOW TO CHANGE WITHOUT WILLPOWER* (2019)

The challenge with addictive situations isn't to know how to behave so that you can access the good while escaping the bad – but to see that the good *isn't there.*

It's a con. A *lure* to keep you ingesting, to keep you putting up with all the awful consequences, for someone else's financial gain. And through it all, you blame yourself. You view the overeating, the binges, the shame...as some kind of personal behavioral dysfunction. It's a perfect trick.

Lift your eyes from the negative consequences. Turn attention toward *what it appears to give* and notice that *none of the purported benefits are true.* Even the so-called delicious taste *steals your very ability to experience flavor* so that every meal tastes progressively worse. It is a cheap sensory trick.

As it sinks in that there are *only downsides* hiding behind that false signal – that it steals exactly what you seek – the jaws of the trap open and you are free.

There is nothing magical or mystical in addiction. There is nothing to be 'fought' or overcome. There is only *deceit.*

What traps an individual is not sickness or withdrawal. It's not recalibrated bodily systems. It is *the mistaken belief that a deceptive item offers something good.*

Addiction is a *misplaced wanting* whereby the individual attributes positive value where none can be found. When this truth is recognized, the addiction is over because the *wanting* that sustained the seeking behavior is gone.

Prior to this realization, the individual attempts to negotiate, but negotiating with a deceptive item is impossible because it always takes what it pretends to deliver. Each engagement tunes the sensory apparatus toward the counterfeit, like a self-homing navigation device, fooling the individual into continued pursuit. And, as internal systems recalibrate, the individual is wound deeper and deeper into a trap.

But this trap only exists inside the person's own mind – a

web of misinterpretations and misunderstandings provoked by a sensory error.

Addiction is initiated and sustained by *errors of belief* that arise as the result of deception. It is undone by seeing the truth.

No one can go back to the phase of naivety when a deceptive item was perceived as only good. Once a danger is known, it cannot be unknown. You cannot pretend a threat isn't there when you know that it is.

The truth is not that one cigarette compels a smoker to have another, any more than a non-smoker walks into a foul cloud of smoke and suddenly starts puffing for life. The truth is that if someone *wants* one cigarette, they will want another, and another, and there it leads, day after day, year after year...

If someone can justify the first engagement, they are more likely to justify the second, particularly when the effect of the first manipulates the sensory system.

But if you *no longer want* the first engagement, and anticipate the misleading effect it imparts, deceptive signals can be discounted and ignored, just as you can ignore the charming compliments that drip from a salesperson's tongue.

It isn't the small levels of occasional, unavoidable exposure that are the problem...it is the *intentional seeking*. The latter implies a misunderstanding, and this misunderstanding multiplies when the deceptive item interacts with the sensors.

Even Allen Carr, who plainly advocated never smoking again, knew this was true. At one stage, Carr deliberately tried to become re-addicted to nicotine so that he could prove to himself how painless and effortless his method of escape really was. Instead, he found himself unable to become re-addicted, no matter how long or frequently he smoked. This is because he retained an absolute revulsion to what he called the "filthy weed."

Carr went on to say that it *would* be possible to teach people how to have the occasional puff of a cigarette but that there was no point...because if they *wanted* to, they hadn't understood.

Curtailing desire is a nightmare. Alternating between moderation approaches is endless drama. But everything is solved, everything is done, when the perpetrator is finally seen in the right light. This is because when a deceptive item is finally seen for what it is...you *no longer want it.*

We can't wave a wand and make excess weight disappear overnight, but you can see the truth in one fell swoop. You can discover that rather than feeling coerced into change, you are filled with a surging yearning *to be free of it.*

The Capacity for Instant Change

Beliefs can change, even while the senses and bodily systems remain corrupted. This *must* be the case, or no addict would ever break free.

One way to think of the mind is as a collection of voting neurons. As the evidence accumulates, a tipping point is reached. A critical mass of evidence can result in a rapid shift in perspective, allowing you to suddenly see things in a new light. This transformation can feel particularly dramatic when a new interpretation makes sense of a whole swag of anomalies at once. In a whoosh, a better way of viewing the world makes the old one obsolete.

In his book, *The Predictive Mind* (2014), Jakob Hohwy describes experiments in which scientists show a different image to each eye. In such cases, participants don't experience a mishmash of both images at once but alternate between seeing one image and then the other. If scientists add sensory data that supports one image but not the other (for example, if they add the smell of roses and one of the images depicts roses), the brain preferentially shows the image with the most supporting data.

In other words, just as in the fake arm experiments, when two ways of viewing the world are possible, the interpretation that appears to be accurate, given the balance of evidence, is experienced as true. When new data is obtained, it can feel like a new viewpoint is suddenly revealed.

Clinical psychologist Marc Lewis, who refers to addiction as "a corrupted form of learning," described the moment before he quit narcotics as "a switch being flipped."[15]

The right mindset can be acquired even by those who are not deliberately looking for it – or those who don't believe escape is possible. Participants of Allen Carr's stop-smoking seminars often arrive under various levels of duress, compelled to attend by loved ones – and may turn up with no intention of changing. Yet, even these people often report quitting effortlessly, describing how unbelievable it feels to be free.

One of the most pervasive incorrect beliefs about addiction is that escape is necessarily a tortuous or protracted affair. Reading reviews of Allen Carr's books helped me realize that it didn't have to be this way. Here are two examples:

> Do you remember being in algebra class in highschool? The teacher could explain how to solve a problem a million times over and maybe you still didn't understand? But then some godsend person (classmate, teachers assistant, maybe even a substitute teacher) came in and explained it in an entirely different way and all of a sudden it clicked?? That is this book.
>
> — KELSEY MALIK, AMAZON REVIEW (2016) OF *ALLEN CARR'S EASY WAY FOR WOMEN TO STOP SMOKING*

> Upon turning the final page, I felt like Keanu Reeves after he's been unplugged from the Matrix. I saw nicotine as it really is: a malevolent Wizard of Oz frantically manipulating the levers of my neural machinery in order to aggrandise itself. And Allen Carr was Toto, tugging back the curtain to reveal the true, pathetic nature of what he called "the little monster".
>
> — LAURENCE PHELAN, INDEPENDENT, *HOW ALLEN CARR SAVED MY LUNGS* (2012)

Some people say that after attending Allen Carr's clinics, they don't even really know how it worked or what happened. What happened is that the illusion collapsed. They suddenly saw that rather than giving up something wonderful, they were escaping something terrible.

James Desena describes quitting alcohol like this:

> I finally came to my senses after engaging in the mental free-for-all argument raging in my head that went on for years. What am I doing? The answer, when it came to me, was so clear: Quit engaging the enemy.
>
> — JAMES DESENA, *OVERCOMING YOUR ALCOHOL, DRUG & RECOVERY HABITS* (2002)

Freedom

To help cement these ideas, let's run through a final analogy. Imagine you work for a company that delivers your salary in a little cardboard box with a dollar sign on the top, and at random intervals during the week, the box appears on your desk. Let's also imagine that the size of the box varies to reflect the amount of money within (the bigger the box, the bigger the bonus).

Now imagine that some cruel individual plays a trick on you by periodically placing a counterfeit box on your desk. This box looks identical to the original box and also has a dollar sign on it, but it is empty. To make matters worse, the fake box contains sharp protrusions, so you scratch your hands opening it.

Whenever you see a counterfeit box on your desk, a bit larger than usual, you get a thrill of excitement, because it seems that you have earned a bonus. Then you open it, scratch your hands, and get zero money.

If there were only ever counterfeit boxes on your desk, you would quickly catch on and throw them in the trash whenever you saw them, wondering who would bother with such an idiotic ploy. But, because the fake boxes are indistinguishable from the genuine item, you cannot just throw them away – because to do so risks discarding real money. Whenever you see a box, you don't know whether it is the genuine item or not, so there is always a little burst of excitement in anticipation of the money it might contain. Yet, as the weeks and months pass, you begin to feel increasingly despondent because your hands are getting scratched raw. To make matters worse, opening either box becomes less and less enjoyable because the average amount of money expected per box declines.

Further complicating matters, the counterfeit boxes are sometimes cunningly taped on top of the genuine item, so in addition to scratching your hands, there is a bit of real money at the bottom (inside the genuine box). However, even when this cunning mixing of genuine and counterfeit boxes occurs, the *good* is always found in the genuine item, and *the harm is always attached to the counterfeit.*

In this scenario, you have a desperate problem. You need the money. But you don't want the scratches. You cannot throw away *all* boxes because to do so eliminates the money. But you wish you could because you hate the scratches.

This is the problem that all addicts face. The counterfeit appears to be something that is desperately needed, and every time the fake item is set down, it feels like discarding a genuine reward.

The box-opening dilemma is solved the moment you have a reliable method for *distinguishing between the two types of boxes.* The moment you can see how to differentiate between the genuine and counterfeit item (and are confident this method does not eliminate any boxes containing a reward), you can safely discard the counterfeit without worrying that you have discarded something of value.

Once you can reliably *recognize the counterfeit*, you have *no desire to open the deceptive boxes*. Why would you? No one wants to scratch their hands opening a box that contains nothing.

The moment you can recognize the counterfeit and see that it contains *nothing good,* no effort is needed to resist opening the fake box.

In this scenario, there would be *zero* jealousy of those poor souls who have not yet worked out how to distinguish between the boxes. Even if some people were at the early phase of the process and had no visible scratch marks on their hands, you wouldn't feel jealous of them *because there is nothing in the box.* Even if, by some miracle, some people were born with exceptionally resilient hands and thus could open the counterfeit boxes without scarring their skin, you still wouldn't feel jealous of them because *there's nothing in the box.*

These individuals waste time and energy carrying out an activity that only ever delivers a survival loss. Even those who keep their counterfeit box exposure to a carefully controlled minimum, and hence limit the damage to their hands, *still get nothing good from the box.* Even the 'thrill' of opening the box is not itself a benefit because by experiencing the thrill in error, each box-opening experience becomes more and more depressing as the average predicted reward declines. In other words, those who open fake boxes continue to waste time, energy, and effort pursuing a harmful activity that offers no benefits at all.

By this stage in the book, some readers may still have doubts and suspect there might remain a mystical benefit tied up in consuming deceptive food. Before proceeding, these individuals should think carefully about the benefits they suspect they are receiving and reread the appropriate section of the book. For example, those who still believe that deceptive foods provide an emotional pick-me-up should reread chapter 10: *Stress and Emotional Eating*, until it becomes clear that deceptive foods dysregulate emotions and make it incrementally more challenging to cope with anything. Those who still believe deceptive foods offer an enticing flavor should reread chapter 10: *Delicious Taste,* until it becomes clear that these items systematically diminish flavor sensitivity and reduce the pleasure experienced while eating, so all flavors taste worse.

During beta reader rounds of this book, a number of individuals reported reading the manuscript several times before the full understanding clicked into place. A significant percentage of those who succeed with Allen Carr's method also report reading his books more than once. I myself have read his books about twenty times.

Keep reading and rereading until you finally see the truth: that you are *normal* and nothing is wrong *except the food.*

Addictive items are a threat disguised as a survival win. If something is perceived as a benefit, the natural inclination is to seek that thing out in order to obtain the expected beneficial outcome. It is the *perception of a benefit* that sustains the *seeking* and perpetuates the pattern of behavior that we call addiction.

Every purported benefit associated with deceptive food is an illusion founded upon false sensory signals. As this truth materializes and the deceptive item is finally recognized (as an imposter that threatens survival), a desire to *avoid* emerges as a natural consequence.

This change in perception and the subsequent change in desire go hand in hand – one is contingent upon the other. *Avoidance* is the natural consequence of *learning the truth* – because the urge to *move away from a survival threat* is an unbreakable, foundational rule in this survival game.

As it becomes evident that *nothing beneficial resides within deceptive food* – that this whole situation was the result of misleading chemical mimicry – you discover that there is an *escape clause*. You find what you have been looking for all of this time: *an easy way out.*

Whereas prior quit attempts involved unpleasant variations of *moderation* and *never,* recognition of the counterfeit transforms everything. Seeing the truth brings with it a profound sense of relief and liberation. You suddenly feel *free* of the deceptive item – as though it has lost its grip on you. This is because the one who was holding on to it was *you.*

As this change in mindset takes hold, the process of escape is revealed to be *exciting* because finally recognizing a deceptive survival threat (particularly one that has derailed your life for so long) is itself *a great survival reward.*

Take a moment to think back to the first time you binge ate after a restrictive diet (or any early overeating memory). Close your eyes and imagine that, right at that moment, when you were desperately *hungry* and irritable, someone had emerged and laid down a beautiful, nourishing, flavor-honest feast: a lavish spread of fruit, berries, tubers, meats, fish, dairy, vegetables, nuts, grains, herbs, spices, natural condiments, and so on – every delicious genuine food you could imagine.

Instead, right at that moment, an imposter stepped in.

That's it. That's all it was.

And as this scenario replayed, over and over again, you were seduced by a counterfeit that pretended to offer what you needed.

Some people fear that their overeating might be too hard to change, that the behaviors are too entrenched, too difficult to turn around. They fear that salvation might be for others, not for them – that something inside them might be permanently ruined, something that can never be fixed.

It can.

You are a normal human being caught in the crosshairs of the food industry, with a sensory system manipulated by those whose survival goals conflict with your own.

The beauty of this situation is that, unlike a personal flaw, deception can be escaped the moment it is understood.

Once an imposter is identified and discarded, sensory systems fall back into line, hunger resets to normal levels, and the problem is *gone*.

Not coped with; not endured. *Gone*.

12

THE ESCAPE METHOD

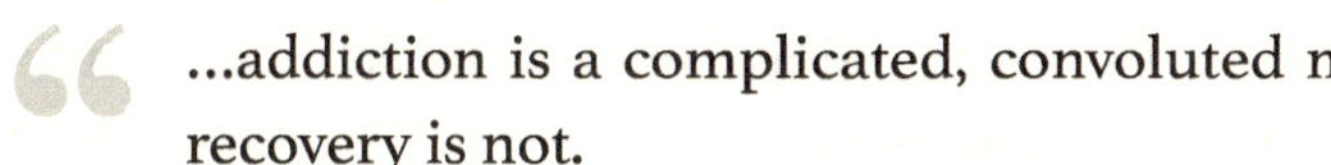

> ...addiction is a complicated, convoluted mess, but recovery is not.
>
> — JAMES DESENA, *OVERCOMING YOUR ALCOHOL, DRUG & RECOVERY HABITS* (2002)

PLEASE NOTE: *If you have skipped ahead to this chapter, hoping to read the magical solution, you will not find it here. As with escaping nicotine, the important part is not so much what to do but achieving the mindset whereby you view the deceptive item in the right light. Although key insights remain in these final pages, these build upon ideas discussed throughout the book. Reading this chapter alone is unlikely to achieve the desired goal.*

What is the goal? This might seem obvious: *to reach a healthy body weight*. But this is not entirely correct. There is no joy in temporarily losing weight if it boomerangs back. Nor is there any joy in losing weight if one must desperately cling to this state, enduring food obsession and constant cravings.

Rather, the goal is to initiate a set of behaviors that naturally lead to a healthy physique. The goal is to be able to eat until full, without it being a drama, leaving the table satisfied and content, with food-related thoughts vacating your mind until hunger rises again sometime later. The goal is to reach the point where you can trust the body to manage food intake rather than micromanaging the task and constantly fighting appetite.

When someone has struggled with overeating for an extended period, various aspects of life often unravel. Overeating can lead to social withdrawal, impede professional development, and leave the consumer feeling depressed and ashamed. Poor health can drain energy to the point where daily tasks feel overwhelming and exhausting. Deceptive food can disrupt the microbiome, prompt insulin resistance, elevate blood pressure, and leave the entire body aching and unwell.

Past efforts to fix these things may have felt futile and challenging. How does one rekindle social relationships while feeling hopeless and ashamed? How does one sustain a vigorous exercise program while aching and weary? The problem can seem enormous and multi-faceted, with so many things to do and fix.

Valuable insights can be drawn from observing how other complex networks recover in the face of rolling collapse. If an electricity network has many substations down and is on the brink of catastrophic system-wide failure, attempting to repair random substations in the heart of the affected area is the wrong approach. Not only is it more challenging to access supplies, transportation, and tools in the midst of a blackout region, but even once repaired, an isolated substation cannot be reconnected to the live grid. A far more effective approach is to strategically repair only those substations on the boundary of the functioning portion of the network. Once restored, these can be immediately reconnected to the live grid, helping to share the load and reverse the collapse.[1]

When a roof is leaking, it is pointless to run around replacing the wallpaper or frantically repairing the timber frames. Such methods only offer temporary reprieve while exhausting energy and resources. *Targeting repairs toward the right place* dramatically improves the odds of saving the system, whereas a broad scatter-gun approach does not.

The method outlined in this book focuses solely on *rectifying the foundational error.* It immediately stems the inflow of misleading molecules, replacing these with a stream of reliable flavor-nutrition relationships. As a result, the sensory apparatus quickly reboots, hunger and satiety systems return to normal, and *all related downstream effects* begin to self-correct on their own.

Your body has all of the necessary recovery systems built in, ready and waiting. Every single cell within the body wants to survive. The only problem was that the raw materials used to repair and restore your survival machine were *falsely labeled.* When this foundational error is corrected, every bodily system begins to function as intended. One by one, internal systems fall back into alignment, and each part of the biological network reaches out and restores another. This positive effect ripples outwards, triggering a cascade of improvements that transforms your entire life.

Alleviating Hunger

One of the most important concepts to understand is that intermittent reinforcement of flavor *increases hunger.* This increase in appetite is the *optimal response* the body can make in this situation.

As has been discussed, the rise in appetite occurs for the following reasons:

1. *Less nutrition, on average, is received per unit of flavor.* When flavor molecules are added to a food, the strength of the flavor increases, but the nutrition received does not. This means that, on average, the expected nutrition per unit of flavor diminishes.
2. *Intermittent reinforcement of flavor increases the need for nutrition.* When nutrients do not arrive as expected, deficiencies can develop despite the influx of calories, resulting in a heightened demand for nutrition. Furthermore, because it is unclear when each nutrient will arrive or in what quantity, the body often needs to endure long stretches without adequate nutrition coming in. To improve the odds of surviving these periods, the body must build up an emergency buffer – an extra store of nutrition over and above what is ordinarily required.

Both the reduction in nutrition per unit of flavor *and* the heightened need for nutrition cause appetite to climb. When both of these factors occur in unison, the effect is multiplied and dramatic, as illustrated in chapter 6: *Tolerance and Escalation*.

To remedy this situation and return hunger to normal levels, *both* these factors must be reset. It is not enough, for example, to return to a flavor-honest diet if this simultaneously restricts food groups or the quantity consumed – such as by consuming a *limited* flavor-honest diet (i.e., a whole-food vegan diet or a whole-food carnivore diet). Although a limited diet may restore reliable flavor-nutrition relationships and deliver an influx of *some* nutrients, it makes it almost impossible to meet *all* nutritional needs – particularly when pre-existing needs are high. As such, hunger must remain elevated or soon re-emerge.

Similarly, there is no long-term relief in alleviating nutritional needs without restoring reliable flavor-nutrition relationships – such as by attempting to reduce needs via supplementation or fortified foods. Even if you could somehow deliver the perfect infusion of nutrients such that the body was restored to an optimally nourished state today, a heightened appetite would return tomorrow when new nutritional needs arrive. This is because delivering nutrients via supplementation does nothing to correct the existing relationships between flavor and nutrition.

Just as handing a wad of cash to a gambler is an ineffective long-term solution, the sudden appearance of nutrition in the digestive tract does not re-establish a reliable relationship between action and outcome (and is hence likely to exacerbate the problem – see chapter 4: *Supplements and Fortification*).

The only way to normalize appetite and restore hunger and satiety systems to their factory settings is to address both of these things in unison. In other words, we must give the body what it has wanted all along: not only a good supply of nutrients *but a reliable way to find them.*

The practical approach detailed on the following pages achieves both of these aims. It rapidly recoups lost nutrition while restoring reliable flavor-nutrition relationships.

The method can be summarized as follows:

- Prioritize nourishment;
- Eat until completely full;
- Eat at regular mealtimes;
- Fast between meals (unless ravenous);
- Disregard deceptive signals;
- Imagine you are normal.

Prioritize Nourishment

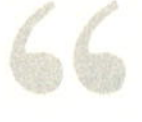

> [When] there is a surfeit of food, its allurement effect sinks so low that the animal will be disinclined to walk even a few steps to get it...
>
> — KONRAD LORENZ, *CIVILIZED MAN'S EIGHT DEADLY SINS* (1974)

Intermittent reinforcement of flavor plunges the body into a kind of starvation – a state in which there is an elevated need for nutrition yet a shortage of incoming nutrients. Unlike ordinary starvation, the deprivation is not of calories, but of individual nutrients. To return appetite to normal levels, these nutritional deficits must be eliminated and the heightened need for nutrition *met*.

To illustrate this point, let's return to B.F. Skinner's pigeon experiments. As described in chapter 5: *Intermittent Reinforcement*, these experiments rewarded hungry pigeons with a pellet of food when they pecked a lever. If the relationship between the lever and the pellet was intermittent – that is, if pecking the lever sometimes delivered a pellet and sometimes did not – the birds pecked at a dramatically increased rate. If the pellets were subsequently withdrawn completely (so no pecks were rewarded) after previously experiencing intermittent reinforcement, the pigeons kept on fruitlessly pecking the lever, sometimes for years on end.

As depressing as this sounds, there is some very good news. B.F. Skinner also discovered something else. He found that the tendency to keep pecking could be brought to a rapid halt.

How?

By *feeding* the pigeon.

You see, the only reason the pigeon *started* pecking the lever was that it was hungry and was trying different behaviors to see if it could locate more food. The only reason it *kept* pecking the lever was that it learned to associate this action with the arrival of additional food pellets.

In case it is not obvious, the pigeon does not peck the lever because it has a behavioral problem or an emotional issue. It does not peck the lever because it has a maladaptive desire to exhaust energy supplies or blunt its beak. It does not peck the lever because it has an 'unbreakable habit' or has 'lost control' over this particular behavior. The pigeon most certainly *is* bored, but boredom is *not why it pecks that one particular spot* over and over again.

It pecks that spot because it is *hungry,* and it has associated this behavior with finding more food.[2]

Every time the pigeon pecks the lever without reward, it seems less and less likely that doing so will deliver the nutrition it needs. But even a low chance is better than zero. Nutrition is essential for life and that pigeon, like you, is a survivor. The very best thing the pigeon can do in this circumstance is *keep pecking.*

Yet, when a *full* bowl of pellets is placed in the cage so that, day after day, nutrition is predictably and reliably available, the pigeon quickly stops pecking the lever. Why would it bother?

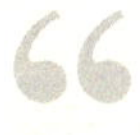

> ...a want that is satisfied is no longer a want. The organism is dominated and its behavior organized only by unsatisfied needs. If hunger is satisfied, it becomes unimportant in the current dynamics of the individual.
>
> — ABRAHAM H. MASLOW, *A THEORY OF HUMAN MOTIVATION* (1943)

Just as nutrient infusion rapidly halts sham eating in animal experiments (see chapter 3: *Sham Eating*), the search for food ceases when the *necessary nutrition arrives*. Skinner found that it didn't matter how deprived the pigeons were during the period when they learned to peck the lever and were exposed to intermittent reinforcement. What influenced how long it took them to *extinguish* the behavior was *how deprived they were when he tried to get them to stop.*[3]

This is unbelievably wonderful news because it means that it doesn't matter how long or tortuous your dieting history has been. The speed at which you escape – the time it takes for hunger and satiety systems to return to normal – depends only upon *how rapidly and reliably your hunger needs are met now*.

You, like the pigeon, just want a reliable way to be fed.

With this in mind, the first strategy detailed here is to *prioritize the most nourishing, flavor-honest foods available*, inundating the body with a rich supply of nutrients. This rapidly meets heightened nutritional needs and swiftly reduces appetite, allowing the healing process to commence.

What, precisely, should you eat?

Paul Jaminet and Shou-Ching Jaminet, authors of the *Perfect Health Diet* (2012), argue that the optimal macronutrient ratio for humans is approximately 30% carbohydrates, 55% fat, and 15% protein.[4] They reached these conclusions after examining the diets of traditional populations – and also noted that breastmilk contains a similar balance of macronutrients. To avoid the inefficiency and metabolic stress of forcing the body to create glucose from ketones or amino acids, the Jaminets suggest that the most sensible approach is to feed the body roughly this ratio of raw materials to begin with. This is not to be taken as an indication that macronutrients should be measured or consumed according to carefully predefined percentages (nothing of the sort is required). These figures are simply included as another broad-brush reminder that the optimal long-term human diet almost certainly contains a *balance of carbohydrates, fats, and protein* (as well as, of course, vitamins, minerals, and other plant compounds). This general guidance, however, still doesn't help you know precisely what to eat at any given moment.

Luckily, you don't need to know.

Just as you don't require detailed guidance about how much air to breathe, or how many mouthfuls of water to drink, or how many times to relieve your bladder, you don't need someone to micromanage your food intake. Every single one of your ancestors managed this task *without formal guidance.* Your body contains a sophisticated biological system that automatically monitors relationships between flavor and nutrition. The optimal method of choosing what to eat is always the same: *eat those genuine foods that taste the best.* When a reliable flavor-nutrition environment returns, food preferences accurately lead you in the right direction.

At each meal, fill your plate with the most delicious, nourishing flavor-honest foods you can find: fresh fruit, vegetables, berries, tubers, meats, fish, dairy, legumes, nuts, and so on – seasoned with herbs, spices, salt, lemon juice, etc. Drink water, whole milk, freshly squeezed juices, or homemade bone broth – whatever you desire. Of course, those with allergies or sensitivities can make adjustments as required.

Aim for nourishment from *all food groups* (including both animal and plant foods) – and prioritize fresh produce where possible. It may help to think of this as the best of a vegan diet and carnivore diet thrown together – a flexible whole food extravaganza, but without obsessive concern about basic processing, such as peeling, chopping, squeezing, scraping, polishing, or grinding. Eat the highest-quality foods you can afford.

> Just pile Real Food you like on your plate or in your bowl. Remember, you want to eat high-quality foods to satisfaction, in order to normalize your appetite and eating behavior.
>
> — JEAN ANTONELLO, *BREAKING OUT OF FOOD JAIL* (1996)

Select foods that taste good together, according to your preferences. Many popular food combinations naturally enhance nutrient absorption and bioavailability. For example, eating vitamin C-rich foods alongside those high in iron can boost iron absorption, which explains why many people desire sweet fruit after an evening meal. Similarly, combinations of beans and corn can provide a more balanced mix of amino acids than either item eaten alone. Do not attempt to intellectually optimize any of these combinations – trust the body to work it out, and simply let flavor preferences guide you toward food combinations that you enjoy.

This method of eating embraces *every single genuine food on Earth*. Right from the outset, meals of highly nourishing genuine foods taste wonderful, even before the sensory system has reset. This is because these foods *naturally contain a high concentration of flavor molecules*, signaling the fact that they *really are potent sources of nutrition*. Because this nutrition arrives as anticipated, these meals leave you *full* and *peaceful*, with an all-encompassing satisfaction that you may not have experienced after eating for a very long time.

It is critical to note that high nourishment does *not* mean low-calorie. Many of the most nourishing foods are also high in calories. What is important is *not* the number of calories eaten at a single meal – or even within a single day or week – but the effect this has on appetite across time. The aim is not to consciously reduce calories but to *meet nutritional needs* so that, as a consequence, calorie intake normalizes of its own accord. The body can only achieve this outcome if it actually *receives the nutrition it needs* – and it tells you what it needs via *flavor preferences.*

If you love the taste of chicken skin, eat it. Chicken skin, like pork crackling, is packed full of nutrients and is rich in collagen (see chapter 8: *Animal Products and Saturated Fat*). Similarly, butter from grass-fed cows, natural cheeses, fatty cuts of meat, eggs, salted corn on the cob, potatoes baked in lard, and raw honey are high-calorie yet *brimming with nourishment.* The emphasis is not on reducing calories but on consuming the most delicious, nourishing diet possible so that an *abundant supply of nutrition* is received, resetting appetite and restoring health quickly.

As part of this process, it is important to eat foods you legitimately *enjoy.* Sally K. Norton, author of *Toxic Superfoods* (2023), writes about the risk of oxalate overload that can come from excessive consumption of spinach smoothies, for example, and other foods such as beets, almond flour, and almond milk that are often consumed in excess by dieters in the name of 'health.' Many of the foods Norton describes as potentially problematic in this regard would never be eaten in excess if a 'healthy diet' was not undertaken or existing flavors were not disguised and distorted in some way. In other words, unless you are new to a food (remember it can take several exposures before a new flavor-nutrition relationship is learned), don't eat something simply because you believe it is good for you; eat foods you *like.*

It is also worth noting that prioritizing nourishment does *not* mean complete elimination of *low-nourishment* genuine foods – such as white rice, white pasta, or white flour. These items are also flavor-honest (see chapter 8: *Grains, Nuts, Seeds, and*

Legumes). However, it is important to note that *the more nutrient-dense the diet is, the faster weight loss will be* – and the faster the body will heal. More nourishing carbohydrate sources, such as sweetcorn, pumpkin, potatoes, sweet fruits, and so on, deliver an influx of nutrition as well as calories, killing two birds with one stone. In other words, a reduction in appetite (and hence weight loss) is *faster* when more nutritionally-dense foods are consumed. The sooner nutritional deficits are alleviated, the faster appetite will reset. Prioritizing *nourishment* is thus recommended where possible.

Note: Photographs illustrating what high-nourishment eating might look like can be accessed here: www.eatlikeanormalperson.com/flavor-honest-food/

Eat Until Completely Full

In avoiding deceptive food, one must not make the critical error of simultaneously limiting genuine food. To achieve optimal health, the body must receive the amount of nutrition it requires. If intake is arbitrarily curbed, weight loss can feel like an ongoing battle – a war against the body – because elevated hunger remains.

Those who maintained a healthy weight as a child might have some sense that eating to appetite while remaining lean is possible. Similarly, if you have previously lost weight following a whole food diet, paleo diet, carnivore diet, or some other diet in which flavor-honest foods are eaten until satiation, you might know that eating to appetite is a plausible weight loss strategy. However, those who have not followed one of the aforementioned diets for any length of time, or who were overweight as children, may have no personal experience that eating to appetite is a viable method of weight loss. This approach can seem particularly dubious if prior attempts to eat intuitively caused appetite and waistline to grow.

It is critical to remember that intuitive eating is doomed to fail while the role of deception is misunderstood. Without an understanding of intermittent reinforcement, intuition naturally leads people toward foods with the highest concentrations of flavor molecules – which are often artificially manipulated foods. The more deceptive food one consumes, the less nutrition is received, and the greater the need becomes – explaining why intuitive eating often fails (see chapter 9: *Intuitive Eating*). Even a century ago, it was recognized that deceptive items have this appetitive effect, whereas *genuine* foods do not. A school textbook from this period notes the following:

> If we eat a sufficient amount of wholesome food to-day, we do not care for a larger amount of the same food to-morrow. Not so with alcohol; the appetite for it grows with using.
>
> — WILLIAM KROHN, *GRADED LESSONS IN PHYSIOLOGY AND HYGIENE* (1906)

Some individuals may nonetheless fear that if they gave their appetite free rein, they would blow up like a balloon – perhaps recalling times when they *did* overeat genuine foods. It is vital to see that overeating genuine food only occurs for a few logical reasons.

Firstly, if someone restricts the *quantity* of food consumed, they are far more likely to eat a larger amount when the restriction abates – regardless of whether the food consumed is genuine or not. This is particularly the case if another restrictive diet is looming. If a lifeform predicts a dietary shortage in the imminent future, it is rational to stock up on nutrition today.

Secondly, if someone limits a particular food group, they may find themselves eating larger volumes of 'permitted' foods to obtain nutrients that are in short supply. For example, recall Provenza's discussion of Arctic explorers who consumed rabbit meat until their stomachs were bloated (see chapter 8: *Animal Products and Saturated Fat*). This was a desperate attempt to obtain fat from the low-fat rabbit meat. Consuming a wide range of foods from all food groups ensures this type of overeating does not occur.

Thirdly, it is critical to remember that the food industry goes to extraordinary lengths to manipulate food in underhand ways. Even meals that *appear* 'non-junk-like' can be heavily spiked with deceptive flavors – promoting the consumption of larger volumes than anticipated.

Finally, and most importantly, eating deceptive foods *also affects the intake of genuine foods.* If someone eats deceptive food today and then consumes flavor-honest food tomorrow, *the influence of that deceptive fodder temporarily remains.* In this way, alternating between deceptive and genuine items prompts an increased consumption of *both* – because the counterfeit and genuine flavors slot into the same sensory receptors and are treated by the body as the same thing.

In short, there are many logical reasons why someone might have previously eaten large volumes of genuine food, but none of these reasons apply when following the method outlined in this book.

When appetite is reliably satisfied using a wide variety of nourishing, flavor-honest foods from all food groups, appetite soon diminishes, and a blessed sense of satiety returns. This does *not* mean, however, that the goal is to eventually arrive at tiny, diet-like portions.

Joey Lott, author of *No More Perfect Diets* (2015), offers the following figures as a broad guideline for how many calories healthy people eat each day, on average:

- Men under 25 years: 3,500 calories
- Women under 25 years: 3,000 calories
- Men 25 years and over: 3,000 calories
- Women 25 years and over: 2,500 calories
- Women pregnant and lactating: 3,500 calories

Kathryn Hansen presents similar figures in *The Brain Over Binge Recovery Guide* (2016). Hansen also notes that the FDA's official figures regarding calorie intake were originally rounded down.

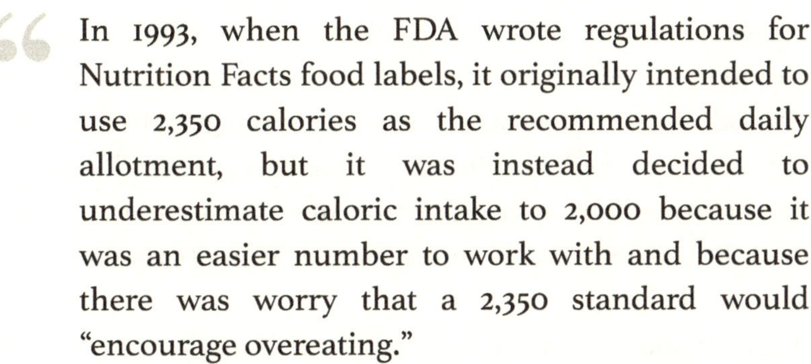

> In 1993, when the FDA wrote regulations for Nutrition Facts food labels, it originally intended to use 2,350 calories as the recommended daily allotment, but it was instead decided to underestimate caloric intake to 2,000 because it was an easier number to work with and because there was worry that a 2,350 standard would "encourage overeating."
>
> — KATHRYN HANSEN, *THE BRAIN OVER BINGE RECOVERY GUIDE* (2016)

Hansen goes on to explain that even the 2,350-calorie figure was later found to be too low. Note that these estimations are *averages*, meaning half the population typically consumes *more* than this.

It is also important to realize that after a period of sustained restrictive eating, individuals may need to temporarily eat more than usual – particularly those who are underweight or have been severely limiting a particular food group for some time. When Ancel Keys re-fed participants in the Minnesota Starvation Experiment, he found that the underweight men needed approximately 4,000 calories per day for several months,[5] sometimes up to 10,000 calories in a single day, before health and weight were restored.

After being sold the notion that 1,200-1,500 calories might be an ideal daily target when losing weight, it can be hard to fathom that an optimal calorie intake might be *anywhere near* these figures – particularly if following a low-calorie diet *still* results in stagnated weight loss. Weight loss often plateaus on conventional diets because the body remains poorly nourished and rations energy carefully, so that incoming nutrition supports only the most essential bodily functions. The dieter is thus left exhausted, cold, and miserable, with poor skin, brittle hair, and weight that refuses to budge.

To undo this unpleasant state, a new strategy called 'reverse dieting' has emerged, in which the dieter is gradually re-fed, upping calories inch by inch, until a new maintenance level is reached. Reverse dieting requires months of meticulous calorie tracking while battling hunger.

A much more pleasant and effective strategy is to *feed the body what it needs* from the outset.

The only way to end this drama and return the body to an optimal physique is to provide it with a reliable stream of sensory data, so that it can *find what it needs.*

It is futile to abandon deceptive flavors and *still* ignore the body's requests. The brain's task is to navigate the deceptive traps that fool the bodily sensors...and then get out of the way so that the body can do its job.

No expert in the world can know what you need to eat, or how much, better than your own body. How could they? Once deceptive influences are removed, internal systems can competently gauge and direct food intake without needing to envision 'fullness scales,' 'hunger charts,' or chewing each mouthful in a meditative trance. Eating until full does not mean 80% full, almost full, or 'maybe-I'll-stop-and-see-in-20-minutes' full. What kind of hopeless design flaw would it be if full did *not* mean full?

To step off this dietary treadmill once and for all, you must aim to satisfy appetite at every meal (where circumstances make this possible). Eating until full means *eating until you have no desire left to eat.*

There is no need to second-guess this process or panic about getting fullness 'right' down to the exact mouthful. If you eat too much at one meal, you will be less hungry at the next and vice versa – the body will sort it out. If you have large energy reserves stored on the body, appetite will factor this in. If you are pregnant, run marathons, or sloth on the couch, appetite will factor this in.

Your body is a master at this survival game. But in order for it to do its job and return your biological survival machine to health, you must *give it the raw materials it needs.*

Some may find this process daunting at first (although you will soon realize how easy it is). This is one reason why establishing a regular meal pattern can be so helpful.

Eat at Regular Mealtimes

Growing evidence suggests that aligning nutritional intake with daylight hours promotes health (see chapter 7: *Disruption of Circadian Rhythm*) – at least in geographic regions where this is possible.

Evidence also suggests that consuming *regular* meals at predictable times is advantageous. This helps to synchronize circadian rhythm and regulate metabolism, sleep, and hormone production. Stephen C. Woods, professor of psychiatry and behavioral neuroscience at the University of Cincinnati, argues that lifeforms adapt to the timing of meal consumption, preparing for nutrient intake by scheduling insulin release and other physiological responses accordingly.[6]

Outside of the advantage of consuming regular meals and aligning food intake roughly with the active part of the day, however, there appears to be no precise consensus about *how many* meals per day is optimal. The science surrounding meal timing is conflicting, inconsistent, and unclear. In fact, it appears that meal frequency is not so much governed by biological need but practical convenience.

Neil Rowland, professor of psychology at the University of Florida, argues that feeding patterns are not an "intrinsic biological property" but are the result of "social and economic imperatives."[7] Rowland notes that animals in the wild and captivity primarily feed in ways that are opportunistic, with eating episodes determined by how readily available food is, how hungry the animal is, and the costs involved in seeking that food – such as whether or not there are risks from predators, and so on. Rowland makes the observation that when rats in captivity have continuous access to grain, they feed approximately ten times per day. Yet, when access to grain is more difficult – i.e., requiring the pressing of buttons or levers in certain combinations before the food bowl becomes available – they eat less frequently. Importantly, however, the overall *amount* consumed remains the same. In other words, if the 'access cost' is high, an animal will eat fewer meals but consume more at each meal. If the access cost is low, an animal will consume a greater number of smaller meals. Rowland also references the work of George Collier, who noted that meal frequency drove meal size in a number of species. It makes sense that this would be the case: if a lifeform eats less frequently, they must consume more each time.

Where does this leave us when it comes to human meal timing? In the absence of firm data, a sensible approach appears to be to select an eating routine that allows you to best fit in with society and your life – minimizing 'access costs' to a reasonable degree.

Eating three meals per day is the most common eating pattern followed by humans all over the world. Whether this approach is biologically superior to one, two, four, five, or six meals per day remains unclear. What *is* clear, however, is that three meals per day did *not* result in vast numbers of the population becoming obese until deceptive foods were involved.

Returning to the ordinary meal pattern of society has several practical advantages. Firstly, this lets you enjoy the convenience of sharing meals with others. Rather than preparing meals alone or being forced to endure the smell and appearance of foods at times when others are eating, you can simply join in. This allows you to strengthen social ties, converse with loved ones around the table, and share cooking and dishwashing chores.

Eating three times a day is also more efficient than preparing four, five, or six meals and avoids continually interrupting the day to prepare snacks. If you only consume three meals per day, you are more likely to make an effort and prepare a delicious, nourishing meal than if eating numerous snacks.

Many eating disorder specialists have found that returning to an ordinary, structured meal pattern plays an important role in re-establishing normal eating. Christopher G. Fairburn, Emeritus Professor of Psychiatry at the University of Oxford, goes so far as to say that, "Establishing a pattern of regular eating is the single most significant change you can make when tackling a binge eating problem."[8]

> Before recovery, my life was dictated by where, when, how, and what I could or couldn't eat. Finally surrendering to eating three meals a day, every day, was both the scariest and most freeing step I had to take toward getting back a life worth living.
>
> — BENAZIR RADMANESH, MINDBODYGREEN, *IT WAS RADICALLY SIMPLE BUT HUGE* (2015)

Another advantage of eating at regular mealtimes is that it acts as a stepping stone to intuitive eating. If someone fears that eating to appetite might result in weight gain, a structured eating pattern offers a reassuring middle ground. You eat until satiety at certain times of day and then set food down to get on with other things, reassured that you can soon eat to appetite again.

Centering food intake around regular mealtimes also reduces the number of food-related decisions to be made. In short, eating three times a day means you don't need to constantly contemplate whether or what to eat.

Finally, eating three meals per day restores the natural balance between eating and fasting.

Fast between meals (unless ravenous)

Hunger is a vital signal, without which we would die, but this does not mean that listening at the *first hint* of hunger is advisable – just as running to the bathroom at the slightest sign of pressure on the bladder is not always the best approach.

Disassembling food into its molecular components and transporting the resulting chemicals from one part of the body to another is a resource-intensive task. Food must be broken down within the gut into smaller, absorbable molecular components, with beneficial nutrients absorbed through the intestine walls and transported into the bloodstream. The circulatory system then distributes these nutrients to various tissues and organs throughout the body. Toxins and other waste products must also be prepared for excretion or elimination, typically involving processing by the liver, kidneys, intestines, and other organs. All of these tasks involve considerable effort.

In contrast, during fasting periods, the body shifts its focus to *healing and restorative functions*, such as repairing damaged tissues and breaking down and recycling old or damaged cellular components via autophagy. While some healing and restorative functions occur at all times, these are more pronounced during fasting periods when the body is not preoccupied with digestion and assimilation. As a consequence, fasting is useful for treating a wide range of health conditions, including certain cancers.[9] As Hereward Carrington notes in his book *Vitality, Fasting and Nutrition* (1922), the first thing one should do when any machine breaks down is "stop the machine."

In *The Pleasure Trap* (2006), Douglas Lisle and Alan Goldhamer describe supervising over 5,000 patients at the TrueNorth Health Center in California. They found that water fasting effectively treats numerous conditions, including Type 2 diabetes, heart disease, high blood pressure, and obesity. One of their most interesting findings, however, is this:

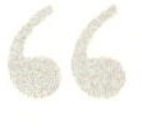

> In our clinical experience, we have seen nothing that can even remotely approach the effectiveness of water-only fasting to encourage the adoption of a healthy diet.
>
> — DOUGLAS J. LISLE AND ALAN GOLDHAMER, *THE PLEASURE TRAP* (2006)

The reason fasting promotes the uptake of a healthy diet is that it helps to reset taste and smell receptors. If a lifeform *needs* food, but food is unavailable in the environment, the mechanism for *detecting* food must improve. You can imagine the brain saying, "I need nutrients, but I can't sense them anywhere. Perhaps food is here, but I'm just not finding it. *Dial the sensors up higher!*"

As with the return to a flavor-honest diet, fasting improves flavor sensitivity, which is why hunger is commonly described as the 'best sauce.' This also explains why intermittent fasting has recently climbed in popularity. Fasting periods provide a way to partially undo the damage from a deceptive environment – rapidly resetting taste and smell receptors. Even short durations of fasting, such as the few hours between meals, boost your ability to detect and experience flavor.

The benefits of fasting are particularly accessible when the last meal of the day is eaten early, and the overnight fast is long. In fact, eating early and going to bed at sunset was a common experience for humans before the invention of electric lights and the distraction of 24-hour digital information streams.

> When I was growing up, all the kids on my block had an early supper around 5:30 p.m. After supper, we played outside and then came in, washed up and went to bed. There were no bedtime snacks—the kitchen closed at 6 p.m. sharp.
>
> — JOHN DOUILLARD, *EAT WHEAT* (2017)

Many studies demonstrate that eating food within a shorter daily feeding window improves metabolic functioning. One study found a shorter and earlier feeding window improved insulin sensitivity, blood pressure, and appetite, even when body weight was held constant.[10] Other studies suggest those who eat their largest meal earlier in the day lose more weight.[11] [12]

Given these benefits of fasting, some might suspect that an even *longer* fast might be ideal. In fact, many people utilize such approaches. Herbert M. Shelton, an American naturopath who supervised over 30,000 extended fasts, sets out the compelling arguments for fasting within his book, *The Science and Fine Art of Fasting* (1934), making it clear that far more medical professionals should investigate fasting protocols when treating various health conditions.

Yet, utilizing fasting as a home treatment for weight loss is more complicated than it might seem. Firstly, it involves non-trivial risks, including electrolyte imbalances, nutritional deficiencies, and, in severe cases, acute kidney injury[13] and death. The refeeding process following an extended fast is the most dangerous period, bringing with it the potential for serious health complications if not managed correctly.

It is also worth noting that although Shelton praises fasting extensively and views it as a cure for almost every ailment, his comments about weight loss are particularly revealing. He notes that when animals undergo extended fasts, they quickly regain the lost weight in the following period. He also describes how those who "refuse to control their eating" during the refeeding process often put on weight very rapidly.

> The inability of the undisciplined individuals of our country and age to control themselves means that they should not undertake to feed themselves at all after a fast. They should be controlled by a man of experience.
>
> — HERBERT M. SHELTON, *THE SCIENCE AND FINE ART OF FASTING* (1934)

Shelton provides numerous sobering case studies, such as a woman who lost 12 pounds (5.4 kg) in a ten-day water fast and then regained 22 pounds (10 kg) in the following weeks. Her husband, who regained a similar amount of weight, described himself as becoming "round as a butter-ball, and so brown and rosy in the face that I was a joke to all who saw me."[14] I confess I can attest to this rebound phenomenon following fasting with grim familiarity.

If an individual has severe health conditions that modern medicine has not remedied, investigating extended fasting with medical supervision may be a wise proposition. However, as a general weight loss strategy, extended fasting can sometimes hinder and unnecessarily complicate progress.

You see, although fasting can initiate dramatic health improvements, it simultaneously *drives the need for nutrition higher*. Even a morbidly obese person needs a regular supply of nutrients (in fact, those who are overweight often have a *heightened* need for nutrition, despite the oversupply of calories, as has been explained within this book). Shelton himself found that overweight patients often coped with fasting much more poorly. He mused that this may be because although "the fat person has a large store of fat on his frame, he is deficient in other food requisites."

We are then left with a question. If fasting offers a superior opportunity for accelerated healing yet comes with non-trivial risks, while eating provides essential nutrition, what is the correct balance?

At one end of the spectrum, an individual could undertake a supervised water fast for several weeks; at the other end, a person could choose to eat whenever they feel the first twinge of hunger. Somewhere in the middle of this enormous range of options lies the simple prospect of what we might call *going back to normal.*

Imagine you were the caregiver of a child who was kidnapped and taken to a vicious land where they were fed only flavor-manipulated foods. When this child is finally rescued and returned, they are obese and sick. What is your inclination?

Should you immediately place the child on an extended water fast, knowing this will undo the damage the quickest while potentially introducing risk? Or can you see that simply returning to a normal meal pattern of nourishing, flavor-honest foods would achieve the same end goal via a route that is far less risky and much more peaceful? Can you also see that subjecting the child to an extended water fast might cause the child to suspect that the previous environment was actually *better?*

You, of course, are not a child. And it is certainly possible to initiate longer fasting periods if you wish. Many adults do, and sometimes an aggressive approach is warranted. Those who find themselves so devoid of energy that the prospect of preparing a single nourishing meal seems so daunting as to be impossible might find that a short fasting period provides sufficient incentive.

However, rest assured that returning to three nourishing meals per day is all that is needed. This still provides the body with reasonable downtime from eating – particularly when the overnight fast is long. A normal meal pattern of three meals is an enjoyable and sustainable approach that can be *maintained for the rest of your life.*

It is worth noting that following a three-meal-per-day routine does not mean one should *never* snack between meals. Children – who have smaller stomachs – must, of course, eat more often. Similarly, those who are pregnant, underweight, or have exceptionally high energy needs for some other reason may also benefit from more frequent meals. There may also be times when food is available at odd times or when you have limited access to food and cannot fully satisfy hunger at an ordinary meal. If someone is so distracted by hunger that it is difficult to concentrate on anything else, it makes sense to have a snack: a piece of fruit, a slice of cheese, a glass of milk, or some other nourishing, flavor-honest food.

There might also be occasions when eating *less* often is optimal. Illness, for example, can result in a lack of appetite. There are also people who may prefer a two-meal-a-day routine – this is fine.

In short, the aim is not to initiate a rigid, inflexible regime but to return to an *ordinary, regular meal pattern* – a pattern that fits in with your life.

Disregard Deceptive Signals

Avoidance is the act of minimizing exposure to a survival threat while accepting that complete elimination of danger is not always possible (see chapter 11: *Avoidance*). Unlike the unyielding stance of *never*, avoidance acknowledges the complexities of competing goals and priorities, recognizing the potential for both accidental and unavoidable exposure.

What does avoidance look like in practice? How does one know when engaging with a misleading survival threat is appropriate? Luckily, avoiding a *known* source of deception is far simpler than it may seem.

Suppose a salesperson compliments you while you are considering a purchase, offering a glowing product review. This information, itself, does not have to complicate the decision-making process. If you understand that a salesperson cannot be relied upon to be truthful in this circumstance – that their incentives directly conflict with your own – the solution is straightforward: *ignore what they say*.

The risk of interacting with a salesperson is not that you *hear* their misleading words. It's not that sound waves emanate from their mouth, vibrate the cochlear membrane, and sway the minuscule, hairlike projections inside your ears, triggering the production of electrical signals that convey this auditory information to the brain. All that matters is *whether you believe them.*

If an individual gives credence to the salesperson's words and lets the misleading information *influence their decision*, they are far more likely to make a poor choice – a choice they might not otherwise have made.

The correct response in this scenario is not to *fear* salespeople. It's not to enter a shop with earmuffs or erect a barricade so that you never encounter a salesperson before a purchase takes place. The correct response is to *exclude the deceptive information* from the decision-making process – to *disregard the unreliable data.*

If the flavor of deceptive foods *accurately signaled what was to come* (obesity, sickness, and death), these items would *not* taste pleasant. Modern manufacturing processes conceal unpleasant flavors, uplift positive flavors, and apply flavor signals where they do not belong (see chapter 4: *Deceptive Flavor*). These misleading sensory messages manipulate consumers into eating these products for someone else's financial gain.

Mentally correct the error. Discount the deceptive signal.

If you find yourself in a situation where it is unclear whether a deceptive item can reasonably be avoided, ask yourself what you would do, in that precise situation, *if that misleading signal was corrected.* In other words, ask yourself what you would do *if you didn't like the taste of that thing.*

Of course, there *are* times when you *might* eat something unpleasant. In this heavily flavor-manipulated world, there are almost certain to be occasions when concessions must be made.

Let's run through how this might work. Imagine you attend a dinner party, and your host serves a meal that contains several genuine ingredients, such as meat, vegetables, fruit, and cheese. However, you notice the sauce is contaminated with deceptive flavors. Should you eat the meal?

When reaching a decision, you need to consider not only the consequences of consuming the meal but the consequences of *not* consuming it. For example, by refusing the food, you may offend your host – particularly if they have spent considerable time and energy preparing the meal. Rejecting the meal also rejects the genuine ingredients – and the nourishment these contain. If you don't eat now, you may have to cook something late at night when you get home, incurring several other negative survival consequences, such as disruption to sleep, microbiome, and circadian rhythm. When all is said and done, perhaps eating the slightly contaminated meal is the best option.

To resolve the uncertainty, ask yourself what you would do, in this precise situation, *if the sauce had an unpleasant flavor.* In other words: what would you do if your host had worked hard to prepare a meal that contained an ingredient you didn't like? When contemplated in this way, several straightforward solutions immediately reveal themselves. Perhaps you might eat the surrounding items while subtly avoiding the majority of the sauce. Perhaps you could pile your plate with meat, vegetables, fruit, and cheese while bypassing the sauce. If the sauce is served to you, perhaps you could force down a small portion yet not request seconds. When the deceptive signal is *discounted from the decision* and the error signal corrected, what appears to be a complicated decision suddenly feels much more like an ordinary choice.

What about a highly deceptive item? For example, suppose someone suggests ordering an ultra-sweetened, flavor-manipulated dessert after eating a meal. Apply the same strategy. Ask yourself what you would do if someone offered you something *highly unpleasant* after you had just eaten a meal. When considered from this perspective, numerous handy, polite refusals come to mind. Unlike a slightly tainted meal, there are likely to be far fewer occasions – if any – when a heavily deceptive item is taken on board – just as there are far fewer occasions when you are prepared to cross a highway teeming with trucks in contrast to a quiet street with bicycles.

Whatever the case, when the misleading flavor signal is mentally corrected, the decision feels much simpler – and the natural outcome is to consume the bare minimum you can get away with.

Correcting a deceptive signal does not mean decision-making is always perfect. As in all areas of life, choices sometimes turn out to be wrong. Sometimes, the relevant data is not at hand. But when a manipulative signal is *recognized and discounted at the outset,* you can make the best possible decision with the information available.

Deceptive foods *always deliver a survival loss*, no matter how slight. Whether this loss is deemed tolerable in any particular situation is up to you.

As an example, when initiating this way of eating, I was a single mother with limited funds. I needed something simple for school lunches, and did not have time to bake homemade bread. Because organic sourdough was outside my budget at the time, I continued to purchase a small amount of manufactured bread (which contains tiny quantities of refined sugar and other additives – I found a brand of pita bread that appeared to have far fewer additives than others). Although I ate this rarely, I decided the practical advantages of purchasing manufactured bread offset the survival loss at that time. In other words, do the best you can, given the circumstance.

On any occasions where a deceptive item cannot reasonably be avoided, accompany or follow the ingestion with a liberal dose of genuine foods (keeping the ratio of genuine to deceptive as high as possible, with zero deception always best). Following ingestion, do not implement compensatory tactics, such as punitive fasting or restriction. Instead, reassure the body that the reliable flavor environment has not departed and continue to eat until satiety at regular meals, ensuring that flavor-nutrition relationships are rapidly pulled back into alignment.

Most importantly, remember that on any rare occasions when deceptive ingredients cannot be avoided, *taste and smell receptors will remain fooled.* The sensory system cannot discern the genuine item from the imposter – this is the whole problem. If a deceptive flavor molecule slots into the taste or smell receptors, a signal is transmitted. The mouth and nose will send the misleading message that the deceptive item is *good.*

Mentally counter the error. Notice how intense and artificial the flavor is – how the flavors try a little too hard. Remind yourself *you know its tricks.* Remind yourself that though the tongue is fooled, *you are not.*

Be aware, too, that a few individuals who escape nicotine using Allen Carr's method find the process so remarkably easy that they begin to adopt a relaxed, lackadaisical attitude.

As health and confidence returns, they begin to forget what all the fuss was about. In curiosity, they one day pick up a cigarette and take a puff before putting it back down.

With sensory systems reset, this process of occasional engagement feels effortless. They find themselves thinking: *It doesn't seem to have a hold on me anymore – perhaps I can smoke now and again.* Inch by inch, avoidance switches to *pursuit*, and the individual slides back into the very same trap.

Protect yourself from this eventuality by *never forgetting what the deceptive item is.* Be aware that others who are still in the trap will try and convince you that there is no harm in swallowing these things now and again.

Cement this firmly in your mind: the error is not in occasional, unavoidable consumption, but in *seeking it out.* Seeking rests upon the mistaken perception that the counterfeit *offers something good.*

There is a tremendous financial incentive for food manufacturers to have the general population believe that nothing is wrong with these substances and that these innocent delicacies might offer a benefit.

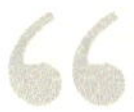

> It's like a trap that is sprung by using a hologram, something ethereal that does not exist.
>
> — WILLIAM PORTER, *ALCOHOL EXPLAINED 2* (2019)

I always imagine how it must have felt for those who first discovered that smoking was addictive and caused lung cancer. Everyone around them would have thought that inhaling tobacco smoke was normal and stopping was unnecessary. But this didn't knock them because *they knew it was true.*

The only way for society-wide change to happen is for one person to alter their beliefs and then another. It can be more challenging for those at the start, but it is also more important because without these people leading the way, larger change won't occur.

Meals with others can be used as an opportunity to demonstrate via your actions that the *reason* you are becoming increasingly vibrant, happy, and energetic is *not* because you are blessed with great genes (we all are) or because you have stumbled upon a perfect life circumstance – but because you have worked out a very simple truth: that to build a thriving survival machine you must feed it the delicious, nourishing, flavor-honest foods it needs.

Imagine You Are Normal

When I first contemplated these ideas about flavor, I could see that the argument had merit. I could see there was a lot of logic to it. I could also see that the flavor-nutrition patterns in the modern food supply varied in such a way that they mimicked the unpredictable delivery of rewards in a slot machine.

As this concept swirled around my head, there emerged the tiny sliver of possibility that this whole dietary debacle was not indicative of my own personal failing but was rather the *expected response to intermittent reinforcement of flavor.* In other words, contemplation of these ideas opened up the tiny possibility that all of this was the *expected outcome* of some kind of horrible sensory trick.

I thought about the girl I had once been, full of hope and potential. I thought of all the wasted years between then and now: the endless diets, the relentless researching, the career opportunities squandered, the love forsaken. I thought about my declining health and how these items had brought me to my knees.

And, in that moment, the hopelessness, disgust, and rage that had previously been directed toward myself lifted and turned instead toward the crinkly packages on the kitchen shelves. In that moment, I became receptive to the tiny possibility that all of this was driven by an external flavor error, *not by an error in me.*

Wondering if it was true, I stood and walked to the bathroom mirror (something I was not in the habit of doing) and went right up to the glass, inches from the reflection. I stared into my eyes as if checking who was in there.

I noticed, as I did so, that my eyes looked exactly like they had when I was a young child – sparkling and green. It felt as if my younger self was looking out at me, and we watched each other, considering.

I thought about that healthy, sun-browned girl, that *normal* girl, and how her eyes and my eyes were the same. I wondered if there was a chance we were *still* the same – that I was normal, just like her, but had forgotten.

We seemed to come to a consensus, her and I, that it really might be true.

This mirror-madness introduced a crucial follow-up question: "If I *were* normal, what would I do?"

I didn't understand the importance of this question at the time, but it had the rather dramatic effect of changing the simulations running through my head. Previously, at every juncture, decisions were prefaced with thoughts about dietary failures and reminders that someone with a track record like mine was going to struggle. Decisions were made alongside the background premise that I was *not normal*, that I really couldn't be trusted to navigate my way sensibly out of this situation – and that this was probably not going to work.

You see, the crux of the issue is that addiction is believed to be a *corruption in decision-making capacity*. It is the belief that, in this one specific arena, decision-making is *no longer normal* – that, in some undefinable way, the individual is compromised and different.

The reason there is a stigma attached to being labeled an alcoholic or a drug addict is that something in the label itself implies that even the individual believes they may one day fly off the wagon again – that they accept they have an inherent, intrinsic *condition*. It is as though they fear there is an uncontrollable aspect hiding inside themselves, shut off behind a locked doorway, and if that doorway opens, all hell will burst through.

But *nowhere* in the theory of intermittent reinforcement is there *anything* about corruption of the decision-maker. Yes, the *data* is misleading; and yes, the *bodily signals* transferring this data from the sensory apparatus to the brain are misleading; and yes, if this deception is undetected, unrecognized, and misunderstood, it provokes faulty beliefs that temporarily misdirect behavior. But once the truth is seen and the erroneous beliefs dismantled, the decision-maker is revealed to remain whole, fully functioning, *as you always were.* That life-seeking, survival-orientated, goal-striving force is always within you. The only thing missing was *the right information.*

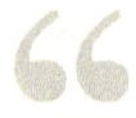

> You cannot react appropriately if the information you act on is faulty or misunderstood.
>
> — MAXWELL MALTZ, *PSYCHO-CYBERNETICS, UPDATED AND EXPANDED* (2016)

In asking myself what I would do if I were normal, I inadvertently set aside any residual fear that I might be suffering from an undefinable, perhaps incurable condition – and imagined instead what I would do if I were *not.*

To be clear, this question does not mean what would *others* normally do in this circumstance...or what is average for society. It means what would *I* do in this precise situation (knowing what I now know about deceptive food) *if I were not afflicted with something unnameable.* What would I do, right here, right now, if I were a *normal human being with a normal capability* like everyone else? In other words, what would I do if I woke up in my own body, in my own life, with a *fully functioning mind and will?*

Funnily enough, when I asked this question, the previously complicated circumstance no longer felt so. Instead, I saw a simple, straightforward path.

First of all, I knew that if I were normal, I wouldn't waste time. I wouldn't pander about. Just as I attacked my first dietary attempts with enthusiasm, I would go all-in, consuming highly nourishing foods, prioritizing nutrient-dense items, pouring in nutrition from all food groups.

At face value, this sounds no different from what I had previously aimed for. But, whereas before this had seemed to be something that I *should* or *must* do, in imagining what I would do if I were normal, I realized I would *choose that anyway.* Even if I imagined myself as having already achieved all of my health and weight loss goals, I realized I would *still* want to feed myself beautiful, nourishing, flavor-honest foods – the true foods of the Earth. I would not want to eat deceptive manmade monstrosities.

In other words, asking this question facilitated a subtle shift from *must* to *want* – the difference between being *forced into something* and being *free to choose.*

Secondly, I realized that if I were normal, I wouldn't panic about occasional infiltration – just as I don't worry about occasionally breathing in second-hand cigarette smoke. Of course, I wouldn't seek it out, but *nor would I fear it.* I wouldn't fret about every little unavoidable encounter. I knew there would be numerous times, such as when having meals out with others, that I would have no way of knowing whether I was eating 100% flavor-honest food or not. I couldn't eliminate deception in every single circumstance, but I *was* certain that I knew which foods were genuine. I knew that as long as I piled my plate with fruits, vegetables, tubers, meats, dairy, and so on – ensuring that almost everything I ate *tasted like it should*, everything would be fine.

In short, in asking myself this question, I temporarily set aside any remaining uncertainties and began to pretend *the problem wasn't me.*

I could see that these ideas about flavor *really might provide a compelling explanation* of what had gone wrong, and I decided to take a chance that it might be true.

At every moment of indecision, I asked myself, "If I were normal, what would I do now?" This question became an unspoken mantra in almost all situations. In response, a clear simulation would arise in my mind, running through a sensible course of action, and I would decide, "Oh, yes, I'll just do that."

And, as a consequence of asking what I would do if I were normal and then *acting* that way, I quickly learned the following:

- I am *not* powerless around these things.
- I really *am* normal, and always was.

And, before long, asking what I would do if I were normal was no longer necessary because there was no *if* about it.

You see, you can *read* that you are not powerless, and know in theory that you *could* have a teaspoonful and not consume a bucketful, but if your experience contradicts this, it just doesn't really seem true – or it seems feasible, but so difficult that it may as well be impossible.

But by grasping the glimmer of hope that I might be normal – and then asking myself what I would do if this were true – I *imagined* myself as normal, acted in that way, and then received evidence that confirmed it was true.

You see, proof only ever comes in the doing. The only way to discover for *sure* whether this hypothesis is right is to test it out in your own life and observe the consequences.

Is there a chance that you started out as a normal human being whose taste and smell receptors were simply led astray by deceptive foods and recalibrated without your knowledge? Is it possible that the conventional 'solutions' (restrictive diets) exacerbated the need for the very thing the counterfeit pretended to deliver, making it more likely that you would overeat these things? And is it possible that this circumstance locked you into a repeating cycle that you couldn't see how to get out of because no one yet had the right information?

And whether you believe in God or evolution (or both), is it really feasible that either of these amazing processes could have ever resulted in such a blundering, monumental error as a lifeform that *didn't know how to accurately find the raw materials it needs to build its own body?*

And can you see that if three-quarters of a population struggles with their weight, the problem *cannot* be the individual and must be the food?

Weight Loss and Healing

The marvelous news is that when molecular trickery is set down, you quickly discover the body can fix this thing on its own. Just as a broken bone mends, a cut heals, and bruises fade, excess weight begins to steadily melt away. The body is a self-healing, self-repairing, self-maintaining survival machine. Inside the nucleus of every cell resides the perfect set of instructions for building you anew.

As a reliable supply of nutrition pours in, taste and smell receptors reset, dietary obsession fades away, energy increases, and peace returns. Hunger stops screaming like a child finally put to sleep at a reasonable hour. Even the gut and microbiome adapt to reflect the anticipated timing of nutrition.[15]

Reliable flavor-nutrition relationships recalibrate the entire bodily system. As nourishment flows in, every aspect of health and mood transforms. If you've ever watered a dying pot plant and watched it come back to life – that's what it feels like. It's like green seeping along your limbs.

When it becomes evident that overeating was *the logical*

outcome of engaging with intermittent reinforcement of flavor – that you are not and never were broken or flawed – an exhilaration swells within you because it means that this thing is finally fixed, remedied, done.

Rather than the fear that comes with seeing a body lurch upward through the clothing sizes, there is a joy in knowing that you have finally *cracked this thing* – that you have thrown your head clear of the water after drowning for so long.

Whereas ordinary diets require ongoing hunger and deprivation, eating to appetite of genuine, nourishing food leaves you feeling even more wonderful with each passing day. As the genuine reward flows in unimpeded, the situation dramatically *improves*. As time passes, you thus receive *more and more evidence* that this approach is *right*.

It will be obvious when appetite has returned to normal levels because your mind will feel light and free, as though a great burden has lifted. When a problem is solved, the working space in the mind clears; the endless pool of theories set down. Food will disappear from your thoughts for great tracts of time until you suddenly remember, with shock, how long it has been since you contemplated eating.

Those who are underweight or have recently ended a severely restrictive diet may find it takes time for appetite to reset. However, those who are overweight and have not recently undergone extreme dietary restriction, are likely to find that appetite noticeably subsides within 3-5 days.

On the fourth day after discarding deceptive foods, I realized that even the muscles in my legs felt different. I was standing at the sink and washing the dishes when I noticed that it felt as though every cell in my body was coming alive.

When I woke on the sixth day, I noticed that my mind felt empty and peaceful, as though the whole issue had been lifted from me. It occurred to me, with some wonderment, that I hadn't felt this way since I was a child.

I had spent almost every moment from age 19 either enduring a restrictive diet (in which I underate or limited access to certain food groups) or implementing 'non-dieting' approaches that unwittingly included deceptive foods. Thus, whether I was dieting or not dieting, hunger was a constant companion and was so omnipresent that I don't think I ever really consciously observed it was there.

But when the relentless, nagging aggravation disappeared – and *peace* swept back in – I realized I felt the same way I used to before this whole drama began. Although I understood it would take time for the excess weight to disappear, I somehow knew *the problem was solved.*

> " The door opened and he stood there, fresh-skinned and glowing. There was something about his eyes. He was inexplicably different. What had happened?
>
> — ALCOHOLICS ANONYMOUS, *THE BIG BOOK* (1939)

When the body has a reliable supply of genuine, nourishing food, excess weight begins to disappear like a snake shedding its skin. Those who are very overweight, like I was, may find this process starts almost immediately. In fact, you may find it happens far faster than expected.

Those who are close to an optimal weight or who have recently undergone extreme dietary restriction may experience a short stabilization period during which nutritional deficits are recouped before the journey to an optimal weight begins. However, in all cases, the speed at which health returns depends upon the concentration of nutrients (see chapter 12: *Prioritize Nourishment*) and the *reliability of flavor-nutrition relationships*.

Eating to appetite of genuine, nourishing foods leads to the return of an optimal weight because it restores hunger to ordinary levels so that less food is consumed than before. Consequently, a larger body size can no longer be maintained, and weight loss is the natural result.

Furthermore, as health and energy return, you will find yourself *doing* more and getting more done. Rather than flogging the body like an old horse, a healthy weight emerges as the natural place to be.

As the weeks pass, this process of weight loss is revealed to be increasingly effortless – and it becomes evident that this is something that can be maintained for the rest of your life.

All at Once

When should this approach be implemented? Are some circumstances more favorable than others? Does it help to ensure that you are well-rested before the escape? Should you spend a few weeks in the sunshine, boosting vitamin D levels, or getting some exercise in before entering the recalibration period?

Is it wise to cultivate friendships and strengthen social ties in advance? Should you clear your schedule, creating external circumstances that are more conducive to change? Surely it is wise to flood the system with beneficial nutrients *before* the escape? Wouldn't all of this put someone in the best position of all to succeed?

At face value, these propositions may sound sensible. But what would you say to a heroin addict who lacks sleep, sunshine, nutrition, fresh air, exercise, and social support? Can you see that for someone to focus on surrounding issues while continuing to dose themselves up to the eyeballs with a toxic, addictive substance is somewhat futile because the main problem is the one they refuse to address? Can you also see that consumption of the deceptive item *exacerbates* these side issues and that almost all of these things will improve once the deceptive influence is gone?

Discarding a deceptive item amidst the chaos and challenges of everyday life is not only possible but, in an odd way, preferable. It provides instant proof that no matter how complicated or stressful life becomes, eating genuine foods doesn't *add* to the difficulty but *makes everything better.*

Nonetheless, mightn't there be circumstances when it is advisable to gradually migrate from a deceptive diet, perhaps changing to reliable flavor-nutrition relationships over several weeks, tapering intake, or reducing different deceptive foods one at a time?

Although reducing the consumption of any deceptive item is advantageous, it is vital to note that partial reduction does not remedy the situation nor result in weight loss. Each time a deceptive item is consumed, it recalibrates bodily systems, leaving the individual perpetually fighting against the tide.

Gradually cutting back delays the recalibration period and prolongs the elevated hunger while never fully relieving withdrawal symptoms. Furthermore, reducing consumption can inadvertently magnify the illusory appeal of the deceptive item.

The moment it becomes evident that *every engagement delivers a loss*, there is zero argument for prolonging the torture. Quitting deceptive foods cold turkey is the best solution there is. It instantly puts the body into healing and reboot mode, initiating a glorious recalibration process that combines the thrill of rapid rewards with immediate action.

> ...something magical happens when one is willing to *go for it.*
>
> — STEVE CHANDLER, *REINVENTING YOURSELF, 20TH ANNIVERSARY EDITION* (2017)

Remember, the quiet aggravation of withdrawal fools people into thinking today is not the right day. This quiet background aggravation seems to imply that it might be easier tomorrow. Yet, when tomorrow comes, it feels exactly like today, and the aggravation caused by the prior ingestion remains and will continue...*until you stop.*

People die waiting for today to be easier than tomorrow, but that day never comes because the easiest option always votes in favor of the counterfeit.

Eating three nourishing meals of flavor-honest foods until satiety provides a delicious and satisfying way of eating that offers access to *every single nutritional reward.* There is no need to wait for the stars to align or for the external circumstances to improve (this is a hopeless game because continuing to engage with a deceptive item makes all circumstances incrementally worse).

Addiction is a recognition problem – set in motion by sensory deception. You have been *deceived.* And you can work that out in one big bang.

Your body has been subjected to an insufficient intake of nutrients and an excessive load of calories for years on end – dancing like a puppet on a flavor string.

You can *stop it.*

Preparation

In the final sub-chapter, we will lay out the ritual of saying goodbye to these deceiving, manipulative substances. Do not turn the page until you are in an excited frame of mind, eager to stop this thing in its tracks.

Overeating can be fixed. In fact, following the method in this book can make it feel almost ridiculously easy. But no one can do it except you. Therefore, before we proceed, I need to ask you a question.

Some individuals may feel they are not ready to answer. Yet, it is a necessary question and we cannot proceed without it.

So, now I ask you: Are you ready to reset taste and smell receptors, restore hunger to ordinary levels, and achieve a healthy weight – surprising all of those who doubt you will ever do it? Are you ready to stand up and walk out of this trap?

When the certainty comes to you, take some time to stock your home with beautiful, nourishing foods. Visit a fruit shop, butcher, organic store, whole food shop – wherever you wish – and fill your kitchen with a spectacular array of nourishing items. Celebrate bringing these wonderful, life-sustaining foods into your home.

While you do so, make sure you retain enough deceptive fodder on hand to see you through a final goodbye. (If you have already discarded deceptive food long ago – you can omit this instruction – and just read the final section.)

When you're ready, turn the page. We're going to rip off the Band-Aid and fix this thing.

The Final Time

> Concentrate on every last syrupy, sickly, poisonous, disgusting mouthful of it. Use it to solidify in your mind the entire pointless miserable cycle...
>
> — WILLIAM PORTER, ALCOHOL EXPLAINED, *REPEATING DAY ONE* (2019)

Allen Carr discovered there is a benefit in saying goodbye to the deceiving entity, not just for the sake of closure, but for fitting all of this new knowledge to the circumstance first-hand – to hearing the lies from the horse's mouth.

When you are ready, sit the deceptive items before you and know this is the final time. Face the deceptive fodder and witness the flimsy trick in person.

This is no final glorious splurge. This is no sad farewell. This is the exposure of the enemy, the final reveal.

Bring the imposter to the entrance of the body, and let the misleading concoction pass your lips and move around the mouth, before sliding down the throat.

Feel the lies as they slip over the tongue. Notice the artificial textures – and think about what this *illusory concoction really is.*

Notice how it dresses up sub-par ingredients and passes them off as something more. Notice the artificial intensity of flavor – how the additives and extracts try so hard to grease and flatter – while never satisfying, never delivering what they promise, always *taking.*

Envision the chemical decoys locking into taste and smell receptors, mislabeling the chemicals that are coming in, seducing the body into taking trash that it does not want.

Notice how the taste and smell receptors are fooled, but *you are not.*

And as these substances enter the body, think of what you have sacrificed on the altar of this particular deception. Think of what this devious little ploy has cost you. Roll the little molecular liars around the tongue – and think of those who quietly fill their coffers at your demise.

And if negative feelings come, relish in them. Fan the flames. You might even find yourself summoning a kind of derision, scorn, fury, or perhaps even *revulsion* toward these misleading substances that masquerade as that which they are not.

And yet, notice, too, how behind all of these emotions, there emerges a slow and burgeoning kind of joy – a sense of relief – as it begins to sink in what all of this means.

And whether this joy makes itself fully known now or in a few days or weeks from now, even though it is hard to fathom, you will think back and recall this moment as the day you truly saw these things for what they are. And the wonderful fact is that once you see the truth, you can't unsee it. And this is exhilarating because it means that even though you may not yet realize it, *this is the moment you were set free.*

Of course, a twinge of hesitancy may bubble up at these words, but time will reveal the truth. Once a trick is exposed, the game is up.

Revel in the dawning of truth. Savor the moment the wool was pulled from your eyes, the curtain thrown down, the pathetic trick laid bare.

And when finally the body is done with this misleading gunk, and you cannot bear to swallow another mouthful, cast any remainder from your home. Hurl the wrappers and any remaining traces of deception away in a blaze of glory and notice how your whole being begins to thrum with excitement at finally *sensing the desire to avoid.*

And as this excitement begins to flow through your veins, know that in this change of perception, you have undertaken the flicking of a switch that reboots your biological system and brings the survival machine back online.

This is the moment the cue-set split in two; the counterfeit recognized and thrown down.

And as genuine flavor signals pour in over the coming days and weeks, take opportunities to notice how frequently you find yourself feeling *peaceful* and *satisfied.* Notice how the body begins to signal satiety the way it was born to.

And as these observations accumulate, notice how any residual doubt fades away and is replaced with increasing certainty that *this approach works.* And as it becomes clear that you can *trust the body to take care of this thing* – that you no longer need to fret about dietary matters – sense the overwhelming relief that you can just *get on with living the rest of your life.*

Like escaping cigarettes, this is a once-and-done thing. No ongoing support is needed. In escaping deception, only the truth is required – nothing else.

If any moments of indecision arise during the first few days or weeks – and you may not experience these at all – remember to ask yourself what you would do if you were normal (which, of course, you will soon discover you are – in fact, you may have worked this out already). And in circumstances where you are surrounded by deceptive food, enjoy these social occasions for the glorious reminders that you are free.

You might not realize it yet, but soon you will. It's hard to believe, I know. But this thing is done.

13

END NOTES

> As you read this someone is no doubt advancing yet another bright idea to make inferior food taste better and look better.
>
> — GIRAUD W. CAMPBELL, *A DOCTOR'S PROVEN NEW HOME CURE FOR ARTHRITIS* (1979)

WE CAN TURN this situation around, one person at a time. But for this to happen, the truth must spread. Food manufacturers don't want us to cotton on to their game because if people only buy foods that look, smell, and taste the way nature intended, there is very little left for them to do. Their entire money-making venture involves adding the illusion of value where it doesn't belong.

If these ideas spread, corporations will go to great lengths to convince people that the concept of intermittent reinforcement of flavor is false. But you will soon have irrefutable evidence in your own life and the lives of those around you that it is true.

It is harder for people to recognize the truth when 99% of the population is fooled. However, a groundswell of popular opinion can turn. It begins with a change of mind in each individual, and whether or not another person changes their mind depends partly on you.

If you have found some of these ideas helpful, please consider taking a moment to write an honest review on Amazon. Even a short review can have a significant impact. While reading reviews of Allen Carr's books, I frequently discovered new insights and ways of interpreting the material that helped me better understand the message. Reviews play a key role in reassuring others that these ideas might be worth their time. Your review could be the one that helps another break free.

I wish to extend my deepest gratitude to all beta readers who provided invaluable feedback on earlier drafts of this book and to all of those who have sent messages through my website over the years. Thank you, too, to every single person who has read this book. All the very best to you.

Now, it's time to lift your arms and race across the hilltops. *You're free.*

REFERENCES

1. Behavior Change Requires a Change of Mind

1. *Calories Needed Each Day*, National Institutes of Health (2010) https://www.nhlbi.nih.gov/health/educational/wecan/downloads/calreqtips.pdf

2. Behavior

1. N.A.A Rahman, A Fazilah, M.E Effarizah, *Toxicity of Nutmeg (Myristicin): A Review* (2015) https://www.researchgate.net/publication/278850055_Toxicity_of_Nutmeg_Myristicin_A_Review
2. Olumayokun A. Olajide, Franklin F. Ajayi, Ambrose I. Ekhelar, S. Olubusayo Awe, J. Modupe Makinde, A. R. Akinola Alada, *Biological effects of Myristica fragrans (nutmeg) extract* (1999) https://onlinelibrary.wiley.com/doi/abs/10.1002/(SICI)1099-1573(199906)13:4%3C344::AID-PTR436%3E3.0.CO;2-E
3. Jessica Elizabeth De La Torre Torres, Fatma Gassara, Anne Patricia Kouassi, Satinder Kaur Brar, Khaled Belkacemi, *Spice Use in Food: Properties and Benefits, Critical Reviews in Food Science and Nutrition* (2015) https://espace.inrs.ca/id/eprint/3833/1/P2789_PP.pdf
4. S.H. Nasr, Y. Kashtanova, V. Levchuk, G.S. Markowitz, *Secondary oxalosis due to excess vitamin C intake* (2006) https://www.kidney-international.org/article/S0085-2538(15)51777-8/fulltext
5. Vasu Sunkara, Timothy D. Pelkowski, Darren Dreyfus, Anjali Satoskar, *Acute Kidney Disease Due to Excessive Vitamin C Ingestion and Remote Roux-en-Y Gastric Bypass Surgery Superimposed on CKD* (2015) https://www.sciencedirect.com/science/article/abs/pii/S0272638615009531
6. R. Weindruch, R. Walford, D. Guthrie, *The retardation of aging in mice by dietary restriction: longevity, cancer, immunity and lifetime energy intake* (1986) https://pdfs.semanticscholar.org/222a/5a6b9165191fec34b1ef4c174198c9bc5f97.pdf
7. Clara M. Davis, *Self Selection of Diet by Newly Weaned Infants: An Experimental Study* (1928) https://www.medicine.mcgill.ca/epidemiology/hanley/reprints/claradavis1928.pdf
8. Stephen Strauss, *Clara M. Davis and the wisdom of letting children choose their own diets* (2006) https://www.ncbi.nlm.nih.gov/pmc/articles/PMC1626509/
9. Fred Provenza, *Nourishment: What Animals Can Teach Us about Rediscovering Our Nutritional Wisdom* (2018)

10. Fred Provenza, *Nourishment: What Animals Can Teach Us about Rediscovering Our Nutritional Wisdom* (2018)
11. "Nutrition is such a new science that we've barely touched the surface as to the power it has over our health and well-being. As scientific studies reveal more, we realize that we have mislabeled good things as bad and bad things as good." – Kate Deering, *How to Heal Your Metabolism* (2015)
12. Louis Rosenfeld, *Vitamine – Vitamin. The early years of discovery* (1997) https://academic.oup.com/clinchem/article/43/4/680/5640821
13. "...it is largely an organism's behavior that determines whether it will survive, that is, live long enough to pass on its genes." – W. David Pierce, Carl D. Cheney, *Behavior Analysis and Learning: A Biobehavioral Approach, Sixth Edition* (2017)
14. "Single-celled organisms, such as Escherichia coli, developed multiple chemical receptors critical for such survival. The rotatory direction of their flagellae – whip-like appendages used to propel them through their environment – is altered by the type of chemical encountered. Thus, chemicals important for sustenance induce a counterclockwise rotation of the flagella, facilitating a smooth and somewhat linear swimming path, whereas toxic chemicals provoke a clockwise flagellar rotation, resulting in tumbling and turning away from the offending stimulus (Larsen et al., 1974)." – Christopher H Hawkes, *Smell and Taste Disorders* (2018)
15. "Happiness is the result of making progress and of goal-attainment at any of the diverse aspects of life that are inherently important: romance, friendships, health, material comfort, security, family, and social regard. These are inherently important because each has been intimately related to successful DNA reproduction throughout the history of our species." – Douglas J. Lisle, Alan Goldhamer, *The Pleasure Trap* (2003)
16. "Medieval water torture exploited the punishing effects of forcing a person to drink water beyond capacity. These tendencies for reinforcers to wax and wane and even turn to punishers evolved because individuals that possessed them survived and reproduced better than those that lacked them." – William M. Baum, *Understanding Behaviorism: Behavior, Culture, and Evolution*, Third Edition (2017)
17. "Toxicologists view all chemicals as potentially poisonous—the key issue is determining the relationship between dosage and lethality." – Danielle Renee Reed, Antti Knaapila, *Genetics of Taste and Smell: Poisons and Pleasures* (2012) https://www.ncbi.nlm.nih.gov/pmc/articles/PMC3342754/
18. "Since information is costly, rational decision makers can be expected to look for ways to reduce the average costs of attention, computation, calculation, and search." – James G. March, *A Primer on Decision Making: How Decisions Happen* (2009)
19. "For instance, animals that startle and run in response to a sudden noise may escape a predator, hence the startle reflex may have provided an adaptive advantage over organisms that did not run, or that ran less quickly in response to the noise. Thus, reflexes are selected across the history of the

species." – W. David Pierce, Carl D. Cheney, *Behavior Analysis and Learning: A Biobehavioral Approach, Sixth Edition* (2017)

20. "Model parameters are continually updated until prediction error is minimised, up to expected levels of noise. This is learning (Friston 2003; Friston and Stephan 2007)." – Jacob Hohwy, *The hypothesis testing brain: Some philosophical applications* (2010) https://www.academia.edu/1989353/The_hypothesis_testing_brain_Some_philosophical_applications
21. "All species that have been tested, including humans, show this kind of conditioning." – W. David Pierce, Carl D. Cheney, *Behavior Analysis and Learning: A Biobehavioral Approach, Sixth Edition* (2017)
22. "The sequences animals learn in some serial pattern experiments seem to extend well beyond the limits of working memory. They would thus appear to require an ability to compare what is going on now with what has gone on in the past." – Claude G. Čech, *Chapter 6: Resistance to Extinction* (1999) https://userweb.ucs.louisiana.edu/~cgc2646/LRN/Chap6.html
23. "...present behavior depends not only on present events, but on many past events. These past events affect behavior as an aggregate, not as momentary happenings." – William M. Baum, *Understanding Behaviorism: Behavior, Culture, and Evolution*, Third Edition (2017)
24. "Many scientists now believe that the brain is basically a Bayesian hypothesis tester. One of its primary activities is making predictions about what input it expects to receive and then updating these predictions in the light of the actual input." – Neil Levy, Addiction as a disorder of belief (2014) https://www.ncbi.nlm.nih.gov/pmc/articles/PMC3991824/
25. "...the goal of the brain is to explore the world and register the consequences of successful exploratory actions to improve the efficacy of future actions." – György Buzsáki, *The Brain from Inside Out* (2019)
26. "...[the brain] computes a weighted running average of all rewards received previously in the presence of the stimulus, with the most recent reward weighted most heavily and the weight for prior rewards declining exponentially in their lag." – Nathaniel D. Daw, Philippe N. Tobler, *Neuroeconomics: Chapter 15. Value Learning through Reinforcement: The Basics of Dopamine and Reinforcement Learning* (2014)
27. Deirdre Barrett, *Supernormal Stimuli: How Primal Urges Overran Their Evolutionary Purpose* (2010)

3. The Role of Flavor

1. James Kennedy, *Ingredients of an All-Natural Banana* (2013) https://jameskennedymonash.wordpress.com/2013/12/12/ingredients-of-an-all-natural-banana/
2. Paul A.S. Breslin, *An Evolutionary Perspective on Food and Human Taste* (2013) https://www.sciencedirect.com/science/article/pii/S0960982213004181
3. Paul A.S. Breslin, Alan C. Spector, *Mammalian taste perception* (2008) https://www.cell.com/current-biology/fulltext/S0960-9822(07)02370-6

4. Paul A.S. Breslin, *An Evolutionary Perspective on Food and Human Taste* (2013) https://www.sciencedirect.com/science/article/pii/S0960982213004181
5. Scott Herness, Fang-li Zhao, *The neuropeptides CCK and NPY and the changing view of cell-to-cell communication in the taste bud* (2009) https://www.sciencedirect.com/science/article/abs/pii/S0031938409001188
6. Linda A. Barlow, Ophir D. Klein, *Developing and regenerating a sense of taste* (2016) https://www.ncbi.nlm.nih.gov/pmc/articles/PMC4435577/
7. Mirre Viskaal van Dongen, Marjolijn C van den Berg, Nicole Vink, Frans J Kok, Cees de Graaf, *Taste-nutrient relationships in commonly consumed foods* (2011) https://www.ncbi.nlm.nih.gov/pubmed/22018329
8. Paul A.S. Breslin, *An Evolutionary Perspective on Food and Human Taste* (2013) https://www.sciencedirect.com/science/article/pii/S0960982213004181
9. Institute for Quality and Efficiency in Health Care, *How does our sense of taste work?* (Updated 2016) https://www.ncbi.nlm.nih.gov/books/NBK279408/?report=reader
10. "In addition to the five canonical taste qualities, there is growing evidence that many vertebrates and invertebrates use their gustatory systems to detect the presence of other compounds, that may include Ca2+, CO2, water and fats..." – Emily R. Liman, Yali V. Zhang, Craig Montell, *Peripheral coding of taste* (2014) https://www.ncbi.nlm.nih.gov/pmc/articles/PMC3994536/
11. Andrea Rinaldi, *The scent of life. The exquisite complexity of the sense of smell in animals and humans* (2007) https://www.ncbi.nlm.nih.gov/pmc/articles/PMC1905909/
12. "Whereas humans are able to distinguish between only five or six primary taste qualities, people are able to differentiate more than a trillion odors..." – Cees de Graaf, Sanne Boesveldt, *Flavor, Satiety and Food Intake* (2017)
13. Stephen A. Goff, Harry J. Klee, *Plant Volatile Compounds: Sensory Cues for Health and Nutritional Value?* (2006) http://science.sciencemag.org/content/311/5762/815
14. Gordon Shepherd, *Neurogastronomy: How the Brain Creates Flavor and Why It Matters* (2013)
15. Institute for Quality and Efficiency in Health Care, *How does our sense of taste work?* (Updated 2016) https://www.ncbi.nlm.nih.gov/books/NBK279408/
16. "It is now estimated that there are between 500-1000 odorant receptor genes in both humans and mice. This number of genes, specific to the olfactory system, comprises 1-2% of the 50,000 to 100,000 genes thought to make up the human genome. This number is second only to the receptors of the immune system." – John C. Leffingwell, *Olfaction* (2001) https://www.leffingwell.com/download/olfaction2.pdf
17. "Nonhuman species provide evidence that the sense of taste has been shaped by evolution; for instance, cats and some other carnivorous species, in addition to chickens, have lost the function of their sweet receptor—they no longer need to taste "sweet" because the foods they eat, the flesh of other animals or starchy grains, contain little sugar." – Danielle Renee Reed, Antti Knaapila, *Genetics of Taste and Smell: Poisons and Pleasures* (2012) https://www.ncbi.nlm.nih.gov/pmc/articles/PMC3342754/

18. "Compared to mammals, chickens have fewer genes for taste receptors, e.g., lacking the taste receptor T1R2 for sweet..." – Hong-Xiang Liu, Prasangi Rajapaksha, Zhonghou Wang, Naomi E Kramer, Brett J Marshall, *An Update on the Sense of Taste in Chickens: A Better Developed System than Previously Appreciated* (2018) https://www.ncbi.nlm.nih.gov/pmc/articles/PMC5951165/
19. "Aquatic carnivorous mammals, such as sea lions [...] appear to have lost a large number of taste receptors, perhaps because most of their prey are swallowed whole and would not be tasted. In this case, the identification of swimming fish via visual recognition and the body and kinetic senses of pursuing prey may have replaced taste." – Paul A.S. Breslin, *An Evolutionary Perspective on Food and Human Taste* (2013) https://www.sciencedirect.com/science/article/pii/S0960982213004181
20. Danielle Renee Reed, Antti Knaapila, *Genetics of Taste and Smell: Poisons and Pleasures* (2012) https://www.ncbi.nlm.nih.gov/pmc/articles/PMC3342754/
21. Richard D. Mattes, *Orosensory Considerations* (2012) https://onlinelibrary.wiley.com/doi/full/10.1038/oby.2006.299
22. "Flavor is information. Compounds like phosphorus and vitamin C are stable. They don't waft off food. So the body senses what it can—those unstable floaty aromas—and associates them with the post-ingestive effects on our bodies." – Mark Schatzker, *The Dorito Effect: The Surprising New Truth About Food and Flavor* (2016
23. "Flavor evaluation is influenced by learning from experience with foods. One main influence is flavor-nutrient learning (FNL), a Pavlovian process whereby a flavor acts as a conditioned stimulus (CS) that becomes associated with the postingestive effects of ingested nutrients (the US)." – Kevin P. Myers, *The convergence of psychology and neurobiology in flavor-nutrient learning* (2018) https://core.ac.uk/download/pdf/216950922.pdf
24. "Sheep can make multiple flavor-feedback associations with minerals. We designed a study in which we made lambs deficient in one of three minerals – phosphorus, calcium or sodium – and gave them a choice of the three differently flavored foods. The lambs had previously ingested these flavored foods with one of the three minerals. Lambs preferred the flavor previously paired with repletion of the mineral – phosphorus, calcium, or sodium – they were lacking." – Fred Provenza, *Nourishment: What Animals Can Teach Us about Rediscovering Our Nutritional Wisdom* (2018)
25. "He wanted to set up an "association" between the flavor of maple and the nutritional payload of phosphorus. A few days later, when these same phosphorus-deficient sheep were offered maple-flavored feed, they gobbled it up, even though there wasn't so much as a speck of phosphorus in it. To their bodies, maple flavor meant one thing: phosphorus." – Mark Schatzker, *The Dorito Effect: The Surprising New Truth About Food and Flavor* (2016)
26. "...sheep trained to avoid cinnamon-flavored rice [previously paired with mild dose of lithium chloride] also avoid any cinnamon flavored food." – Fred Provenza, *Nourishment: What Animals Can Teach Us about Rediscovering Our Nutritional Wisdom* (2018)

27. "When sheep eat a meal of four familiar foods (alfalfa, barley, oats, and corn) and one novel food (rye), and then get an orally administered nauseating capsule of lithium chloride, they subsequently ignore the novel food, but not the familiar foods." – Fred Provenza, *Nourishment: What Animals Can Teach Us about Rediscovering Our Nutritional Wisdom* (2018)
28. Emily R. Liman, Yali V. Zhang, Craig Montell, *Peripheral coding of taste* (2015) https://www.ncbi.nlm.nih.gov/pmc/articles/PMC3994536/
29. "You can get along with other people only if you can accurately gauge whether their intentions are benign or dangerous. Even a slight misreading can lead to painful misunderstandings in relationships at home and at work." – Bessel van der Kolk, *The Body Keeps the Score* (2015)
30. "Our own studies have shown that sniffing in a smell gives rise to a spatial pattern of activity in the brain. These patterns function as images of smell, with different images for different smells, much as different faces form different images in our visual system. Human brains are very good at recognizing faces, which can be thought of as a highly developed form of pattern recognition. From our studies we think that the same ability occurs with the patterns laid down by smells—that is, the ability to recognize many different patterns representing as many different smells." – Gordon Shepherd, *Neurogastronomy: How the Brain Creates Flavor and Why It Matters* (2013)
31. "Importantly, flavor evaluation is neither innate nor fixed." – Kevin P. Myers, *The convergence of psychology and neurobiology in flavor-nutrient learning* (2018) https://core.ac.uk/download/pdf/216950922.pdf
32. "Our likes and wants are subjective properties we assign to food based on our past experiences, and our current state of satiation and satiety." – J. Stanton, *What Is Hunger, and Why Are We Hungry?* (2012) https://www.youtube.com/watch?v=254L_Gr9s-4
33. Zata Vickers, Flavor, *Satiety and Food Intake* (2017)
34. Cees de Graaf, Sanne Boesveldt, *Flavor, Satiety and Food Intake* (2017)
35. "In the orbitofrontal cortex, feeding to satiety with one food decreases the responses of these neurons to that food, but not to other foods, showing that sensory-specific satiety is computed in the primate (including human) orbitofrontal cortex." – Edmund Rolls, *Brain mechanisms underlying flavour and appetite* (2006) https://www.ncbi.nlm.nih.gov/pubmed/16815796
36. "...dopamine neurons come to respond with bursts to stimuli that immediately precede and reliably predict the reward..." – Roy A. Wise, Mykel A. Robble, *Dopamine and Addiction* (2020) https://www.annualreviews.org/doi/full/10.1146/annurev-psych-010418-103337
37. Richard D. Mattes, *Orosensory Considerations* (2012) https://onlinelibrary.wiley.com/doi/full/10.1038/oby.2006.299
38. Keri McCrickerd, *Flavor, Satiety and Food Intake* (2017)
39. Paul A.S. Breslin, *An Evolutionary Perspective on Food and Human Taste* (2013) https://www.sciencedirect.com/science/article/pii/S0960982213004181
40. Christopher H Hawkes, *Smell and Taste Disorders* (2018)

41. "As ingestion continues, the various inhibitory effects of the ingested food and digestive products accumulating in the stomach and small intestine begin to slow the rate of eating and finally stop it. Since orosensory and postingestional stimuli act concurrently shortly after a meal begins..." John D. Davis, Gerard P. Smith, *The conditioned satiating effect of orosensory stimuli* (2009) https://www.sciencedirect.com/science/article/abs/pii/S0031938409001401
42. "Eating two oranges made participants feel physically full, but they were still mentally hungry – looking for or wanting something else to eat." – Zata Vickers, *Flavor, Satiety and Food Intake* (2017)
43. "The behavioural sequence of satiety occurred after the first sham-fed meal, but meal size doubled and the intermeal interval was about 50% shorter than was observed in the preceding real feeding test." – Gerard P. Smith, *Satiation: From Gut to Brain* (1998)
44. "...after 17 hours of food deprivation, sham feeding continued for 7.5 hours in rats without the occurrence of the behavioural sequence of satiety (Young et al.,). Continuous sham feeding has also been observed in rhesus monkeys after overnight food deprivation." – Gerard P. Smith, *Satiation: From Gut to Brain* (1998)
45. "The observation of absence of satiety when food drained out of the upper small intestine has been confirmed in monkeys..." – Danielle Greenberg, *Satiation: From Gut to Brain* (1998)
46. "Both experiments confirmed previous results – intake was equivalent to the volume of gastric contents withdrawn." – Gerard P. Smith, *Satiation: From Gut to Brain* (1998)
47. "The infusions elicited the complete behavioral sequence for satiety, and the reductions in sham feeding were related to the chemical concentration of the nutrient infusions." – Danielle Greenberg, *Satiation: From Gut to Brain* (1998)
48. "The duodenal infusion had been shown to stop sham feeding and elicit the behavioural sequence of satiety after 17 hours of food deprivation (Liebling et al., 1975)." – *Gerard P. Smith, Satiation: From Gut to Brain* (1998)
49. "The satiating effect of intestinal nutrient infusions in the sham-feeding preparation indicates, however, that gastric distention is not necessary for the inhibition of meal size." – Danielle Greenberg, *Satiation: From Gut to Brain* (1998)
50. "Equivolumetric infusions of saline did not suppress sham feeding and did not elicit behaviors typical of satiety. Thus, in the monkey as well as in the rat and humans, the mechanical stimuli produced by the volume of saline infusions did not produce a satiating effect." – Danielle Greenberg, *Satiation: From Gut to Brain* (1998)
51. "If intestinal infusions were given 6-12 minutes before sham feeding was initiated, no suppression of intake was observed. Maximal suppression of sham feeding was obtained when the [nutrient] infusion began 12 minutes after the onset of sham feeding." – Danielle Greenberg, *Satiation: From Gut to Brain* (1998)

52. "...a synergistic interaction between post-pyloric and gastric stimuli in the control of compensatory intake..." – Gerard P. Smith, *Satiation: From Gut to Brain* (1998)
53. "Roux-en-Y gastric bypass surgery (RYGB) and other bariatric procedures alter gastrointestinal processing of food in a number of ways. Thus, it is plausible that these procedures alter post-oral unconditioned stimuli that support flavor-consequence learning, leading to altered food selection, amount eaten, and affect. Surprisingly, however, there is almost no research on the role of flavor-consequence learning in the effects of bariatric surgery on appetite. This issue urgently warrants investigation." – Lori Asarian, Nori Geary, *RYGB and flavor-consequence learning* (2020) https://www.sciencedirect.com/science/article/abs/pii/S0195666319305732
54. "...total subdiaphragmatic vagotomy abolished the suppression of sham feeding elicited by intestinal infusion of sodium oleate." – *Danielle Greenberg, Satiation: From Gut to Brain* (1998)
55. "When the caloric density of their food was cut in half, after a few days rats doubled the volume of food that they ate. Other labs found similar results." – Seth Roberts, *What makes food fattening* (2005) https://sethroberts.net/wp-content/uploads/2018/12/whatmakesfoodfattening.pdf
56. "However, studies in which food has been calorically diluted (i.e., by the addition of nonnutritive bulk so that more volume must be eaten to achieve the same caloric load) have shown that animals easily adapt to this manipulation by increasing their meal size (Adolph, 1947; Janowitz & Grossman, 1949). They readily consume a larger volume to get their calories, which suggests that gastric capacity is rarely a factor in normal consumption." – Stephen C. Woods, *The Eating Paradox: How We Tolerate Food* (1991)
    https://www.appstate.edu/~steelekm/classes/psy5150/Documents/Woods1991.pdf

4. Deceptive Flavor

1. "A soft drink with low natural juice content may require a clouding agent to boost the turbidity in order for it to resemble the cloudy natural juice of the fruit it is named after." – Joanna Blythman, *Swallow This: Serving Up the Food Industry's Darkest Secrets* (2015)
2. Avery Gilbert, *What the Nose Knows* (2015)
3. "When they see something they like, they extract its flavor molecules from the fruit on the tree. Then, back in the lab, they mimic mother nature's molecules with chemicals." – Morley Safer, CBS News, *Tweaking tastes and creating cravings* (2011) https://www.youtube.com/watch?v=a7Wh3uq1yTc [2:30]
4. Glanbia Nutritionals, *Flavor Masking Challenges and How to Solve Them* https://www.glanbianutritionals.com/en/nutri-knowledge-center/nutritional-resources/flavor-masking-challenges-and-how-solve-them

5. Jeff Gelski, *Eliminating the pea flavor in pea protein*, (2018) https://www.foodbusinessnews.net/articles/11344-eliminating-the-pea-flavor-in-pea-protein
6. "Sweetness is used to mask not only bitter but also acidic tastes. This is important in wines or fruit juices, especially citrus juices that can contain strong-flavored volatile oils from pith, seeds, and peels that are the result of large-scale juice operations." – Florentine Hilty-Vancura, *New Strategies For Masking And Modifying Flavor* (2017) https://www.preparedfoods.com/articles/120329-new-strategies-for-masking-and-modifying-flavor
7. "The biggest challenge in plant-based protein product development today is overcoming the unwanted or off flavor that comes from these sources. For example, a beany soy flavor or bitter pea protein flavor can deter consumers from craving plant-based products." – Innova Flavors, *Understanding Flavor Masking Agents: 5 Things You Need to Know* (2021) https://www.innovaflavors.com/blog/understanding-flavor-masking-agents-5-things-you-need-to-know
8. Innova Flavors, *Understanding Flavor Masking Agents: 5 Things You Need to Know* (2021) https://www.innovaflavors.com/blog/understanding-flavor-masking-agents-5-things-you-need-to-know
9. "Trying to block bitter flavours is far more practical than, say, trying to remove any of the vast range of compounds that can make food taste unpleasant. And only tiny amounts of bitter blockers are required to stop the bitter signal reaching the brain." – Celeste Biever, *Bitter pills banished by taste-blocking compounds* (2003) https://www.newscientist.com/article/dn3433-bitter-pills-banished-by-taste-blocking-compounds/
10. Danielle Andrews, Smita Salunke, Anne Cram, Joanne Bennett, Robert S. Ives, Abdul W. Basit, Catherine Tuleu, *Bitter-blockers as a taste masking strategy: A systematic review towards their utility in pharmaceuticals* (2021) https://www.sciencedirect.com/science/article/abs/pii/S0939641120303179
11. Celeste Biever, *Bitter pills banished by taste-blocking compounds* (2003) https://www.newscientist.com/article/dn3433-bitter-pills-banished-by-taste-blocking-compounds/
12. "Microencapsulation is a technology that is extensively used in foods..." – Nitamani Choudhury, Murlidhar Meghwal, Kalyan Das, *Microencapsulation: An overview on concepts, methods, properties and applications in foods* (2021) https://onlinelibrary.wiley.com/doi/10.1002/fft2.94
13. Florentine Hilty-Vancura, *New Strategies For Masking And Modifying Flavor* (2017) https://www.preparedfoods.com/articles/120329-new-strategies-for-masking-and-modifying-flavor
14. Mark Schatzker, *The Dorito Effect: The Surprising New Truth About Food and Flavor* (2016)
15. "Dutch chemists soon discovered that the compound diacetyl, produced either synthetically or by microorganisms, could add a "buttery" flavor to foods. Creameries then started adding a chemical that doesn't naturally occur in butter to actual butter in order to make it taste more like...butter." – Alison Herman, *The Absurd History of Artificial Flavors* (2015) https://amp.firstwefeast.com/drink/2015/06/the-absurd-history-of-artificial-flavors

16. "Enhanced or value-added meat and poultry products are raw products that contain flavor solutions added through marinating, needle injecting, soaking, etc. The presence and amount of the solution will be featured as part of the product name, for example, "Chicken Thighs Flavored with up to 10% of a Solution" or "Beef Steak Marinated with 6% of a Flavor Solution."" – United States Department of Agriculture, *Water in Meat and Poultry* (2013) https://www.fsis.usda.gov/food-safety/safe-food-handling-and-preparation/food-safety-basics/water-meat-poultry
17. "Monosodium glutamate (MSG) is perhaps the most common of the glutamates added to foods. Many consumers, however, have been avoiding MSG when it appears on a label. But extracts and concentrations of tomatoes and mushrooms, rich in natural glutamic acid compounds, are stepping up to take MSG's place." – Florentine Hilty-Vancura, *New Strategies For Masking And Modifying Flavor* (2017) https://www.preparedfoods.com/articles/120329-new-strategies-for-masking-and-modifying-flavor
18. "MSG enhancement of flavour appears to require some existing umami-like element to be present: thus when MSG is added to boiled rice alone, it elicits either neutral or negative palatability ratings, but when added to fried rice, palatability ratings increase." – Martin R Yeomans, *Flavor, Satiety and Food Intake* (2017)
19. "The perfect illusion is one that does not depart too much from reality, but has a touch of the unreal to it, like a waking dream. Lead the seduced to a point of confusion in which they can no longer tell the difference between illusion and reality." – Robert Greene, *The Art of Seduction* (2003)
20. "...the most often selected foods were chocolate (selected by 54 % of participants), candy (46 %), cookies (25 %), chips (25 %), pastries (21 %), cake (21 %), pasta (18 %), pizza (18 %), ice cream (16 %), and French fries (14 %). These foods correspond to the most often craved foods identified in previous studies on food craving." – Adrian Meule, Ashley N. Gearhardt, *Five years of the Yale Food Addiction Scale: Taking stock and moving forward* (2014) https://link.springer.com/article/10.1007/s40429-014-0021-z
21. *Pizza Hut Ingredient Listing* (2014) https://web.archive.org/web/20201112013723/https://d3ixjveba7l33q.cloudfront.net/mobilem8-php/wp-content/uploads/2015/01/PH-Ingredient-Listings-English-June-2014.pdf
22. Tod Cooperman, *Which supplements should be taken with food?* (2021) https://www.consumerlab.com/answers/which-supplements-should-be-taken-with-food/supplements_taken_with_food/
23. Ranjani R. Starr, *Too Little, Too Late: Ineffective Regulation of Dietary Supplements in the United States* (2015) https://www.ncbi.nlm.nih.gov/pmc/articles/PMC4330859/
24. Fred Provenza, *Nourishment: What Animals Can Teach Us about Rediscovering Our Nutritional Wisdom* (2018)
25. "When questioned about cravings, sensory properties are the attributes most commonly reported." – Richard D. Mattes, *Orosensory Considerations* (2012) https://onlinelibrary.wiley.com/doi/full/10.1038/oby.2006.299

26. "More intelligent individuals, who were better at spotting contradictions, would have been at an evolutionary advantage as they would be less readily duped. The better they were at detecting lies, the better they would have also been at preventing any of their own lies from being spotted and thus at manipulating others. The standards of lying and storytelling would then increase, driving the need to be even more intelligent and linguistically able to stay ahead." – Enrico Coen, *The storytelling arms race: origin of human intelligence and the scientific mind* (2019) https://www.nature.com/articles/s41437-019-0214-2.epdf
27. "Once one agent learns how to become more competitive by sacrificing a common value, all its competitors must also sacrifice that value or be outcompeted and replaced by the less scrupulous." – Scott Alexander, *Meditations on Moloch* (2014) https://slatestarcodex.com/2014/07/30/meditations-on-moloch/
28. "The smallest package, the machine-made cigarette, blended shredded tobacco, flavoring agents, and humectants to create a product that was cheap, addictive, and universal, cutting across class and occupational lines." – David T. Courtwright, *The Age of Addiction* (2019)
29. "In 1910 German health officials complained that certain shopkeepers were selling morphine-laced candies, along with discount morphine injections for "delicate nerves."" – David T. Courtwright, *The Age of Addiction* (2019)
30. William Krohn, *Graded Lessons in Physiology and Hygiene* (1906) https://www.google.co.nz/books/edition/Graded_Lessons_in_Physiology_and_Hygiene/TNM4AAAAMAAJ
31. Jonathan Rees, *Food Adulteration and Food Fraud* (2020)
32. Larry Olmsted, *Real Food/Fake Food: Why You Don't Know What You're Eating and What You Can Do About It* (2017)

5. Intermittent Reinforcement

1. B.F. Skinner, *Science and Human Behavior* (1965)
2. Robert Sapolsky, excerpt from Stanford University lecture on Human Sexual Behavior https://www.youtube.com/watch?v=ZIRZu1dRp8Q
3. "In PG, accumbens DA is maximal during a gambling task when the probability of winning and losing money is identical—a 50% chance for a two-outcome event representing maximal uncertainty (Linnet et al., 2012)." – Patrick Anselme, Mike J. F. Robinson, *What motivates gambling behavior? Insight into dopamine's role* (2013) https://www.ncbi.nlm.nih.gov/pmc/articles/PMC3845016/
4. "...only in the presence of uncertainty is it anticipated that there will be information available in the outcome. If reward (P = 1) or no reward (P = 0) occurs exactly as predicted, that event contains no information beyond that already given by the conditioned stimulus; that is, it is redundant. However, when the prediction of reward is uncertain, the outcome (reward or no reward) always contains information. The outcome at P = 0.5 contains, on

average, the maximal amount of information (one bit) of any probability." – Christopher D. Fiorillo, Philippe N. Tobler, Wolfram Schultz, *Discrete Coding of Reward Probability and Uncertainty by Dopamine Neurons* (2003) https://www.hms.harvard.edu/bss/neuro/bornlab/nb204/exam/FiorilloSchultz_Science.pdf

5. "...Martha Weiss and her students let these butterflies loose on a field of yellow and magenta flowers. Sometimes only the yellow flowers had nectar, sometimes only the magenta ones (Weiss and company had fun arranging this). The butterflies quickly learned which color signaled the consequence they wanted." – Susan Schneider, *The Science of Consequences: How They Affect Genes, Change the Brain, and Impact Our World* (2012)
6. "At the start of training, before the animal has learned to discriminate among stimuli, it ought to treat all stimuli along the relevant dimension as equivalent. So, rather than exhibit a tent-shaped gradient, animals at this point ought to have a flat-line gradient in which the same proportion of responses is given to all similar stimuli." – Claude G. Čech, *Chapter 7: Attention & Categorization* (1998) https://userweb.ucs.louisiana.edu/~cgc2646/LRN/Chap7.html
7. "By reinforcing responses to a circular red spot while extinguishing responses to circular spots of all other colors, we may give the red spot exclusive control over the behavior. This is discrimination." – B.F. Skinner, *Science and Human Behavior* (1965)
8. "Each time the system is recalculated, the posterior becomes the prior of the new iteration. It was an evolving system, which each new bit of information pushed closer and closer to certitude." – Sharon Bertsch McGrayne, *The Theory That Would Not Die: How Bayes' Rule Cracked the Enigma Code, Hunted Down Russian Submarines, and Emerged Triumphant from Two Centuries of Controversy* (2012)
9. "Some birds plagued by the cuckoo do eventually evolve a detector and begin to reject the intruder's egg after centuries of victimization." – Deirdre Barrett, *Supernormal Stimuli: How Primal Urges Overran Their Evolutionary Purpose* (2010)
10. "...many behavioral experiments have shown that contingencies of reinforcement generalize across species, type of reinforcement, diverse settings, and different operants." – W. David Pierce, Carl D. Cheney, *Behavior Analysis and Learning: A Biobehavioral Approach, Sixth Edition* (2017)
11. "This general result has been obtained with goldfish (Igaki & Sakagami, 2004), rats (e.g., Blackman, 1968; Shahan & Burke, 2004), pigeons (e.g., Nevin, 1974; Nevin, Tota, Torquato, & Shull, 1990), normal children (Tota-Faucette, 1991), children with developmental disabilities (Ahearn et al., 2003; Mace et al., 2010), college students (Cohen, 1996), and adults with mental retardation (Mace et al., 1990). These studies have employed different sorts of responses and reinforcers, and have evaluated resistance to change by presenting various disruptors including response-independent reinforcers between schedule components, pre-session feeding to devalue reinforcers, response-contingent punishment, conditioned suppression, concurrent distraction,

and extinction – i.e., withholding all reinforcers…" – John A. Nevin, *Resistance to extinction and behavioral momentum* (2012) https://www.ncbi.nlm.nih.gov/pmc/articles/PMC3335979/

6. Addiction

1. "Fentanyl selectively binds to the mu-receptor in the central nervous system (CNS) thereby mimicking the effects of endogenous opiates." – US National Library of Medicine, *Fentanyl, Compound Summary* https://pubchem.ncbi.nlm.nih.gov/compound/fentanyl
2. US National Library of Medicine, *Caffeine, Compound Summary* https://pubchem.ncbi.nlm.nih.gov/compound/2519
3. J P Boulenger, J Patel, R M Post, A M Parma, P J Marangos, *Chronic caffeine consumption increases the number of brain adenosine receptors* (1983) https://pubmed.ncbi.nlm.nih.gov/6298543/
4. Paul J. Marangos, Jean-Philippe Boulenger, Jitendra Patel, *Effects of chronic caffeine on brain adenosine receptors: Regional and ontogenetic studies* (1984) https://www.sciencedirect.com/science/article/abs/pii/0024320584902078
5. "Individuals who regularly consume caffeine have increased the number of adenosine receptors in their central nervous system (CNS) and become more sensitive to normal physiologic effects of adenosine." – Karima R. Sajadi-Ernazarova, Jackie Anderson, Aayush Dhakal, Richard J. Hamilton, *Caffeine Withdrawal* (2023) https://www.ncbi.nlm.nih.gov/books/NBK430790/
6. Britannica, *Acetylcholine, chemical compound* (2024) https://www.britannica.com/science/acetylcholine
7. Marina R. Picciotto, Michael J. Higley, Yann S. Mineur, *Acetylcholine as a neuromodulator: cholinergic signaling shapes nervous system function and behavior* (2012) https://www.ncbi.nlm.nih.gov/pmc/articles/PMC3466476/
8. "…compatible with the idea that the brain transforms all rewards onto a single scale of value that facilitates decision making when different actions may procure different types of rewards…" – Kelly Diederen, Paul Fletcher, *Dopamine, Prediction Error and Beyond* (2020) https://journals.sagepub.com/doi/full/10.1177/1073858420907591
9. Armin Lak, William R. Stauffer, Wolfram Schultz, *Dopamine prediction error responses integrate subjective value from different reward dimensions* (2014) https://www.pnas.org/doi/abs/10.1073/pnas.1321596111
10. "According to the now canonical theory, reward predictions are represented as a single scalar quantity, which supports learning about the expectation, or mean, of stochastic outcomes." – Will Dabney, Zeb Kurth-Nelson, Naoshige Uchida, Clara Kwon Starkweather, Demis Hassabis, Rémi Munos, Matthew Botvinick, *A distributional code for value in dopamine-based reinforcement learning* (2020) https://www.nature.com/articles/s41586-019-1924-6
11. Abraham H. Maslow, *A Theory of Human Motivation* (1943) https://psychclassics.yorku.ca/Maslow/motivation.htm

12. "Negative prospection and even depression itself is not inherently dysfunctional, maladaptive, or problematic; indeed, both could be essential for adaptive functioning, because incessant optimism would have serious costs (Nesse, 2004; Norem & Chang, 2002)." – Martin Seligman, Peter Railton, Roy Baumeister, Chandra Sripada, *Homo Prospectus* (2016)
13. Rajita Sinha, *Chronic Stress, Drug Use, and Vulnerability to Addiction* (2008) https://nyaspubs.onlinelibrary.wiley.com/doi/abs/10.1196/annals.1441.030
14. George F. Koob, A Role for Brain Stress Systems in Addiction (2008) https://www.sciencedirect.com/science/article/pii/S0896627308005308
15. Jean Lud Cadet, *Epigenetics of Stress, Addiction, and Resilience: Therapeutic Implications* (2014) https://link.springer.com/article/10.1007/s12035-014-9040-y
16. Nick E. Goeders, *The impact of stress on addiction* (2003) https://www.sciencedirect.com/science/article/pii/S0924977X03001779
17. Rajita Sinha, Ania M. Jastreboff, Stress as a Common Risk Factor for Obesity and Addiction (2013) https://www.sciencedirect.com/science/article/pii/S0006322313001340
18. "Cortisol levels rise during any kind of exercise. If the exercise is moderate and enjoyable, cortisol drops below its normal level soon after we stop exercising. If the exercise is extreme or unpleasant, cortisol levels stay high for a long time." – Russell Farris, Per Marin, *The Potbelly Syndrome: How Common Germs Cause Obesity, Diabetes, and Heart Disease* (2005)
19. Kevin Laland, *Darwin's Unfinished Symphony: How Culture Made the Human Mind* (2017)
20. "The first individuals to solve the mazes are those driven to find novel foraging solutions by hunger, or by the metabolic costs of growth, or pregnancy. [...] Motivation, rather than cleverness or ability, is what explains patterns of innovation here. Fishes are typically reluctant to swim into dark holes and through dark compartments, since predators might be lurking behind them. The hungrier an individual, the more likely it will be to take risks and try out new solutions to find food." – Kevin Laland, *Darwin's Unfinished Symphony: How Culture Made the Human Mind* (2017)
21. "As David Sloan Wilson discovered, a group usually solves problems better than the individuals within it. Pit one socially networked problem-solving web against another—a constant occurrence in nature—and the one which most successfully takes advantage of complex adaptive system rules, that which is the most powerful cooperative learning contraption, will almost always win." – Howard Bloom, *Global Brain: The Evolution of Mass Mind from the Big Bang to the 21st Century* (2001)
22. "The striking technologies that characterize our species, from the kayaks and compound bows used by hunter-gatherers to the antibiotics and airplanes of the modern world, emerge not from singular geniuses but from the flow and recombination of ideas, practices, lucky errors, and chance insights among interconnected minds and across generations." – Joseph Henrich, *The Secret of Our Success: How Culture Is Driving Human Evolution, Domesticating Our Species, and Making Us Smarter* (2015)

23. "[Heyes, Jaldow, and Dawson] did an experiment on observational learning in which one group of rats saw another go through extinction (i.e., our group saw the others perform a response they had also learned, but they also saw that the response [no] longer resulted in reinforcement). As you might expect [...] the observational group exhibited faster extinction." – Claude G. Čech, *Chapter 6: Resistance to Extinction* (1999) https://userweb.ucs.louisiana.edu/~cgc2646/LRN/Chap6.html
24. "...consistent with observational learning and perceptual learning, animals that observe other animals making a discrimination will learn that discrimination more rapidly (the Kohn and Dennis study mentioned in Chapter 5). Also, stimulus differentiation will speed up discrimination learning, as we saw in the Gibson, Walk, and Tighe study." – Claude G. Čech, *Chapter 7: Attention & Categorization* (1998) https://userweb.ucs.louisiana.edu/~cgc2646/LRN/Chap7.html
25. Paul Schmid-Hempel, *Immune defence, parasite evasion strategies and their relevance for 'macroscopic phenomena' such as virulence* (2009) https://www.ncbi.nlm.nih.gov/pmc/articles/PMC2666695/
26. "...one of the most exciting insights of recent years is the gathering evidence for the generality and multitude of mechanisms by which parasites evade the host's immune responses, gain entrance to tissues or by which they manipulate the signalling network of the immune system. Indeed, the mechanisms of immune evasion are mind-boggling in their subtlety and diversity, and have been described for all major parasite groups..." – Paul Schmid-Hempel, *Immune defence, parasite evasion strategies and their relevance for 'macroscopic phenomena' such as virulence* (2009) https://www.ncbi.nlm.nih.gov/pmc/articles/PMC2666695/

7. Bodily recalibration

1. Harvard Health Publishing, *Potassium lowers blood pressure* (2017) https://www.health.harvard.edu/heart-health/potassium-lowers-blood-pressure
2. "Bodies counter nutrient deficits or excesses. To maintain homeostasis, cells can increase (up-regulate) or decrease (down-regulate) the number of receptors on the membrane, thus altering sensitivity to a compound." – Fred Provenza, *Nourishment: What Animals Can Teach Us about Rediscovering Our Nutritional Wisdom* (2018)
3. "Conditioning (also referred to as learning) is a change in behavior due to experience (exposure to stimuli that cause small-scale physical changes to the body that behaves), and a stimulus is anything that can potentially control behavior (Chance, 2009; Fraley, 2008, p. 64)." – James O'Heare, *Changing Problem Behavior* (2010)

   "Conditioning creates changes to the structure of the body of the learner via stimulation from the environment, which change the evocative capacity of the SD on subsequent presentations." – James O'Heare, *Changing Problem Behavior* (2010)

4. "A decrease in olfactory sensitivity can be seen as part of the food intake control mechanism, where appetite regulation hormones may be able to shift olfactory sensitivity to achieve nutritional homeostasis." – Cees de Graaf, Sanne Boesveldt, *Flavor, Satiety and Food Intake* (2017)
5. "The group with higher taste bud densities gave significantly higher average intensity ratings for sucrose (196%), NaCl (135%) and PROP (142%), but not for citric acid (118%) and quinine HCl (110%) than the lower density group. Thus, the subjects with higher fungifrom taste bud densities also reported some tastes as more intense than subjects with fewer fungiform taste buds." – J. Miller, Frank E. Reedy, *Variations in human taste bud density and taste intensity perception* (1990)

   https://www.sciencedirect.com/science/article/abs/pii/003193849090374D
6. Pu Feng, Liquan Huang, Hong Wang, *Taste Bud Homeostasis in Health, Disease, and Aging* (2014) https://www.ncbi.nlm.nih.gov/pmc/articles/PMC3864165/
7. "So critical are taste sensations to the recognition and enjoyment of foods, and the appropriate digestion and utilization of nutrients, that humans who acutely lose their sense of taste, such as following radiotherapy, for example, often will not eat." – Paul A.S. Breslin, Alan C. Spector, *Mammalian taste perception* (2008) https://www.cell.com/current-biology/fulltext/S0960-9822(07)02370-6
8. Pu Feng, Liquan Huang, Hong Wang, *Taste Bud Homeostasis in Health, Disease, and Aging* (2014) https://www.ncbi.nlm.nih.gov/pmc/articles/PMC3864165/
9. "Many people with anosmia are known to skip meals because the appeal for food is not there. Nothing seems to taste good anymore and the flavor is gone. Another reason appetite is affected, is that the aroma of foods does not cause a desire for food because the person cannot detect the luring odors from the food. Not eating results in malnutrition and involuntary weight loss. This can also lead to illness because the proper foods are not being eaten to keep a person healthy." – Lora Muxworthy, *The Dangers and Safety Precautions Related to the Olfactory Dysfunction Anosmia* (1999) https://web.archive.org/web/20031205082740/http://hubel.sfasu.edu/courseinfo/SL99/anosmia.html
10. Annette Heist, *With No Sense Of Smell, The World Can Be A Grayer, Scarier Place* (2016)

    https://www.npr.org/sections/health-shots/2016/10/10/496455192/with-no-sense-of-smell-the-world-can-be-a-grayer-scarier-place
11. "Obese individuals have been reported to display a weakened sense of taste and thus may be driven to consume more calories to attain such reward." – Andrew Kaufman, Ezen Choo, Anna Koh, Robin Dando, *Inflammation arising from obesity reduces taste bud abundance and inhibits renewal* (2018) https://journals.plos.org/plosbiology/article?id=10.1371/journal.pbio.2001959
12. Z. M. Patel, J. M. DelGaudio, S. K. Wise, *Higher Body Mass Index Is Associated with Subjective Olfactory Dysfunction* (2015) https://www.ncbi.nlm.nih.gov/pmc/articles/PMC4496469/

13. "Obese women required higher MSG concentrations to detect a taste and preferred significantly higher MSG concentrations in a soup-like vehicle." – M. Yanina Pepino, Susana Finkbeiner, Gary K. Beauchamp, Julie A. Mennella, *Obese Women Have Lower Monosodium Glutamate Taste Sensitivity and Prefer Higher Concentrations Than Do Normal-weight Women* (2012) https://onlinelibrary.wiley.com/doi/full/10.1038/oby.2009.493
14. Johanna Overberg, Thomas Hummel, Heiko Krude, Susanna Wiegand, *Differences in taste sensitivity between obese and non-obese children and adolescents* (2012) https://adc.bmj.com/content/97/12/1048.short
15. "However, certain eating behaviors may be altered in some cases of chemosensory dysfunction, such as increased seasoning and sugar use in anosmic individuals. Changes in related culinary practices, such increased salt, sugar, and fat use, could complicate issues with hypertension, diabetes and cardiovascular disease, respectively." – Jonathan C. Kershaw, Richard D. Mattes, *Nutrition and taste and smell dysfunction* (2018) https://www.sciencedirect.com/science/article/pii/S2095881118300209
16. "...it is well known that diabetes and obesity affect taste preferences in adults. For example, in diabetic patients, taste responses, especially to sweet, are blunted (Wasalathanthri et al., 2014), and obese individuals also have decreased taste sensitivity (Stewart et al., 2010; Stewart et al., 2011)." – Linda A. Barlow, Ophir D. Klein, *Developing and regenerating a sense of taste* (2015) https://www.ncbi.nlm.nih.gov/pmc/articles/PMC4435577/
17. "Type 2 diabetic patients had a blunted taste response for sweet followed by sour and salt tastes. This taste abnormality may influence the choice of nutrients, with a preference for sweet-tasting foods, thereby exacerbating hyperglycemia." – S.M. Gondivkar, A. Indurkar, S. Degwekar, R. Bhowate, *Evaluation of gustatory function in patients with diabetes mellitus type 2* (2009) https://www.ncbi.nlm.nih.gov/pubmed/19913725/
18. M. Balslev Jørgensen, Nils H. Buch, *Studies on the Sense of Smell and Taste in Diabetics* (1960) https://www.tandfonline.com/doi/abs/10.3109/00016486109126521
19. Brynn E Richardson, Eric A Vander Woude, Ranjan Sudan, Jon S Thompson, Donald A Leopold, *Altered Olfactory Acuity in the Morbidly Obese* (2004) https://link.springer.com/article/10.1381/0960892041719617
20. "Smell dysfunction is associated with age and degenerative complications of diabetes, suggesting a degenerative mechanism related to diabetes." – J.P. Le Floch, G. Le Lièvre, M. Labroue, M. Paul, R. Peynegre, L. Perlemuter, *Smell dysfunction and related factors in diabetic patients* (1993) https://www.ncbi.nlm.nih.gov/pubmed/8325211
21. "Mortality for anosmic older adults was four times that of normosmic individuals while hyposmic individuals had intermediate mortality (p<0.001), a "dose-dependent" effect present across the age range." – Jayant M Pinto, Kristen E Wroblewski, David W Kern, L Philip Schumm, Martha K McClintock, *Olfactory dysfunction predicts 5-year mortality in older adults* (2014) https://pubmed.ncbi.nlm.nih.gov/25271633/

22. "Olfactory dysfunction has been associated with diabetes mellitus. Furthermore, it has been proposed to be a diabetic complication, given that it has been linked with microvascular complications, such as diabetic peripheral neuropathy. Interestingly, it has been suggested that olfactory dysfunction is a manifestation of central neuropathy in diabetes, a hypothesis based on the observation that diabetes, olfactory dysfunction, and cognitive decline often coexist. However, evidence is limited and inconsistent." – Evanthia Gouveri, Nikolaos Papanas, *Olfactory Dysfunction: A Complication of Diabetes or a Factor That Complicates Glucose Metabolism? A Narrative Review* (2021) https://www.ncbi.nlm.nih.gov/pmc/articles/PMC8658580/
23. "Kaufman has found that heavier mice have fewer taste buds present in their tongues. In addition, he has observed slower taste bud cell regeneration in these heavier mice, which may be a reason for why they have fewer cells. [...] Promisingly, if the heavier mice are switched back to a lean diet, there appears to be a reversal of this effect." – Ava Fan, *Obesity, Could it be Taste Buds?* (2016) https://web.archive.org/web/20221126200419/https://research.cornell.edu/news-features/obesity-could-it-be-taste-buds
24. L. Graham, G. Murty, D. J. Bowrey, *Taste, Smell and Appetite Change After Roux-en-Y Gastric Bypass Surgery* (2014) https://link.springer.com/article/10.1007/s11695-014-1221-2
25. National Institutes of Health, *Overweight & Obesity Statistics* (2021) https://www.niddk.nih.gov/health-information/health-statistics/overweight-obesity
26. Maja Divjak, *Insulin Receptor and Type 2 Diabetes*, Part 2 (2015) https://www.youtube.com/watch?v=VbwRYFMPZS4
27. "Upon binding to its receptor, insulin triggers a chain of molecular interactions inside the cell. The signal propagates through the cytoplasm and eventually renders glucose uptake (the response)." – Guanyu Wang, *Raison d'être of insulin resistance: the adjustable threshold hypothesis* (2014) https://www.ncbi.nlm.nih.gov/pmc/articles/PMC4223910/
28. "The predominate pathologies of hyperinsulinemia, type 2 diabetes are athero-arteriosclerosis, cardiovascular disease, cerebral vascular disease, hypertension, nephropathy, retinopathy, peripheral and central neuropathy, and penile erectile dysfunction." – Joseph R. Kraft, *Diabetes Epidemic & You* (2008)
29. "During pregnancy, for example, the thresholds increase consistently to strengthen the mother's insulin resistance to meet the increasing glucose demand of the expanding fetal brain." – Guanyu Wang, *Raison d'être of insulin resistance: the adjustable threshold hypothesis* (2014) https://www.ncbi.nlm.nih.gov/pmc/articles/PMC4223910/
30. "Contrary to the common belief that insulin promotes glucose disposal, the results imply that insulin is the body's 'ration stamp' to restricting glucose utilization by peripheral tissues and that insulin resistance is primarily a well-evolved mechanism." – Guanyu Wang, *Raison d'être of insulin resistance: the adjustable threshold hypothesis* (2014) https://www.ncbi.nlm.nih.gov/pmc/articles/PMC4223910/

31. "According to the hypothesis, a typical cell exhibits an all-or-none response to insulin (figure 2b). The switching between *all* and *none* occurs at two threshold insulin concentrations I_{on} and I_{off}, which render hysteresis: the delayed switch-on to spare glucose for the brain and the delayed switch-off to avoid hyperglycaemia." – Guanyu Wang, *Raison d'être of insulin resistance: the adjustable threshold hypothesis* (2014) https://www.ncbi.nlm.nih.gov/pmc/articles/PMC4223910/
32. "By varying the levels of insulin and the degree of insulin sensitivity of tissues the energy budget allocation to different organs can be finely manipulated." – Milind Watve and Chittaranjan Yajnik, *Evolutionary origins of insulin resistance: a behavioral switch hypothesis* (2007)
    https://www.ncbi.nlm.nih.gov/pmc/articles/PMC1868084/
33. "Longer-term studies of the Atkins diet failed to confirm the much hoped-for benefits. Dr. Gary Foster from Temple University published two-year results showing that both the low-fat and the Atkins groups had lost but then regained weight at virtually the same rate." – Jason Fung, *The Obesity Code* (2016)
34. Stephan Guyenet, *Interview with Chris Voigt of 20 Potatoes a Day* (2010) https://wholehealthsource.blogspot.com/2010/12/interview-with-chris-voigt-of-20.html
35. "This was (for me) the instant cure to a life-long battle with binge eating disorder. [...] I was eating to "satisfied" and finding satisfied well before "painfully gorged" which was something I had never experienced in my life. A switch had been flipped.
    That scoreboard is getting recalibrated!" – M. Stone, Amazon Review of *The Potato Hack* by Tim Steel (2016) *https://www.amazon.com/gp/customer-reviews/RNUGWX6S217K3/*
36. "In comparison with sucrose alone, ingestion of sucrose with whole berries resulted in reduced glucose and insulin concentrations during the first 30 min and a slower decline during the second hour and a significantly improved glycemic profile. Berries prevented the sucrose-induced late postprandial hypoglycemic response and the compensatory free fatty acid rebound. Nearly similar effects were observed when sucrose was consumed with berry nectars. The improved responses were evident despite the higher content of available carbohydrate in the berry and nectar meals, because of the natural sugars present in berries." – Riitta Törrönen, Marjukka Kolehmainen, Essi Sarkkinen, Hannu Mykkänen, Leo Niskanen, *Postprandial glucose, insulin, and free fatty acid responses to sucrose consumed with blackcurrants and lingonberries in healthy women* (2012) https://www.ncbi.nlm.nih.gov/pubmed/22854401
37. "Weight loss was higher in the moderate natural fructose group (4.19 ± 0.30 kg) than the low-fructose group (2.83 ± 0.29 kg) (P = .0016)." – Magdalena Madero, Julio C Arriaga, Diana Jalal, Christopher Rivard, Kim McFann, Oscar Pérez-Méndez, Armando Vázquez, Arturo Ruiz, Miguel A Lanaspa, Carlos Roncal Jimenez, Richard J Johnson, Laura-Gabriela Sánchez Lozada, *The effect of two energy-restricted diets, a low-fructose diet versus a moderate*

natural fructose diet, on weight loss and metabolic syndrome parameters: a randomized controlled trial (2011) https://www.ncbi.nlm.nih.gov/pubmed/21621801

38. "The incretin effect describes the phenomenon whereby oral glucose elicits higher insulin secretory responses than does intravenous glucose, despite inducing similar levels of glycaemia, in healthy individuals. This effect, which is uniformly defective in patients with type 2 diabetes, is mediated by the gut-derived incretin hormones glucose-dependent insulinotropic polypeptide (GIP) and glucagon-like peptide-1 (GLP-1)." – Michael A Nauck, Juris J Meier, *The incretin effect in healthy individuals and those with type 2 diabetes: physiology, pathophysiology, and response to therapeutic interventions* (2016) https://www.ncbi.nlm.nih.gov/pubmed/26876794
39. "Although a PIR [pre-absorptive insulin release] comprises a tiny portion of the overall insulin secreted, it is responsible for decreasing blood sugar during a meal by 50%. When the PIR is experimentally blocked in humans during feeding, dysregulation of blood sugar (dysglycemia) ensues and high levels of plasma insulin are attained. A blunted PIR is associated with obesity, exacerbating if not causing metabolic problems." – Paul A.S. Breslin, *An Evolutionary Perspective on Food and Human Taste* (2013) https://www.sciencedirect.com/science/article/pii/S0960982213004181
40. "The proof of this is easily demonstrable. When an animal is prevented from secreting insulin cephalically (typically accomplished by the cutting of the neural link between the brain and the pancreas, the vagus nerve) and then the animal is given the same caloric load as that given to a control animal, the animal is glucose intolerant (Berthoud, Bereiter, Trimble, Siegel, & Jeanrenaud, 1981; Louis-Sylvestre, 1978b). This means that the amount of glucose detectable in the blood after a test meal attains significantly higher levels when there is no cephalic insulin. Another way of saying this is that without cephalic insulin, animals secrete insufficient insulin during a meal to eliminate the ingested glucose from the blood in the normal time, and they therefore appear diabetic after meals (see Berthoud et al., 1981; Nicolaidis, 1977)." – Stephen C. Woods, *The Eating Paradox: How We Tolerate Food* (1991) https://www.appstate.edu/~steelekm/classes/psy5150/Documents/Woods1991.pdf
41. "Comparable results in terms of abnormally elevated blood glucose levels occur if food is simply put into the stomach so that the mouth-to-brain-to-pancreas reflex is circumvented (Proietto, Rohner-Jeanrenaud, Ionescu, & Jeanrenaud, 1987; Steffens, 1976)." – Stephen C. Woods, *The Eating Paradox: How We Tolerate Food* (1991) https://www.appstate.edu/~steelekm/classes/psy5150/Documents/Woods1991.pdf
42. "A key factor in anticipating incoming nutrients, particularly sugars, is the taste receptor responses. It is well established that humans show a PIR [pre-absorptive insulin release] to oral glucose, activated presumably via a carbohydrate taste receptor, such as T1R2/T1R3 25, 54, 55." – Paul A.S. Breslin, *An Evolutionary Perspective on Food and Human Taste* (2013) https://www.sciencedirect.com/science/article/pii/S0960982213004181

"The taste buds also serve as endocrine organs and secrete regulatory hormones in response to nutrient stimulation, including glucagon like peptide-1 (GLP-1) and glucagon, among other endocrine peptides [52]. The secretory responses of digestive hormones by peripheral tissues would signal to digestive organs, such as the pancreas, that nutrients are being ingested and prepare metabolic systems to respond, such as insulin secretion to control elevated blood glucose. These anticipatory processes are essential to optimal metabolism during and after feeding." – Paul A.S. Breslin, *An Evolutionary Perspective on Food and Human Taste* (2013) https://www.sciencedirect.com/science/article/pii/S0960982213004181

43. Tino Just, Hans Wilhelm Pau, Ulrike Engel, Thomas Hummel, *Cephalic phase insulin release in healthy humans after taste stimulation?* (2008) https://www.ncbi.nlm.nih.gov/m/pubmed/18556090/
44. "It is well established that animals, including people, begin secreting insulin as soon as they start eating, before any increase of ingested fuels into the blood. Such insulin is called *cephalic insulin* because its secretion is triggered more by food-related stimuli such as tastes or smells..." – Stephen C. Woods, *The Eating Paradox: How We Tolerate Food* (1991) https://www.appstate.edu/~steelekm/classes/psy5150/Documents/Woods1991.pdf

    "After first demonstrating that animals can be trained to secrete insulin (Woods, Alexander, & Porte, 1972; Woods, Hutton, & Makous, 1970), my colleagues and I found that arbitrary stimuli associated with food presentation can develop the ability to elicit insulin secretion (Woods, 1976; Woods et al., 1977). These stimuli included specific sounds, odors, and even the time of day (Woods et al., 1977). Anything that informed the animals that food was imminent seemed capable of acquiring this ability. – Stephen C. Woods, *The Eating Paradox: How We Tolerate Food* (1991) https://www.appstate.edu/~steelekm/classes/psy5150/Documents/Woods1991.pdf
45. "...a two- to three-fold higher insulin secretory response to oral as compared to intravenous glucose administration. In subjects with type 2 diabetes, this incretin effect is diminished or no longer present." – Michael A. Nauck, Juris J. Meier, *Incretin hormones: Their role in health and disease* (2018) https://onlinelibrary.wiley.com/doi/full/10.1111/dom.13129
46. "...the ones who used AS had a higher insulin resistance. The study also showed that the duration of use of artificial sweeteners had a direct impact on insulin resistance." – Kushagra Mathur, Rajat Kumar Agrawal, Shailesh Nagpure, Deepali Deshpande, *Effect of artificial sweeteners on insulin resistance among type-2 diabetes mellitus patients* (2020) https://www.ncbi.nlm.nih.gov/pmc/articles/PMC7014832/
47. "Recent results from both human epidemiological and experimental studies with animals suggest that intake of noncaloric sweeteners may promote, rather than protect against, weight gain and other disturbances of energy regulation. [...] Using a rat model, the present research showed that intake of noncaloric sweeteners reduces the effectiveness of learned associations between sweet tastes and postingestive caloric outcomes..." – Terry L. Davidson, Ashley A. Martin, Kiely Clark, Susan E. Swithers, *Intake of high-*

intensity sweeteners alters the ability of sweet taste to signal caloric consequences (2010) https://www.tandfonline.com/doi/abs/10.1080/17470218.2011.552729

48. "When we reviewed eating patterns from the myCircadianClock app, we found that the traditional breakfast-lunch-dinner pattern is no longer observed, even among healthy non–shift-working adults. In fact, the number of eating occasions ranged from 4.2 times a day to 10.5 times a day." – Satchin Panda, *The Circadian Code* (2018)
49. Satchin Panda, *The Circadian Code* (2018)
50. "Just like our plumbing gets weaker and leaks after a while, we have hundreds of miles of blood vessels that need to be checked for leakage and repaired. Similarly, our gut lining and skin needs daily repair to keep bacteria, chemicals, and toxins from entering our body. Inside every organ, many cells die and need to be replaced. Our blood cells also need replacement. This repair, through the production of new replacement cells, does not happen randomly; rather it occurs at a specific time of the day: at night, when we're asleep." – Satchin Panda, *The Circadian Code* (2018)
51. Carlos López-Otín, Lorenzo Galluzzi, José M.P. Freije, Frank Madeo, Guido Kroemer, *Metabolic Control of Longevity* (2016) https://www.sciencedirect.com/science/article/pii/S0092867416309813
52. Shubhroz Gill, Satchidananda Panda, *A smartphone app reveals erratic diurnal eating patterns in humans that can be modulated for health benefits* (2016) https://www.ncbi.nlm.nih.gov/pmc/articles/PMC4635036/
53. "We also learned from this experiment that a daily eating– fasting cycle drives almost every rhythm in the liver. Instead of thinking that all timing information comes from the outside world through the eye's blue light sensor, we learned that just like the first light of the morning resets our brain clock, the first bite of the morning resets all other organ clocks." – Satchin Panda, *The Circadian Code* (2018)
54. "The absorption of glucose, amino acids, and fat is strongly circadian. Nutrient absorption requires a lot of energy, which is why it can't happen all the time. Gut cells that absorb these nutrients and other chemicals in food have different channels or doors that allow only certain types of molecules to go through, and the opening and closing of these doors is circadian." – Satchin Panda, *The Circadian Code* (2018)
55. John Nash Ott, *The Effects of Natural and Artificial Light on Living Organisms* (1975) https://www.youtube.com/watch?v=BOUA8UAEAdY
56. Kylie A. Robert, John A. Lesku, Jesko Partecke, Brian Chambers, *Artificial light at night desynchronizes strictly seasonal reproduction in a wild mammal* (2015) https://www.ncbi.nlm.nih.gov/pmc/articles/PMC4614780/
57. Jeff T. Bowles, *The Miraculous Results of Extremely High Doses of the Sunshine Hormone Vitamin D3* (2013)
58. "[Yvonne] Foss believes that vitamin D is the cause of common obesity through a survival strategy developed by the organism during the evolutionary pathway to protect the organism from a cold climate. She theorises that vitamin D originated as a photoreceptor system in primitive organisms, which were responsible to inform and defend the body against

lower climates. The body would respond to lower UV radiation with reduced skin production of vitamin D that would signal the increase of fat tissue accumulation, enhancing organism protection from the cold weather by reducing heat conduction and increasing its thermogenic capacity." - Fernanda Reis de Azevedo, Bruno Caramelli, *Hypovitaminosis D and Obesity – Coincidence or Consequence?* (2013) https://www.ncbi.nlm.nih.gov/pmc/articles/PMC6003590/

59. Rosa M Ortega, Aránzazu Aparicio, Elena Rodríguez-Rodríguez, Laura M Bermejo, José M Perea, Ana M López-Sobaler, Baltasar Ruiz-Roso, Pedro Andrés, *Preliminary data about the influence of vitamin D status on the loss of body fat in young overweight/obese women following two types of hypocaloric diet* (2008) https://www.ncbi.nlm.nih.gov/pubmed/18279549/
60. "Compared to reading a printed book, reading on an iPad suppressed melatonin release by over 50 percent at night. Indeed, iPad reading delayed the rise of melatonin by up to three hours, relative to the natural rise in these same individuals when reading a printed book." – Matthew Walker, *Why We Sleep* (2017)
61. "Worse, should you attempt to diet but don't get enough sleep while doing so, it is futile, since most of the weight you lose will come from lean body mass, not fat." – Matthew Walker, *Why We Sleep* (2017)
62. "...short sleep was associated with lower fat loss during caloric restriction in overweight subjects." – Omar Mesarwi, Jan Polak, Jonathan Jun, Vsevolod Y. Polotsky, *Sleep disorders and the development of insulin resistance and obesity* (2014) https://www.ncbi.nlm.nih.gov/pmc/articles/PMC3767932/
63. "From the output, computers calculated the size of the microbiota community—the sum total of viruses, bacteria, fungi, protozoa, and other organisms that dwell within each of us. The final tally came to more than one hundred trillion organisms, dwarfing the population of human cells by a factor of 10. The amount of genetic material of microbial origin surpassed our own by 150 times." – Kathleen McAuliffe, *This is Your Brain on Parasites: How Tiny Creatures Manipulate Our Behavior and Shape Society* (2017)
64. "In the gut, resident microbes take a share of every meal you eat, but in return they aid in digestion, synthesizing vitamins and disarming dangerous bacteria that you ingest. They also churn out virtually every major neurotransmitter that tunes our emotions—notably, GABA, dopamine, serotonin, acetylcholine, and noradrenaline—as well as hormones with psychoactive properties." – Kathleen McAuliffe, *This is Your Brain on Parasites: How Tiny Creatures Manipulate Our Behavior and Shape Society* (2017)
65. "Regress evolutionary time still further and we have discovered that the very simplest forms of unicellular organisms that survive for periods exceeding twenty-four hours, such as bacteria, have active and passive phases that correspond to the light-dark cycle of our planet. It is a pattern that we now believe to be the precursor of our own circadian rhythm, and with it, wake and sleep." – Matthew Walker, *Why We Sleep* (2017)
66. "Plentiful sleep maintains a flourishing microbiome within your gut from which we know so much of our nutritional health begins." – Matthew

Walker, *Why We Sleep* (2017)

67. Mahesh S. Desai, Anna M. Seekatz, Nicole M. Koropatkin, Thaddeus S. Stappenbeck, Gabriel Núñez, Eric C. Martens, *A Dietary Fiber-Deprived Gut Microbiota Degrades the Colonic Mucus Barrier and Enhances Pathogen Susceptibility* (2016) https://www.cell.com/cell/fulltext/S0092-8674(16)31464-7
68. "The same species of bacteria may be a helper (a symbiont), a harmless freeloader (a commensal), or a hurter (a parasite), depending on circumstances that are constantly in flux." – Kathleen McAuliffe, *This is Your Brain on Parasites: How Tiny Creatures Manipulate Our Behavior and Shape Society* (2017)
69. "Additives found in many health foods have also been implicated in killing beneficial gut microbes and they can irritate and damage the intestinal wall directly." – John Douillard, *Eat Wheat: A Scientific and Clinically-Proven Approach to Safely Bringing Wheat and Dairy Back Into Your Diet* (2017)
70. Satchin Panda, *The Circadian Code* (2018)
71. "Emulsifiers are used to improve a food's texture and to prevent mixtures from separating, particularly in ice cream. Last year, Benoit Chassaing of Georgia State University showed that mice that drank water containing one of two emulsifiers underwent changes in gut bacteria and inflammation of the gut – changes that led to obesity and diabetes in these animals." – Michael Le Page, *Surge in obesity and diabetes could be linked to food additives* (2016)
    https://www.newscientist.com/article/2076906-surge-in-obesity-and-diabetes-could-be-linked-to-food-additives/
72. "In ecology, *biome* refers to the sets of plants and animals in a community such as a jungle, forest, or coral reef. An enormous diversity of species, large and small, interact to form complex webs of mutual support. When a keystone species (think wolves in Scotland) disappears or goes extinct the ecology suffers. It can even collapse." – Martin J. Blaser, *Missing Microbes: How the Overuse of Antibiotics Is Fueling Our Modern Plagues* (2014)
73. Fred Provenza, *Nourishment: What Animals Can Teach Us about Rediscovering Our Nutritional Wisdom* (2018)
74. "Intestinal bacteria regulate hormones your own body makes to stoke or suppress your appetite—for example, ghrelin, the molecule that goads you to get a second serving at the buffet, and leptin, which tells you to push your plate away. It's also suspected that gut bacteria may themselves synthesize chemicals that signal brain regions governing satiety." – Kathleen McAuliffe, *This is Your Brain on Parasites: How Tiny Creatures Manipulate Our Behavior and Shape Society* (2017)
75. "Diet strongly affects human health, partly by modulating gut microbiome composition. We used diet inventories and 16S rDNA sequencing to characterize fecal samples from 98 individuals. Fecal communities clustered into enterotypes distinguished primarily by levels of Bacteroides and Prevotella. Enterotypes were strongly associated with long-term diets, particularly protein and animal fat (Bacteroides) versus carbohydrates (Prevotella). A controlled-feeding study of 10 subjects showed that

microbiome composition changed detectably within 24 hours of initiating a high-fat/low-fiber or low-fat/high-fiber diet, but that enterotype identity remained stable during the 10-day study. Thus, alternative enterotype states are associated with long-term diet." – Gary D Wu, Jun Chen, Christian Hoffmann, Kyle Bittinger, Ying-Yu Chen, Sue A Keilbaugh, Meenakshi Bewtra, Dan Knights, William A Walters, Rob Knight, Rohini Sinha, Erin Gilroy, Kernika Gupta, Robert Baldassano, Lisa Nessel, Hongzhe Li, Frederic D Bushman, James D Lewis, *Linking long-term dietary patterns with gut microbial enterotypes* (2011) https://www.ncbi.nlm.nih.gov/pubmed/21885731

76. "When the ill mice stopped consuming emulsifiers, their gut bacteria gradually returned to normal." – Michael Le Page, *Surge in obesity and diabetes could be linked to food additives* (2016) https://www.newscientist.com/article/2076906-surge-in-obesity-and-diabetes-could-be-linked-to-food-additives/
77. "Gary Wu, a professor of gastroenterology at the University of Pennsylvania, has shown that diet over the long term—a year or more—correlated very strongly with the overall microbiome." – Rob Knight, Brendan Buhler, *Follow Your Gut* (2015)
78. Diabetes Research Institute Foundation, *Diabetes Statistics* (2022) https://diabetesresearch.org/diabetes-statistics/
79. Centers for Disease Control and Prevention, *National Diabetes Statistics Report: Estimates of Diabetes and Its Burden in the United States* (2023) https://www.cdc.gov/diabetes/data/statistics-report/index.html
80. Centers for Disease Control and Prevention, *Leading Causes of Death*, US (2024) https://www.cdc.gov/nchs/fastats/leading-causes-of-death.htm
81. Timothy A Welborn, Satvinder S Dhaliwal, Stanley A Bennett, *Waist–hip ratio is the dominant risk factor predicting cardiovascular death in Australia* (2003) https://onlinelibrary.wiley.com/doi/abs/10.5694/j.1326-5377.2003.tb05704.x
82. Centers for Disease Control and Prevention, *National Diabetes Statistics Report: Estimates of Diabetes and Its Burden in the United States* (2020) https://www.cdc.gov/diabetes/pdfs/data/statistics/national-diabetes-statistics-report.pdf
83. National Institute of Diabetes and Digestive and Kidney Diseases, *Overweight & Obesity Statistics*, UK (2021) https://www.niddk.nih.gov/health-information/health-statistics/overweight-obesity

8. Genuine Food

1. "Food Processing Externalizes Digestion Compared to other primates, humans have an unusual digestive system. Starting at the top, our mouths, gapes, lips, and teeth are oddly small, and our lip muscles are weak. Our mouths are the size of a squirrel monkey's, a species that weighs less than three pounds." – Joseph Henrich, *The Secret of Our Success* (2015)

   "We also have puny jaw muscles that reach up only to just below our ears. Other primates' jaw muscles stretch to the tops of their heads, where they sometimes even latch onto a bony central ridge. Our stomachs are small, having only a third of the surface area that we'd expect for a primate of our size, and our colons are too short, being only 60% of their expected mass. Our bodies are also poor at detoxifying wild foods. Overall, our guts—stomachs, small intestines, and colons—are much smaller than they ought to be for our overall body size." – Joseph Henrich, *The Secret of Our Success* (2015)

2. U.S. Environmental Protection Agency, *Sugarcane Processing* https://www3.epa.gov/ttn/chief/ap42/ch09/final/c9s10-1a.pdf
3. Robert Lustig, *Sugar: The Bitter Truth* (2009) https://www.youtube.com/watch?v=dBnniua6-oM
4. Thomas Jensen, Manal F. Abdelmalek, Shelby Sullivan, Kristen J. Nadeau, Melanie Green, Carlos Roncal, Takahiko Nakagawa, Masanari Kuwabara, Yuka Sato, Duk-Hee Kang, Dean R. Tolan, Laura G Sanchez-Lozada, Hugo R. Rosen, Miguel A. Lanaspa, Anna Mae Diehl, and Richard J Johnson, *Fructose and Sugar: A Major Mediator of Nonalcoholic Fatty Liver Disease* (2018) https://www.ncbi.nlm.nih.gov/pmc/articles/PMC5893377/
5. "Flavors and phytochemicals decline after harvest, more rapidly in some fruits and vegetables than others. For example, by the time broccoli is purchased at the store, typically ten days to two weeks since harvest, it loses more than 75 to 80 percent of health-promoting phytochemicals, 50 percent of its vitamin C, and most of its sugars and antioxidants. Loss of sugars, due to respiration after picking, reduces palatability." – Fred Provenza, *Nourishment: What Animals Can Teach Us about Rediscovering Our Nutritional Wisdom* (2018)
6. Julia Phillips, *Why Fruit Has a Fake Wax Coating* (2017) https://www.theatlantic.com/technology/archive/2017/04/why-fruit-has-a-fake-wax-coating/524619/
7. "It is a common practice to color the skins of oranges in certain orange growing areas of the country because of climatic or cultural conditions which cause the oranges to mature while still green in color." – US FDA, Compliance Policy Guide, *Sec 550.625 Oranges – Artificial Coloring* (1980) https://www.fda.gov/regulatory-information/search-fda-guidance-documents/cpg-sec-550625-oranges-artificial-coloring
8. "Citrus juices are excellent sources of vitamin C and contribute other key nutrients such as potassium, folate, magnesium, and vitamin A. OJ [orange juice] intake has been associated with better diet quality in children and adults. OJ intake has not been associated with adverse effects on weight or other body measures in observational studies in children and adults." – Gail C. Rampersaud, M. Filomena Valim, *100% citrus juice: Nutritional contribution, dietary benefits, and association with anthropometric measures* (2016) https://www.tandfonline.com/doi/abs/10.1080/10408398.2013.862611
9. Ahmad Adnan, Muhammad Mushtaq, Tanveer ul Islam, Fruit Juices: Extraction, Composition, Quality and Analysis, *Chapter 12 – Fruit Juice Concentrates* (2018) https://www.sciencedirect.com/science/article/pii/B9780128022306000126

10. "Do you remember what canned orange juice tasted like? It was sweet and it had a pleasant acidity, and the color was about right, but it wasn't "orangey"." – Society of Flavor Chemists Inc. and the Chemical Sources Association Inc., *A Short History of the Flavor Industry* (2020) https://flavorchemists.com/wp-content/uploads/2020/07/earlmerwin_flavor_history-1.pdf
11. "Daily consumption of dried fruits is recommended in order to gain full benefit of essential nutrients, health-promoting phytochemicals, and antioxidants that they contain, together with their desirable taste and aroma." – Sui Kiat Chang, Cesarettin Alasalvar, Fereidoon Shahidi, *Review of dried fruits: Phytochemicals, antioxidant efficacies, and health benefits* (2016) https://www.researchgate.net/publication/291015880_Review_of_dried_fruits_Phytochemicals_antioxidant_efficacies_and_health_benefits
12. Gary Williamson, Arianna Carughi, *Polyphenol content and health benefits of raisins* (2010) https://www.sciencedirect.com/science/article/pii/S0271531710001375
13. Lara Pizzorno, *Nothing Boring About Boron* (2015) https://www.ncbi.nlm.nih.gov/pmc/articles/PMC4712861/
14. "The Mbuti pygmies of the Congo obtain as much as 80 YO of their dietary energy from honey during the honey season (Crane, 1983), but this lasts for only 2 months of the year (Turnbull, 1963)." – K A Allsop, J B Miller, *Honey revisited: a reappraisal of honey in pre-industrial diets* (1996) https://pubmed.ncbi.nlm.nih.gov/8672404/
15. "...every drop of honey is packed with up to two hundred beneficial bionutrients such as vitamins, minerals, amino acids, bioflavonoid (plant molecules that are anti-diabetic), disease-fighting antioxidants, organic acids, monosaccharides and obligosaccharides (sugars) and numerous enzymes." – Mike McInnes, *The Honey Diet* (2014)
16. "In North America, maple sap, which is boiled down to syrup, has long been enjoyed as a spring tonic, believed to increase health and vitality." – Joey Lott, *In Defense of Sugar: The Sweet Truth about the Diet Industry's Latest Evil* (2015)
17. "...a number of studies performed by a University of Rhode Island team have shown that maple syrup contains many novel compounds that are antibacterial and that help to modulate the immune system." – Joey Lott, *In Defense of Sugar: The Sweet Truth about the Diet Industry's Latest Evil* (2015)
18. "In addition, total phenol content and phenolic acid composition were also determined. Results indicated a total phenolic content of 26.5, 31.5, 372 and 3837 μg GAE/g for refined, white, brown and jaggery, respectively. The HPLC analysis revealed the presence of different phenolic acids in brown sugar and jaggery." – M.A. Harish Nayaka, U.V. Sathisha, M.P. Manohar, K.B. Chandrashekar, Shylaja M. Dharmesh, *Cytoprotective and antioxidant activity studies of jaggery sugar* (2009) https://www.sciencedirect.com/science/article/pii/S0308814608014167

19. "Ancient medical scriptures, Sushruta Sanhita (Chapter 45, sloka 146), dating back to 2500 years states how Jaggery is useful in purification of blood, prevents rheumatic afflictions and disorders of bile and possess nutritive properties of high order. It supplements the requirement of iron and calcium in women and children, prevents anemia and increases vitality in men and help in digestion. Magnesium in jaggery strengthens the nervous system and potassium conserve the acid balance in the cells and combats acids and acetones. The preventive action of jaggery on smoke-induced lung lesions (Sahu and Saxena 1994) and the presence of micronutrients in jaggery have antitoxic and an anticarcinogenic property..." – M. Esther Magdalene Sharon, Cv Kavitha Abirami, K Alagusundaram, *Energy Losses in Traditional Jaggery Processing* (2013) https://www.researchgate.net/profile/M_Esther_Sharon/publication/256719273_Energy_Losses_in_Traditional_Jaggery_Processing/links/00b49523ae75496f23000000/Energy-Losses-in-Traditional-Jaggery-Processing.pdf
20. Lucía Seguí, Laura Calabuig-Jiménez, Noelia Betoret, Pedro Fito, *Physicochemical and antioxidant properties of non-refined sugarcane alternatives to white sugar* (2015) https://ifst.onlinelibrary.wiley.com/doi/abs/10.1111/ijfs.12926
21. "Several recent meta-analyses have attempted to put human fructose-alone experimentation into a dose-dependent perspective. In a series of papers from the research group of Sievenpiper and Jenkins, isocaloric comparisons of fructose with other carbohydrates (sucrose, HFCS, lactose, starch) were found not to affect weight gain (33) or blood pressure (38), did not increase uric acid in nondiabetic and diabetic subjects (39), and improved glycemic control (40). Some differences were observed with hypercaloric feeding trials, but that was likely due to confounding from extra calories rather than fructose." – John S. White, *Challenging the Fructose Hypothesis: New Perspectives on Fructose Consumption and Metabolism* (2013) https://www.ncbi.nlm.nih.gov/pmc/articles/PMC3649105/
22. US FDA, Food for Human Consumption, Part 172 – Food Additives Permitted for Direct Addition to Food for Human Consumption, *Subpart F – Flavoring Agents and Related Substances* (2023) https://www.accessdata.fda.gov/scripts/cdrh/cfdocs/cfcfr/CFRSearch.cfm?fr=172.515&SearchTerm=synthetic%20flavoring
23. "...it appears that people who lived in what is now Mozambique may have eaten a diet based on sorghum as far back as 105,000 years ago, Neanderthals apparently consumed grains 44,000 years ago, and there is evidence to suggest that grains were consumed in Europe over 30,000 years ago." – Rosane Oliveira, *Busting the (Whole) Grain Myth* (2016) https://pblife.org/nutrition/busting-whole-grain-myth/
24. "Arguments that the currently consumed wheat has been genetically modified resulting in adverse effects on body weight and illnesses cannot be substantiated. In particular, populations in some countries have obtained the major part of their daily energy intake from wheat-based foods for many years, such as Turkey, without reporting any detrimental effects on body

weight or chronic disease. In line with this is the evidence that grains and grasses have already been consumed and processed throughout Europe during the Mid-Upper Palaeolithic era." – Fred Brouns, Vincent van Buul, and Peter Shewry, *Does wheat make us fat and sick?* (2013) https://www.sciencedirect.com/science/article/pii/S0733521013000969

25. Francisco Bernardino Castillo Rodriguez, Gerardo Alberto Sanchez Olivares, GRUPO ALTEX SA de CV patent, *Process for the production of refined whole wheat flour with low coloration* (2014) https://patents.google.com/patent/US8821954B2/en
26. Francisco Bernardino Castillo Rodriguez, Gerardo Alberto Sanchez Olivares, GRUPO ALTEX SA de CV patent, *Process for the production of refined whole wheat flour with low coloration* (2014) https://patents.google.com/patent/US8821954B2/en
27. Fred Brouns, Vincent van Buul, Peter Shewry, *Does wheat make us fat and sick?* (2013) https://www.sciencedirect.com/science/article/pii/S0733521013000969
28. Carlo Colantuoni, Pedro Rada, Joseph McCarthy, Caroline Patten, Nicole M. Avena, Andrew Chadeayne, Bartley G. Hoebel, *Evidence That Intermittent, Excessive Sugar Intake Causes Endogenous Opioid Dependence* (2012) https://onlinelibrary.wiley.com/doi/full/10.1038/oby.2002.66
29. Fred Provenza, *Nourishment: What Animals Can Teach Us about Rediscovering Our Nutritional Wisdom* (2018)
30. "...mineral intake, except for calcium, was significantly lesser in rats fed the white flour diet than in the other groups. The rats fed the white flour diet had the lowest food intake, weight gain, fecal excretion and intestinal fermentation. The most important result was that Mg and Fe status were drastically lower in rats fed the white flour diet than in those fed whole flour or control diets." – Charles Coudray, Marie A. Levrat-Verny, Jean C. Tressol, Christine Feillet-Coudray, Noëlle M. Horcajada-Molteni, Christian Demigné, Yves Rayssiguier, Christian Rémésy, *Mineral supplementation of white wheat flour is necessary to maintain adequate mineral status and bone characteristics in rats* (2001) https://www.sciencedirect.com/science/article/pii/S0946672X01800560
31. "With three thousand inmates in the institution the annual death-rate from beriberi prior to the use of unpolished rice was 201 per 1,000; this fell to nil in 21 months when unpolished rice was used, and when polished rice was resumed it again rose to 157 per 1, 000, to disappear a second time when the unpolished rice was supplied." – *Beriberi. An Additional Experience* (1915) https://www.cabdirect.org/cabdirect/abstract/19152900222
32. "...the Quarantine Officer, Dr. A. Richardson, has seen six severe cases of beri-beri during the sixteen months up to August, 1923. They were all in white men who had been working in the interior and living exclusively on white flour and corned beef. About six months of this diet seemed sufficient to produce beri-beri." – W.A. Sawyer, *Advantages of Nation-Wide and International Organization for Disease Control with Special Reference to*

Hookworm Disease and Beri-beri (1923) https://nla.gov.au/nla.obj-2567518667/view?partId=nla.obj-2567519895#page/n1/mode/1up

33. "At Trenggalek an epidemic occurred in December, 1918, when only maize was supplied to the prisoners, whereas under the same feeding no beriberi was reported from other prisons in the district. The procuring of unpolished rice put an end to this epidemic." – *Further about Beri-beri and Food* (1922) https://www.cabdirect.org/cabdirect/abstract/19222901716
34. "For centuries, dark bread was considered a sign of poverty, food only for the peasantry; in oriental countries, unpolished rice is consumed only by the poorest of the natives; whole grain cereals, containing the entire kernel including the seed germ, have been considered food fit only for animals, not for civilized man. Yet the peasants maintain a degree of health unknown to their wealthier lords living upon refined foods; the poor oriental, who must of necessity mill his rice by hand, never suffers from beri-beri, an affliction of those who live upon the polished rice from commercial mills; and the animal fed a whole grain ration attains a rapid growth and healthy vigor unexperienced by others fed a more artificial diet." – C. Ulysses Moore and Jessie Laird Brodie, *The Comparative Nutritional Value of White and Whole Wheat Flour* (1925) https://scholarsbank.uoregon.edu/xmlui/bitstream/handle/1794/5535/mscr_3_Comparative_value_of_flours.pdf
35. Mary Spencer, *The behaviour of rats and mice feeding on whole grains* (1953) https://www.ncbi.nlm.nih.gov/pmc/articles/PMC2217681/
36. Sally K. Norton, *Toxic Superfoods: How Oxalate Overload Is Making You Sick – and How to Get Better* (2023)
37. "While there are numerous studies labelling WGA and other lectins as toxic, inflammatory, neurotoxins, cancer-causing and a reason to avoid all grains, some studies are beginning to change our understanding. For example, one study demonstrated that the WGA has beneficial effects on the gastrointestinal tract and have anti-tumor properties." – John Douillard, *Eat Wheat: A Scientific and Clinically-Proven Approach to Safely Bringing Wheat and Dairy Back Into Your Diet* (2017)
38. Ibrahim Abdulwaliyu, Shefiat Olayemi Arekemase, Judy Atabat Adudu, Musa Latayo Batari, Mercy Nwakamaswor Egbule, Stanley Irobekhian Reuben Okoduwa, *Investigation of the medicinal significance of phytic acid as an indispensable anti-nutrient in diseases* (2019) https://www.sciencedirect.com/science/article/pii/S2352939319301216
39. "The chief foods of the Tarahumara are corn and beans, other vegetables and fruits, and small quantities of game, fish, and eggs. If sufficient calories are provided, their diet, which has been the traditional fare of Mesoamerica for several thousand years, is nutritionally adequate." – Martha P. McMurry, Maria Teresa Cerqueira, Sonja L. Connor, and William E. Connor, *Changes in Lipid and Lipoprotein Levels and Body Weight in Tarahumara Indians after Consumption of an Affluent Diet* (1991) https://www.nejm.org/doi/full/10.1056/NEJM199112123252405
40. "Phytates are considered an anti-nutrient because they bind to minerals (e.g. zinc, calcium, and magnesium) and prevent their absorption. However,

when analyzed carefully, the 'anti-nutrient' effect of phytates seems only to appear when a large quantity of phytates are consumed in conjunction with a nutrient-poor diet. Also, cooking, boiling, fermenting, soaking or germinating whole grains will inactivate phytic acid and free minerals up for absorption by the body." – Rosane Oliveira, *Busting the (Whole) Grain Myth* (2016) https://pblife.org/nutrition/busting-whole-grain-myth/

41. "Eating organic, slow fermented sourdough bread with no preservatives or oils is a great option over other breads. The fermented culture of lactic acid and probiotic strains used to make sourdough actually help to break down gluten and, according to some studies, even render the bread gluten-free." – John Douillard, *Eat Wheat: A Scientific and Clinically-Proven Approach to Safely Bringing Wheat and Dairy Back Into Your Diet* (2017)
42. "It should be noted that typical white flour is usually "treated" using a combination of chlorine, benzoyl peroxide and/or azodicarbonamide. These oxidants exert their action by oxidizing the carotenoid pigments that give the yellow color to flour." – Adelmo Monsalve-Gonzalez, Aruna Prakash, General Mills Inc patent, *Bran and bran containing products of improved flavor and methods of preparation* (2001) https://patents.google.com/patent/US8053010B2/en
43. Francisco Bernardino Castillo Rodriguez, Gerardo Alberto Sanchez Olivares, GRUPO ALTEX SA de CV patent, *Process for the production of refined whole wheat flour with low coloration* (2014) https://patents.google.com/patent/US8821954B2/en
44. "Through a particular treatment process, the present invention is able to lighten the darker color of whole wheat flour, and all but eliminate the bitter flavors. As a result, the present invention provides whole wheat flours that can be used to provide finished whole wheat products that look and taste as good as those made with regular white flour." – Lloyd E. Metzger, General Mills Inc patent, *Method of bleaching cereal grains* (2002) https://patents.google.com/patent/US7101580B2/en
45. Adelmo Monsalve-Gonzalez, Aruna Prakash, General Mills Inc patent, *Bran and bran containing products of improved flavor and methods of preparation* (2001) https://patents.google.com/patent/US8053010B2/en
46. US Department of Agriculture, *Wheat flour, white, all-purpose, enriched, bleached* (2018) https://fdc.nal.usda.gov/fdc-app.html#/food-details/168894/nutrients
47. "To compensate for the loss of nutrients, government regulations dictate the addition of vitamins and minerals into these flours and label the modified flour as refined flour. These additives are primarily niacin, reduced iron, thiamine mononitrate, riboflavin and folic acids. As practiced with whole wheat flour, ascorbic acid, amylase and azodicarbonamide are also added." – Lilei Yu, Anne-Laure Nanguet, and Trust Beta, *Comparison of Antioxidant Properties of Refined and Whole Wheat Flour and Bread* (2013) https://www.mdpi.com/2076-3921/2/4/370/htm
48. Lisa Petrison, *A Foodie's Guide to Avoiding Glyphosate (And Other Bad Stuff) – Grain Overview* (2020) https://web.archive.org/web/20201024142439/https://

paradigmchange.me/lc/grain-overview/

49. NZ Ministries for Primary Industries, *The 2015/2016 Report on Pesticides in Fresh and Frozen Produce* (2017) https://www.mpi.govt.nz/dmsdocument/19922-The-20152016-Report-on-Pesticides-in-Fresh-and-Frozen-Produce-A-survey-under-the-Food-Residues-Surveillance-Programme-FRSP-
50. Consumer NZ, *How did a banned herbicide end up in organic grain?* (2019) https://www.consumer.org.nz/articles/organic-claims
51. Surabhi Awasthi, Reshu Chauhan, Sudhakar Srivastava, Rudra D. Tripathi, *The Journey of Arsenic from Soil to Grain in Rice* (2017) https://www.frontiersin.org/articles/10.3389/fpls.2017.01007/full
52. Fred Provenza, *Nourishment: What Animals Can Teach Us about Rediscovering Our Nutritional Wisdom (2018)*
53. D.E. Yen, *The Adaptation of Kumara by the New Zealand Maori* (1961) https://www.jstor.org/stable/20703913
54. "The potato became the major contributor to the European population explosion of 1750–1850 which in turn resulted in increased urbanization and contributed to the underpinning of the Industrial Revolution in England in the nineteenth century. By feeding rapidly growing populations the potato permitted a small number of nations in northern Europe to assert dominion over much of the world between 1750 and 1950." – H. De Jong, *Impact of the Potato on Society* (2016) https://link.springer.com/article/10.1007/s12230-016-9529-1
55. Stanisław Kazimierz Kon, Aniela Klein, *The value of whole potato in human nutrition* (1928) https://www.ncbi.nlm.nih.gov/pmc/articles/PMC1252113/
56. New Zealand Food Safety, Ministry for Primary Industries, *Identifying Food Additives* (2022) https://www.mpi.govt.nz/dmsdocument/3433-Identifying-Food-Additives
57. "Populations who have long been dependent on eating high-starch diets have between 6.5 and 7 copies, on average. The Hadza, African hunter-gatherers who live in savannah woodlands and rely on starchy roots and tubers, have the most, at almost 7 copies, on average, and some Hadza have as many as 15 copies. European-Americans and Japanese are not far behind, at 6.8 and 6.6 copies. By contrast, populations long dependent on low-starch diets have copy counts around 5.5." – Joseph Henrich, *The Secret of Our Success* (2015)
58. Mnason Tweheyo, Kåre A. Lye, Robert B. Weladji, *Chimpanzee diet and habitat selection in the Budongo Forest Reserve, Uganda* (2004) https://www.sciencedirect.com/science/article/abs/pii/S0378112703004122
59. "Potato protein content is fairly low but has an excellent biological value of 90–100. Potatoes are particularly high in vitamin C and are a good source of several B vitamins and potassium. The skins provide substantial dietary fiber. Many compounds in potatoes contribute to antioxidant activity and interest in cultivars with pigmented flesh is growing." – Mary Ellen Camire, Stan Kubow, Danielle J. Donnelly, *Potatoes and Human Health* (2009) https://www.tandfonline.com/doi/abs/10.1080/10408390903041996

60. "Prior efforts to increase the crispiness of snack food products made from dehydrated potato products have included the addition of fibrous cellulosic material to the snack food dough, as described in U.S. Patent No. 4,876,102 issued October 24, 1989 to Feeney et al. U.S. Patent No. 4,219,575, issued August 26, 1980 to Saunders et al, teaches the addition of modified food starch to potato-based dough in order to increase the crispiness of French fries made therefrom." – Maria Dolores Martinez-Serna Villagran, Jianjun Li, David K. Yang, Joel F. Evans, David S. Chang, Procter and Gamble Co patent, *Potato chips based on potato flakes* (2001) https://patents.google.com/patent/EP1303195A2/en
61. "These snack products are largely characterized by a bland potato flavor profile and possibly off-flavors because of the large extent of processing to which the potato material is subjected. For the most part, these snack products are made from dehydrated potatoes which have already been subjected to losses of flavor attributable to leaching, plus changes in flavor due to intensive mixing and dehydration; and they are often subjected further to intensive moist heat treatment and, in most cases, to exposure to a second heat treatment by frying or high temperature extrusion." – Miles Willard, Individual patent, *Potato flavor enhancing composition and method of use* (1987) https://patents.google.com/patent/US4698230
62. "The formed products have less fried potato flavor because the fried outside areas have had much of the soluble flavor precursors extracted, and the internal portions comprise only the relatively flavorless particles that are bound together in a watery mass." – Miles Willard, Individual patent, *Potato flavor enhancing composition and method of use* (1987) https://patents.google.com/patent/US4698230
63. "A process for producing a potato-chip flavor concentrate which comprises the steps of heating a potato material until a browned product is formed; extracting the browned potato material with a solvent; contacting the extract with a cation-exchange resin, thereby to adsorb flavoring compounds onto the resin; and eluting the adsorbed flavoring compounds from the resin by means of a suitable solvent. Preferred process conditions involve heating comminuted potato material, slurrying the browned potato material in a water-and-alcohol extraction solvent, contacting the resulting extract with a cation-exchange resin and eluting the adsorbed flavoring material by addition of a strong base or acid." – M Sevenants, Procter and Gamble Co patent, *Processing for producing potato chip flavor concentrate* (1974) https://patents.google.com/patent/US3857982
64. Norman J. Temple, *Fat, Sugar, Whole Grains and Heart Disease: 50 Years of Confusion* (2018) https://www.ncbi.nlm.nih.gov/pmc/articles/PMC5793267/
65. Rajiv Chowdhury, Samantha Warnakula, Setor Kunutsor, Francesca Crowe, Heather A. Ward, Laura Johnson, Oscar H. Franco, Adam S. Butterworth, Nita G. Forouhi, Simon G. Thompson, Kay-Tee Khaw, Dariush Mozaffarian, John Danesh, Emanuele Di Angelantonio, *Association of Dietary, Circulating, and Supplement Fatty Acids With Coronary Risk: A Systematic Review and Meta-analysis* (2014) https://www.acpjournals.org/doi/10.7326/M13-1788

66. "During 5–23 y of follow-up of 347,747 subjects, 11,006 developed CHD or stroke. Intake of saturated fat was not associated with an increased risk of CHD, stroke, or CVD." – Patty W Siri-Tarino, Qi Sun, Frank B Hu, Ronald M Krauss, *Meta-analysis of prospective cohort studies evaluating the association of saturated fat with cardiovascular disease* (2010) https://www.ncbi.nlm.nih.gov/pmc/articles/PMC2824152/
67. "Despite popular belief among doctors and the public, the conceptual model of dietary saturated fat clogging a pipe is just plain wrong. A landmark systematic review and meta-analysis of observational studies showed no association between saturated fat consumption and (1) all-cause mortality, (2) coronary heart disease (CHD), (3) CHD mortality, (4) ischaemic stroke or (5) type 2 diabetes in healthy adults. Similarly in the secondary prevention of CHD there is no benefit from reduced fat, including saturated fat, on myocardial infarction, cardiovascular or all-cause mortality. It is instructive to note that in an angiographic study of postmenopausal women with CHD, greater intake of saturated fat was associated with less progression of atherosclerosis whereas carbohydrate and polyunsaturated fat intake were associated with greater progression." – Aseem Malhotra, Rita F Redberg, Pascal Meier, *Saturated fat does not clog the arteries: coronary heart disease is a chronic inflammatory condition, the risk of which can be effectively reduced from healthy lifestyle interventions* (2016) https://bjsm.bmj.com/content/51/15/1111
68. "The medical literature is still full of articles arguing opposing positions. For example, in 2017, after a review of the evidence, the American Heart Association Presidential Advisory strongly endorsed that "lowering intake of saturated fat and replacing it with unsaturated fats, especially polyunsaturated fats, will lower the incidence of CVD"." – Nita G Forouhi, Ronald M Krauss, Gary Taubes, Walter Willett, *Dietary fat and cardiometabolic health: evidence, controversies, and consensus for guidance* (2018) https://www.bmj.com/content/361/bmj.k2139
69. Zoe Harcombe, *Dietary fat and cardiometabolic health: evidence, controversies, and consensus for guidance* (2018) https://www.bmj.com/content/361/bmj.k2139/rr-3
70. "The general purpose of hydrogenation is the saturation of double bonds of the unsaturated fatty acids with hydrogen. During the process, several chemical changes take place such as geometric isomerization, positional isomerization, conjugation and the hydrogenation. The catalytic addition of hydrogen to the double bonds in the fatty acids chains provides an effective means for modifying the properties of oils and fats. The reaction product is a saturated compound." – Luidy Alfonso Rodriguez Posada, Adriana Fernanda Cruz Serna, Aceites y Grasas Vegetales SA patent, *Fatty product with low quantity of saturated fat and basically composed of stearic acid* (2007) https://patents.google.com/patent/EP2196094A1/en
71. Robert Lee White, Joseph Mcgrady, Procter and Gamble Co patent, *Hydrogenation process for making rapid melting fats* (1986) https://patents.google.com/patent/EP0246366B1/en

72. Health Canada, *TRANSforming the Food Supply* (2007) https://www.canada.ca/en/health-canada/services/nutrients/fats/task-force-trans-fat/transforming-food-supply-report.html
73. Е.В. Борисенко, Борисенко Елена Викторовна patent, *Fragrance agent imparting butter flavor and fragrance* (2003) https://patents.google.com/patent/RU2207016C2/en
74. Russell J de Souza, Andrew Mente, Adriana Maroleanu, Adrian I Cozma, Vanessa Ha, Teruko Kishibe, Elizabeth Uleryk, Patrick Budylowski, Holger Schünemann, Joseph Beyene, Sonia S Anand, *Intake of saturated and trans unsaturated fatty acids and risk of all cause mortality, cardiovascular disease, and type 2 diabetes: systematic review and meta-analysis of observational studies* (2015) https://www.ncbi.nlm.nih.gov/pmc/articles/PMC4532752/
75. "This current meta-analysis of cohort studies suggested that total fat, SFA, MUFA, and PUFA intake were not associated with the risk of cardiovascular disease. However, we found that higher TFA intake is associated with greater risk of CVDs in a dose-response fashion." – Yongjian Zhu, Yacong Bo, Yanhua Liu, *Dietary total fat, fatty acids intake, and risk of cardiovascular disease: a dose-response meta-analysis of cohort studies* (2019) https://www.ncbi.nlm.nih.gov/pmc/articles/PMC6451787/
76. Kylie Kavanagh, Kate L. Jones, Janet Sawyer, Kathryn Kelley, J. Jeffrey Carr, Janice D. Wagner, Lawrence L. Rudel, *Trans Fat Diet Induces Abdominal Obesity and Changes in Insulin Sensitivity in Monkeys* (2012) https://onlinelibrary.wiley.com/doi/full/10.1038/oby.2007.200
77. US FDA, *Trans Fat* (2023) https://www.fda.gov/food/food-additives-petitions/trans-fat
78. Maurice Halder, Ploingarm Petsophonsakul, Asim Cengiz Akbulut, Angelina Pavlic, Frode Bohan, Eric Anderson, Katarzyna Maresz, Rafael Kramann, Leon Schurgers, *Vitamin K: Double Bonds beyond Coagulation Insights into Differences between Vitamin K1 and K2 in Health and Disease* (2019) https://www.ncbi.nlm.nih.gov/pmc/articles/PMC6413124/
79. Chris Kresser, *Vitamin K2: Are You Consuming Enough?* (2017) https://kresserinstitute.com/vitamin-k2-consuming-enough/
80. Christopher Masterjohn, *On the Trail of the Elusive X-Factor: A Sixty-Two-Year-Old Mystery Finally Solved* (2008) https://www.westonaprice.org/health-topics/abcs-of-nutrition/on-the-trail-of-the-elusive-x-factor-a-sixty-two-year-old-mystery-finally-solved/
81. Laura Laffranchi, Francesca Zotti, Stefano Bonetti, Domenico Dalessandri, P. Fontana, *Oral implications of the vegan diet: observational study* (2010) https://www.researchgate.net/profile/Domenico_Dalessandri/publication/49739421_Oral_implications_of_the_vegan_diet_observational_study/links/0c96051b484ae6396f000000.pdf
82. Chris Kresser, *What Is Nutrient Density and Why Is It Important?* (2008) https://chriskresser.com/what-is-nutrient-density-and-why-is-it-important/
83. "Protein is a key component of diet because it is essential for formation and repair of muscle tissue as well as critical to normal cell function through

production of enzymes, hormones and neurotransmitters." – Martin R Yeomans, *Flavor, Satiety and Food Intake* (2017)

84. E Proksch, D Segger, J Degwert, M Schunck, V Zague, S Oesser, *Oral supplementation of specific collagen peptides has beneficial effects on human skin physiology: a double-blind, placebo-controlled study* (2013) https://www.ncbi.nlm.nih.gov/pubmed/23949208
85. Dinesh D. Jayasena, Dong Uk Ahn, Ki Chang Nam, Cheorun Jo, *Flavour Chemistry of Chicken Meat: A Review* (2013) https://www.ncbi.nlm.nih.gov/pmc/articles/PMC4093335/
86. Dinesh D. Jayasena, Dong Uk Ahn, Ki Chang Nam, Cheorun Jo, *Flavour Chemistry of Chicken Meat: A Review* (2013) https://www.ncbi.nlm.nih.gov/pmc/articles/PMC4093335/
87. "Among indigenous populations from the British Isles and Scandinavia, over 90% of people are lactase persistent, while rates in eastern and southern Europe range from 62% to 86%. In India, the rate is 63% in the north but 23% in the south. In Africa, the patterns are strikingly patchy." – Joseph Henrich, *The Secret of Our Success* (2015)
88. "...hydrogenation leaves the margarine white, so carotene molecules are added to restore the yellow color. Butanedione is added to give it a butter odor." – Gordon Shepherd, *Neurogastronomy: How the Brain Creates Flavor and Why It Matters* (2013)
89. Hasegawa Co Ltd patent, *Milky flavor and enhancer* (2019) https://patents.google.com/patent/JP6449207B2/en
90. Impossible Foods Inc patent, *Methods and compositions for affecting the flavor and aroma profile of consumables* (2015) https://patents.justia.com/patent/9700067
91. Impossible Foods Inc patent, *Ground meat replicas* (2015) https://patents.justia.com/patent/10172380
92. Impossible Foods Inc patent, *Methods for extracting and purifying non-denatured proteins* (2017) https://patents.justia.com/patent/10087434
93. Impossible Foods Inc patent, *Methods and compositions for consumables* (2017) https://patents.justia.com/patent/10172381
94. Impossible Foods Inc patent, *Ground meat replicas* (2015) https://patents.justia.com/patent/10172380
95. Michelle Perro, *Rat Feeding Study Suggests the Impossible Burger May Not Be Safe to Eat* (2019) https://www.gmoscience.org/rat-feeding-studies-suggest-the-impossible-burger-may-not-be-safe-to-eat/
96. Jane Wardle, Lucy Cooke, *Genetic and environmental determinants of children's food preferences* (2008) https://www.cambridge.org/core/journals/british-journal-of-nutrition/article/genetic-and-environmental-determinants-of-childrens-food-preferences/7F704253648453ICAC03BDCEE961CC0A
97. "Recipes appear to use spices in ways that increase their effectiveness. Some spices, like onions and garlic, whose killing power is resistant to heating, are deployed in the cooking process. Other spices, like cilantro, whose antimicrobial properties might be damaged by heating are added fresh in recipes." – Joseph Henrich, *The Secret of Our Success* (2015)

98. US Department of Agriculture, *Salt, table* (2018) https://fdc.nal.usda.gov/fdc-app.html#/food-details/173468/nutrients
99. Ji-Su Kim, Hee-Jee Lee, Seung-Kyu Kim, Hyun-Jung Kim, *Global Pattern of Microplastics (MPs) in Commercial Food-Grade Salts: Sea Salt as an Indicator of Seawater MP Pollution* (2018) https://pubs.acs.org/doi/abs/10.1021/acs.est.8b04180
100. Harriet V. Kuhnlein, *The trace element content of indigenous salts compared with commercially refined substitutes* (1980) https://www.tandfonline.com/doi/abs/10.1080/03670244.1980.9990626
101. "We cry salt, we sweat salt, and the cells in our bodies are bathed in salty fluids. Without salt we would not be able to live." – James DiNicolantonio, *The Salt Fix: Why the Experts Got It All Wrong – and How Eating More Might Save Your Life* (2020)
102. Laurence Finberg, John Kiley, Charles N. Luttrell, *Mass Accidental Salt Poisoning in Infancy: A Study of a Hospital Disaster* (1963) https://jamanetwork.com/journals/jama/article-abstract/664258
103. Jane Higdon, Victoria J. Drake, Barbara Delage, Harry G. Preuss, *Sodium (Chloride)* (2019) https://lpi.oregonstate.edu/mic/minerals/sodium
104. "For many foods, adding salt increases the liking for that food up to a certain point, after which more salt reduces its pleasantness (palatability)." – Institute of Medicine (US), National Academy of Sciences, *Strategies to Reduce Sodium Intake in the United States* (2010) https://www.ncbi.nlm.nih.gov/books/NBK50958/
105. "Sodium chloride—once dissociated into ions (individual atoms that carry an electrical charge)—imparts salt taste. It is now widely accepted that it is the sodium ion (Na^+) that is primarily responsible for saltiness, although the chloride ion (Cl^-) plays a modulatory role (Bartoshuk, 1980). For example, as the negatively charged ion (anion) increases in size (e.g., from chloride to acetate or gluconate), the saltiness declines. Many sodium compounds are not only salty but also bitter; with some anions, the bitterness predominates to such a degree that all saltiness disappears (Murphy et al., 1981)." – Institute of Medicine (US), National Academy of Sciences, *Strategies to Reduce Sodium Intake in the United States* (2010) https://www.ncbi.nlm.nih.gov/books/NBK50958/
106. "However, scientists know that a second salt-sensing receptor also exists, but much about this receptor, including its identity, remains unknown. Like ENaC, the second receptor detects sodium salts, but it also is sensitive to non-sodium salts such as potassium chloride (KCl), which is frequently used to replace sodium in foods." – Monell Chemical Senses Center, *Unraveling the enigma of salty taste detection* (2016) https://www.sciencedaily.com/releases/2016/02/160211142756.htm
107. "The hypothesis for a second receptor is based in part on work showing that some salt taste is perceived even when cations that cannot fit into the ENaC (potassium, calcium, ammonium) are present, rather than sodium or lithium. In addition, salt still elicits a taste in animal model studies, although to a lesser extent and with less specificity, when the ENaC is

blocked by amiloride (DeSimone and Lyall, 2006; McCaughey, 2007)." – Institute of Medicine (US), National Academy of Sciences, *Strategies to Reduce Sodium Intake in the United States* (2010) https://www.ncbi.nlm.nih.gov/books/NBK50958/

108. "Combining glutamic acid with sodium creates the well-known flavoring compound monosodium glutamate, or MSG. MSG imparts a savory taste (called "umami") as well as a salt taste to food. Some studies have shown that it is possible to maintain food palatability with a lowered overall sodium level in a food when MSG is substituted for some of the salt (Ball et al., 2002; Roininen et al., 1996; Yamaguchi, 1987)." – Institute of Medicine (US), National Academy of Sciences, *Strategies to Reduce Sodium Intake in the United States* (2010) https://www.ncbi.nlm.nih.gov/books/NBK50958/
109. "The hypothesized specificity of the salt taste mechanism makes the existence of a true salt taste substitute unlikely, although not impossible. Thus, this differs in principle from a sweet taste, where the receptor mechanisms are more easily mimicked by other molecules; as a consequence, there exist many alternative sweeteners (Beauchamp and Stein, 2008)." – Institute of Medicine (US), National Academy of Sciences, *Strategies to Reduce Sodium Intake in the United States* (2010) https://www.ncbi.nlm.nih.gov/books/NBK50958/
110. Institute of Medicine (US), National Academy of Sciences, *Strategies to Reduce Sodium Intake in the United States* (2010) https://www.ncbi.nlm.nih.gov/books/NBK50958/
111. "The salty taste enhancer itself is a flavor improving agent that does not show salty taste or has a very thin salty taste, but has an effect of strongly feeling the salty taste of sodium chloride by adding a very small amount to sodium chloride..." – Adeka Corp patent, *Flavor improver* (2015) https://patents.google.com/patent/JP6553409B2/en
112. "...one might develop a salt taste enhancer, a compound that magnifies the taste of low levels of salt. Adequate substitutes and enhancers for many uses do not yet exist, but one way to attempt to identify such molecules is to use the salt taste receptor to assay for such effects." – Institute of Medicine (US), National Academy of Sciences, *Strategies to Reduce Sodium Intake in the United States* (2010) https://www.ncbi.nlm.nih.gov/books/NBK50958/
113. Professor H. Douglas Goff, Dairy Science and Technology Education Series, University of Guelph, Canada, The Ice Cream eBook, *Milk Solids-not-fat* https://web.archive.org/web/20210515111939/https://www.uoguelph.ca/foodscience/book-page/milk-solids-not-fat
114. US Food and Drug Administration, *Pure and Highly Concentrated Caffeine* (2023) https://www.fda.gov/food/dietary-supplement-products-ingredients/pure-and-highly-concentrated-caffeine
115. Jon Kole, Anne Barnhill, *Caffeine Content Labeling: A Missed Opportunity for Promoting Personal and Public Health* (2013) https://www.ncbi.nlm.nih.gov/pmc/articles/PMC3777296/
116. Karima R. Sajadi-Ernazarova, Jackie Anderson, Aayush Dhakal, Richard J. Hamilton, *Caffeine Withdrawal* (2023) https://www.ncbi.nlm.nih.gov/books/

NBK430790/

117. "Caffeine is a powerful stimulant and very small amounts of pure or highly concentrated caffeine may have serious effects and could even be deadly." – US Food and Drug Administration, *FDA Warns Consumers About Pure and Highly Concentrated Caffeine* (2018) https://www.fda.gov/food/dietary-supplement-products-ingredients/fda-warns-consumers-about-pure-and-highly-concentrated-caffeine
118. "From 2005 to 2011, the number of emergency room visits due to adverse events from energy drinks increased 10-fold to more than 14,000, with patients typically suffering from caffeine-related symptoms." – Jon Kole, Anne Barnhill, *Caffeine Content Labeling: A Missed Opportunity for Promoting Personal and Public Health* (2013) https://www.ncbi.nlm.nih.gov/pmc/articles/PMC3777296/
119. "Physicians working in the emergency departments (ED) and the hospital must be familiar with this syndrome when they encounter patients with relevant symptoms, as they overlap with symptoms such as anxiety, depression, mood disorders, insomnia." – Karima R. Sajadi-Ernazarova, Jackie Anderson, Aayush Dhakal, Richard J. Hamilton, *Caffeine Withdrawal* (2023) https://www.ncbi.nlm.nih.gov/books/NBK430790/
120. "In December 2019 FSANZ approved the prohibition of the retail sale of foods in which total caffeine is present in a concentration of 5% or more (if the food is a solid or semi-solid food) or 1% or more (if the food is a liquid food). This prohibition came into force on 12 December 2019." – Food Standards Australia New Zealand, *Caffeine* (2023) https://www.foodstandards.govt.nz/consumer/generalissues/Pages/Caffeine.aspx
121. "The 1994 Dietary Supplement Health and Education Act (DSHE Act) defined *dietary supplements* as a distinct category of foods, which are regulated differently than all other foods, classified as *conventional foods*. Many energy drinks are classified as liquid dietary supplements." – Jon Kole, Anne Barnhill, *Caffeine Content Labeling: A Missed Opportunity for Promoting Personal and Public Health* (2013) https://www.ncbi.nlm.nih.gov/pmc/articles/PMC3777296/
122. Food Standards Australia New Zealand, *Pure and highly concentrated caffeine products* (2019) https://web.archive.org/web/20230306214457/https://www.foodstandards.gov.au/Documents/CaffeineReport2019.pdf
123. "Growing evidence in the last decade indicates that theobromine has psychoactive actions in humans that are qualitatively different from those of caffeine (Mitchell et al., 2011; Baggott et al., 2013). The effect of theobromine on blood pressure (van den Bogaard et al., 2010) is also qualitatively different than that of caffeine (Mitchell et al., 2011) but the reasons for these differences are not established." – Eva Martínez-Pinilla, Ainhoa Oñatibia-Astibia, Rafael Franco, *The relevance of theobromine for the beneficial effects of cocoa consumption* (2015) https://www.ncbi.nlm.nih.gov/pmc/articles/PMC4335269/
124. "The analog of theobromine, pentoxifylline, is effective in reducing inflammation and increasing the number of macrophages with wound

repair anti-inflammatory properties (Sunil et al., 2014)." – Eva Martínez-Pinilla, Ainhoa Oñatibia-Astibia, Rafael Franco, *The relevance of theobromine for the beneficial effects of cocoa consumption* (2015) https://www.ncbi.nlm.nih.gov/pmc/articles/PMC4335269/

125. Matthew J. Baggott, Emma Childs, Amy B. Hart, Eveline de Bruin, Abraham A. Palmer, Joy E. Wilkinson, Harriet de Wit, *Psychopharmacology of theobromine in healthy volunteers* (2013) https://link.springer.com/article/10.1007/s00213-013-3021-0
126. E.S. Mitchell, M. Slettenaar, N. vd Meer, C. Transler, L. Jans, F. Quadt, M. Berry, *Differential contributions of theobromine and caffeine on mood, psychomotor performance and blood pressure* (2011) https://www.sciencedirect.com/science/article/abs/pii/S0031938411003799
127. "Surprisingly, we have found that theobromine may counteract the transient increase in blood pressure resulting from caffeine consumption." – Mark John Berry, Andrew Hoddle, Ellen Siobhan Mitchell, Michael William Pleasants, Unilever Nv patent, *Frozen confectionery and beverage products comprising theobromine and caffeine* (2012) [translated from Portuguese] https://patents.google.com/patent/PT2206438E/en
128. "The maximum amount of cocoa powder that may be used in ice confections, such as in chocolate flavored ice cream, is about 12% by weight. If larger amounts of cocoa powder are used, the non-frozen mixture becomes very viscous, therefore difficult to process, and particularly difficult to aerate. This results in a hard, dense and unpleasant iced confectionery product. Similarly, the maximum amount of cocoa powder that can be used in the chocolate / chocolate analog is about 25%. This is because the fat content in the chocolate / chocolate analog has to be at least 45% so that it is sufficiently fluid to be suitable as a coating for ice creams, and the sugar content must be at least about 30 % so that it tastes acceptable." – Mark John Berry, Andrew Hoddle, Ellen Siobhan Mitchell, Michael William Pleasants, Unilever Nv patent, *Frozen confectionery and beverage products comprising theobromine and caffeine* (2012) [translated from Portuguese] https://patents.google.com/patent/PT2206438E/en
129. "Typically, cocoa powder comprises approximately 2% by weight of theobromine and 0.2% caffeine. However, said amounts are too low to have a substantial effect on mood states on the normal levels of cocoa solids found in most food products. Therefore there is a desire to enrich food products with caffeine and theobromine in order to achieve the beneficial effects of said compounds when consumed as ingredients of a food product." – Patent BRPI0905427B1, *Frozen confection and drink* (2012) [translated from Portuguese] https://patents.google.com/patent/BRPI0905427B1/en
130. "None of the samples were considered to have a bitter taste despite high levels of caffeine and theobromine. All testers considered that the products were sensorially acceptable. Due to the size of the nuggets (approximately 3 mm), only a relatively small amount of 14 PE2206438 was bitten when the product was being consumed. Most of them were swallowed whole, so the bitter taste of cocoa was barely perceptible. The nuggets provided

interesting textural contrast to the ice cream, which may also have distracted the tasters from any bitter taste of the product." – Mark John Berry, Andrew Hoddle, Ellen Siobhan Mitchell, Michael William Pleasants, Unilever Nv patent, *Frozen confectionery and beverage products comprising theobromine and caffeine* (2012) [translated from Portuguese] https://patents.google.com/patent/PT2206438E/en

131. "Only 50% of the volunteers were able to eat the full portion of the chocolate because of the very bitter taste of chocolate with high cocoa content. Conversely, 90% of the volunteers ate the full portion of the 17 PE2206438 ice confectionery product. In addition, 100% of the volunteers rated the flavor of the portion of the ice confection product as "acceptable" or "highly acceptable."" – Patent BRPI0905427B1, *Frozen confection and drink* (2012) [translated from Portuguese] https://patents.google.com/patent/BRPI0905427B1/en
132. Mark John Berry, Andrew Hoddle, Ellen Siobhan Mitchell, Michael William Pleasants, Unilever Nv patent, *Frozen confectionery and beverage products comprising theobromine and caffeine* (2012) [translated from Portuguese] https://patents.google.com/patent/PT2206438E/en
133. Matthew J. Baggott, Emma Childs, Amy B. Hart, Eveline de Bruin, Abraham A. Palmer, Joy E. Wilkinson, Harriet de Wit, *Psychopharmacology of theobromine in healthy volunteers* (2013) https://www.ncbi.nlm.nih.gov/pmc/articles/PMC3672386/
134. "If caffeine is listed as part of a "proprietary blend," then the amount of the blend must be listed, but not the amount of caffeine in the blend." – Jon Kole, Anne Barnhill, *Caffeine Content Labeling: A Missed Opportunity for Promoting Personal and Public Health* (2013) https://www.ncbi.nlm.nih.gov/pmc/articles/PMC3777296/
135. Erica M. Schulte, Nicole M. Avena, Ashley N. Gearhardt, *Which Foods May Be Addictive? The Roles of Processing, Fat Content, and Glycemic Load* (2015) https://journals.plos.org/plosone/article?id=10.1371/journal.pone.0117959
136. Alev Keser, Ayşegül Yüksel, Gül Yeşiltepe-Mutlu, Asuman Bayhan, Elif Özsu, Şükrü Hatun, *A new insight into food addiction in childhood obesity* (2015) https://web.archive.org/web/20240216171421/https://www.turkishjournalpediatrics.org/uploads/pdf_TJP_1465.pdf
137. Mark John Berry, Andrew Hoddle, Ellen Siobhan Mitchell, Michael William Pleasants, Unilever Nv patent, *Frozen confectionery and beverage products comprising theobromine and caffeine* (2012) [translated from Portuguese] https://patents.google.com/patent/PT2206438E/en
138. "Cocoa is also rich in minerals: potassium, phosphorus, copper, iron, zinc, and magnesium." – Maria Teresa Montagna, Giusy Diella, Francesco Triggiano, Giusy Rita Caponio, Osvalda De Giglio, Giuseppina Caggiano, Agostino Di Ciaula, Piero Portincasa, *Chocolate, "Food of the Gods": History, Science, and Human Health* (2019) https://www.mdpi.com/1660-4601/16/24/4960/htm
139. "A series of beneficial effects on the cardiovascular system might occur following regular intake of cocoa-containing foods and beverages. Benefits

include effects on blood pressure, insulin resistance, and vascular and platelet function." – Maria Teresa Montagna, Giusy Diella, Francesco Triggiano, Giusy Rita Caponio, Osvalda De Giglio, Giuseppina Caggiano, Agostino Di Ciaula, Piero Portincasa, *Chocolate, "Food of the Gods": History, Science, and Human Health* (2019) https://www.mdpi.com/1660-4601/16/24/4960/htm

140. "In healthy volunteers, consuming 100 g dark chocolate reduced platelet aggregation, an effect not seen after ingestion of white chocolate or milk chocolate." – Roberto Corti, Andreas J. Flammer, Norman K. Hollenberg, Thomas F. Lüscher, *Cocoa and Cardiovascular Health* (2009) https://www.ahajournals.org/doi/full/10.1161/CIRCULATIONAHA.108.827022

141. "A recent meta-analysis of randomized controlled studies of cocoa administration (173 subjects; mean duration, 2 weeks) confirmed a significant reduction in pressure: mean systolic and diastolic blood pressures were reduced by 4.7 mm Hg (95% CI, 7.6 to 1.8; P=0.002) and 2.8 mm Hg (95% CI, 4.8 to 0.8; P=0.006), respectively.85 This finding is remarkable in that the blood pressure–lowering effects of currently used antihypertensive drugs are in the same range." – Roberto Corti, Andreas J. Flammer, Norman K. Hollenberg, Thomas F. Lüscher, *Cocoa and Cardiovascular Health* (2009) https://www.ahajournals.org/doi/full/10.1161/CIRCULATIONAHA.108.827022

142. "On the other hand, a large prospective study exploring data from 83,310 postmenopausal women free of pre-existing major chronic diseases found no association between chocolate consumption and risk of coronary heart disease, stroke, or both combined. Conversely, an increased risk existed among women less than 65 years, in the highest quintile of chocolate consumption." – Maria Teresa Montagna, Giusy Diella, Francesco Triggiano, Giusy Rita Caponio, Osvalda De Giglio, Giuseppina Caggiano, Agostino Di Ciaula, Piero Portincasa, *Chocolate, "Food of the Gods": History, Science, and Human Health* (2019) https://www.mdpi.com/1660-4601/16/24/4960/htm

143. "Appropriately controlled studies show that the effects of caffeine on performance and mood, widely perceived to be net beneficial psychostimulant effects, are almost wholly attributable to reversal of adverse withdrawal effects associated with short periods of abstinence from the drug." – Jack E. James, Peter J. Rogers, *Effects of caffeine on performance and mood: withdrawal reversal is the most plausible explanation* (2005) https://link.springer.com/article/10.1007/s00213-005-0084-6

144. "There is also evidence that avoidance of caffeine

withdrawal determines caffeine consumptions to a greater extent than the positive effects of caffeine." – Md. Sahab Uddin, Mohammad Abu Sufian, Md. Farhad Hossain, Tanvir Kabir, Tanjir Islam, Mosiqur Rahman, Rajdoula Rafe, *Neuropsychological Effects of Caffeine: Is Caffeine Addictive?* (2017) https://www.longdom.org/open-access/neuropsychological-effects-of-caffeine-is-caffeine-addictive-2161-0487-1000295.pdf

145. Abdallah Salem, Wendy Hope, *Effect of Adenosine Receptor Agonists and Antagonists on the Expression of Opiate Withdrawal in Rats* (1997) https://www.

sciencedirect.com/science/article/pii/S0091305796003930
146. Inmaculada Ballesteros-Yáñez, Carlos A. Castillo, Stefania Merighi, Stefania Gessi, *The Role of Adenosine Receptors in Psychostimulant Addiction* (2018) https://www.frontiersin.org/articles/10.3389/fphar.2017.00985/full
147. Jon Kole, Anne Barnhill, *Caffeine Content Labeling: A Missed Opportunity for Promoting Personal and Public Health* (2013) https://www.ncbi.nlm.nih.gov/pmc/articles/PMC3777296/
148. "[Although] theobromine is said to provide a synergistic relaxation effect when present in combination with the GABA, no evidence of this is provided. In fact, the relaxing effect of the GABA could be cancelled out by the stimulatory effect of the theobromine. Without wishing to be limited by theory, the present inventors believe that to optimise the relaxatory effect, a product should in fact be high in GABA and low in theobromine, and preferably also low in caffeine." – Mark John Berry, Andrew Hoddle, Regina Beate Gisela Nicol, Michael William Pleasants, Krassimir Petkov Velikov, Conopco Inc patent, *Frozen confectionery products* (2009) https://patents.google.com/patent/US20090285947
149. Mark John Berry, Andrew Hoddle, Regina Beate Gisela Nicol, Michael William Pleasants, Krassimir Petkov Velikov, Conopco Inc patent, *Frozen confectionery products* (2009) https://patents.google.com/patent/US20090285947
150. Clifford D. May, *How Coca-Cola Obtains Its Coca* (1988) https://www.nytimes.com/1988/07/01/business/how-coca-cola-obtains-its-coca.html
151. "In this early 1900s advertisement, customers enjoy Coca-Cola at a soda fountain. The beverage started out as a medicinal tonic containing cocaine to treat fatigue and stimulate the brain." – Gail Jarrow, *The Poison Eaters* (2019)
152. Jean Friedman-Rudovsky, *Red Bull's New Cola: A Kick from Cocaine?* (2009) https://content.time.com/time/world/article/0,8599,1900849,00.html
153. Warren Buffet, *MBA Talk – Part 5* (2007) https://www.youtube.com/watch?v=sYx-Cr_RVzE 6:27 timestamp
154. Georgia Institute of Technology, College of Computing, *Metabolic Pathways* https://www.cc.gatech.edu/~turk/bio_sim/articles/metabolic_pathways.png
155. Jasmine Rana, Khan Academy, *Overview of metabolism: Anabolism and catabolism | Biomolecules | MCAT* (2013) https://www.youtube.com/watch?v=ST1UWnenOoo&feature=youtu.be
156. Rhonda Patrick, Joe Rogan Episode (2014) https://www.youtube.com/watch?v=qhoxB4OJdpQ&t=3663s 17:00 timestamp

9. Eating Disorders: The Common Path

1. "...there's a misconception that anorexia is wildly different from bulimia, binge eating disorder, an EDNOS diagnosis and so on. The truth is that people with eating disorders – regardless of how they are presenting – often think very similarly." – The Recover Clinic, *Can you go from one eating*

disorder to another? (2021) https://www.therecoverclinic.co.uk/can-you-go-from-one-eating-disorder-to-another/

2. “Research has shown that about one-third of those with anorexia cross over to bulimia and 14 percent of those with bulimia cross over to anorexia (Eddy, Dorer, Franko, et al., 2008). Between anorexia subtypes, up to 62% of patients with restricting-type anorexia later develop the binge eating/purging-type (Eddy, Keel, Dorer, et al., 2002).” – The Emily Program, *Can You Have Anorexia and Bulimia at the Same Time?* (2020) https://www.emilyprogram.com/blog/can-you-have-anorexia-and-bulimia-at-the-same-time/
3. “If a Stone Age girl wasn’t the prettiest in her small tribe, the difference wasn’t likely to be dramatic. Everyone had opportunities to see others looking their worst—tired, bedraggled, sick—as well as on their best days. Now society culls from millions of young women to select the best faces and bodies, and then perfects these with Adobe Photoshop. The difference between the resulting magazine cover and our average modern girl is staggering.” – Deirdre Barrett, *Supernormal Stimuli: How Primal Urges Overran Their Evolutionary Purpose* (2010)
4. Radoslav Detchev, *Actors Give Advice on Diet & Exercise* (2017) https://youtu.be/rF3ixuORPaw
5. “In normal living there is an ebb and flow among drives and impulses, first one dominating, then another. In starvation this pleasant balancing process is upset, and the hunger drive gradually dominates more and more of the person's activities and thoughts.” – Ancel Keys, *Men and Hunger* (1946) https://archive.org/details/MenAndHunger/page/n11
6. “Over eons, the organisms left standing are those with exquisitely tuned strategies for acquiring and spending their calories.” – Herman Pontzer, *Burn: The Misunderstood Science of Metabolism* (2021)
7. Leah M. Kalm, Richard D. Semba, *They Starved So That Others Be Better Fed: Remembering Ancel Keys and the Minnesota Experimen*t (2005) https://www.sciencedirect.com/science/article/pii/S002231662210249X
8. Vicente Javier Clemente-Suárez, Maria Isabel Ramírez-Goerke, Laura Redondo-Flórez, Ana Isabel Beltrán-Velasco, Alexandra Martín-Rodríguez, Domingo Jesús Ramos-Campo, Eduardo Navarro-Jiménez, Rodrigo Yáñez-Sepúlveda, José Francisco Tornero-Aguilera, *The Impact of Anorexia Nervosa and the Basis for Non-Pharmacological Interventions* (2023) https://www.mdpi.com/2072-6643/15/11/2594
9. Carolina Lopez, Daniel Stahl, Kate Tchanturia, *Estimated intelligence quotient in anorexia nervosa: a systematic review and meta-analysis of the literature* (2010) https://annals-general-psychiatry.biomedcentral.com/articles/10.1186/1744-859X-9-40
10. Simona Giordano, *Anorexia Nervosa: A Case for Exceptionalism in Ethical Decision Making* (2019) https://muse.jhu.edu/pub/1/article/743045/summary
11. Simona Giordano, *Secret Hunger: The Case of Anorexia Nervosa* (2020) https://link.springer.com/article/10.1007/s11245-020-09718-x

12. Simona Giordano, *Secret Hunger: The Case of Anorexia Nervosa* (2020) https://link.springer.com/article/10.1007/s11245-020-09718-x
13. Helene Tran, Pierre Poinsot, Sebastien Guillaume, Dominique Delaunay, Marion Bernetiere, Catherine Bégin, Pierre Fourneret, Noel Peretti, Sylvain Iceta, *Food Addiction as a Proxy for Anorexia Nervosa Severity: New Data Based on the Yale Food Addiction Scale 2.0* (2020) https://www.sciencedirect.com/science/article/abs/pii/S0165178120331334
14. "Although it appears that anorectics do not experience hunger because they eat so little, most do get hungry and at times their hunger is so extreme that it frightens them." – Jean Antonello, *Breaking Out of Food Jail* (1996)
15. Lea Muldtofte, *The Grace of my Perfect Skeleton: an Autoethnographic Analysis of the Anorexic Body* (2018) https://capaciousjournal.com/cms/wp-content/uploads/2017/12/capacious-muldtofte-grace-of-my-perfect-skeleton.pdf
16. Vicente Javier Clemente-Suárez, Maria Isabel Ramírez-Goerke, Laura Redondo-Flórez, Ana Isabel Beltrán-Velasco, Alexandra Martín-Rodríguez, Domingo Jesús Ramos-Campo, Eduardo Navarro-Jiménez, Rodrigo Yáñez-Sepúlveda, José Francisco Tornero-Aguilera, *The Impact of Anorexia Nervosa and the Basis for Non-Pharmacological Interventions* (2023) https://www.mdpi.com/2072-6643/15/11/2594
17. Darcy K Groesbeck, Renee M Bluml, Eric H Kossoff, *Long-term use of the ketogenic diet in the treatment of epilepsy* (2006) https://www.cambridge.org/core/journals/developmental-medicine-and-child-neurology/article/longterm-use-of-the-ketogenic-diet-in-the-treatment-of-epilepsy/927405527DC6CCF246FBA057EACA60E3
18. "A 15-month longitudinal prospective study used dual energy X-ray absorptiometry (DEXA) every 3 months to measure bone mineral content (BMC) in children on the KD [ketogenic diet]. Whole body and spine BMC for-age and height declined..." – A.G. Christina Bergqvist, *Long-term monitoring of the ketogenic diet: Do's and Don'ts* (2012) https://pdfs.semanticscholar.org/5031/d6d33d6b4fd2c5a49329e0b920dc8b6ed4ee.pdf
19. "As in humans, animals are assumed to have a limited capacity for noticing or attending things in their environments (indeed, presumably a smaller capacity than we do). Thus, only what the animal pays attention to may be coded as a hypothesis. As a simplifying assumption, most theorists start with a model in which animals attend only a single dimension or feature." – Claude G. Čech, *Chapter 7: Attention & Categorization* (1998) https://pdfs.semanticscholar.org/5031/d6d33d6b4fd2c5a49329e0b920dc8b6ed4ee.pdf
20. "Complications such as heart arrhythmias, cardiac contractile function impairment, sudden death, osteoporosis, kidney damage, increased cancer risk, impairment of physical activity and lipid abnormalities can all be linked to long-term restriction of carbohydrates in the diet." – Shane A. Bilsborough, Timothy C Crowe, *Low Carbohydrate Diets: what are the potential short- and long-term health implications?* (2003) https://pubmed.ncbi.nlm.nih.gov/14672862/
21. Khamael Hasan Obaid, Maysaa Jalal Majeed, *Exploring the Impact of the Ketogenic Diet on Thyroid Function* (2024) https://www.iasj.net/iasj/download/

1deccf98acb3852e

22. Thomas DeLauer, *5 Things Paul Saladino Changed His Mind on After Quitting Carnivore* (2023) https://www.youtube.com/watch?v=RRdkm6-eg-g
23. Claude G. Čech, *Chapter 7: Attention & Categorization* (1998) https://www.ucs.louisiana.edu/~cgc2646/LRN/Chap7.html
24. "...binge eating does occur in children, particularly among those who are overweight. In one sample of 112 overweight children, over 5% met the criteria for binge eating disorder." – Christopher Fairburn, *Overcoming Binge Eating, Second Edition* (2013)
25. William Miller, Janet C'de Baca, *Quantum Change: When Epiphanies and Sudden Insights Transform Ordinary Lives* (2001)

10. Errors of Perception

1. "These beliefs always look very convincing: they have to be in order to fool you. You would not think, for example, that smoking enables you to leap tall buildings in a single bound. That's too absurd." – Gillian Riley, *How to Stop Smoking and Stay Stopped For Good* (2007)
2. "Averaging across several studies, there seems to be no net advantage to having privileged information about ourselves: the amount of accuracy obtained by people about the causes of their responses is nearly identical with the amount of accuracy obtained by strangers." – Timothy D. Wilson, *Strangers to Ourselves: Discovering the Adaptive Unconscious* (2004)
3. Kevin Simler, Robin Hanson (describing studies on split brain patients by Roger Sperry and Michael Gazzaniga), *The Elephant in the Brain: Hidden Motives in Everyday Life* (2020)
4. "The results of a large-scale adoption study in Denmark and of twin studies in the United States and Sweden are noteworthy in this regard (Stunkard 1991). The former study found a high correlation between the body weight of adoptees and those of their biological parents, coupled with little or no correlation between the weights of adoptees and those of their adoptive parents. The twin studies revealed quite high indices of heritability (0.75–0.80) for obesity in monozygotic pairs, even when the twins were raised apart under disparate conditions." – Richard E. Keesey, Matt D. Hirvonen, *Body Weight Set-Points: Determination and Adjustment* (1997) https://www.sciencedirect.com/science/article/pii/S0022316623015900
5. "A gene for growth during pregnancy – once for making insulin-like growth factor 2 or IGF2 – was more active (less methylated) in people conceived during the worst days of starvation. The children and grandchildren were also more susceptible to obesity, diabetes, cardiovascular disease, microalbuminuria (increase in urine alcumin), and other health problems." – Fred Provenza, *Nourishment: What Animals Can Teach Us about Rediscovering Our Nutritional Wisdom* (2018)
6. Fred Provenza, *Nourishment: What Animals Can Teach Us about Rediscovering Our Nutritional Wisdom* (2018)

7. "The thrifty-gene hypothesis assumes chronic food shortages prevented obesity. However, many traditional societies had plentiful food year round. For example, the Tokelau, a remote tribe in the South Pacific, lived on coconut, breadfruit and fish, which were available year round. Regardless, obesity was unknown among them until the onset of industrialization and the Westernization of their traditional diet." – Jason Fung, *The Obesity Code* (2016)
8. Richard E. Keesey, Matt D. Hirvonen, *Body Weight Set-Points: Determination and Adjustment* (1997) https://www.sciencedirect.com/science/article/pii/S0022316623015900
9. Ruth B. S. Harris, *Role of set-point theory in regulation of body weight* (1990) https://faseb.onlinelibrary.wiley.com/doi/10.1096/fasebj.4.15.2253845
10. "Leptin is known to play a key role in appetite and thus weight regulation, and may be important in regulating the set point and regulating body weight towards the set point." – Ruth B. S. Harris, *Role of set-point theory in regulation of body weight* (1990) https://faseb.onlinelibrary.wiley.com/doi/10.1096/fasebj.4.15.2253845
11. "While set point theory has been supported in animals and humans, it may not apply to humans eating a western diet, which may be obesogenic to an extent that it overcomes the homeostatic process set forth in set point theory." – Ruth Harris, *Role of set-point theory in regulation of body weight* (1990) https://faseb.onlinelibrary.wiley.com/doi/10.1096/fasebj.4.15.2253845
12. "By being the most efficient forager it can be, it effectively minimizes the time that it spends in the prey cycle, leaving it free for other activities." – Paul Glimcher, *Decisions, Uncertainty, and the Brain: The Science of Neuroeconomics* (2004)
13. "Since 2005, the genome-wide association study (GWAS) has made it possible to identify 119 independent loci associated with BMI and common obesity status in large populations." – Hélène Huvenne, Béatrice Dubern, Karine Clément, Christine Poitou, *Rare Genetic Forms of Obesity: Clinical Approach and Current Treatments in 2016* (2016) https://www.ncbi.nlm.nih.gov/pmc/articles/PMC5644891/
14. John R. Speakman, David A. Levitsky, David B. Allison, Molly S. Bray, John M. de Castro, Deborah J. Clegg, John C. Clapham, Abdul G. Dulloo, Laurence Gruer, Sally Haw, Johannes Hebebrand, Marion M. Hetherington, Susanne Higgs, Susan A. Jebb, Ruth J. F. Loos, Simon Luckman, Amy Luke, Vidya Mohammed-Ali, Stephen O'Rahilly, Mark Pereira, Louis Perusse, Tom N. Robinson, Barbara Rolls, Michael E. Symonds, Margriet S. Westerterp-Plantenga, *Set points, settling points and some alternative models: theoretical options to understand how genes and environments combine to regulate body adiposity* (2011) https://www.ncbi.nlm.nih.gov/pmc/articles/PMC3209643/
15. "The identified variants mostly have small to very small effect sizes; only 1-2% of the BMI variance is explained. Currently, a consensus explanation for this 'missing heritability' in complex diseases has not yet emerged." – Johannes Hebebrand, Anna-Lena Volckmar, Nadja Knoll, Anke Hinney,

Chipping Away the 'Missing Heritability': GIANT Steps Forward in the Molecular Elucidation of Obesity – but Still Lots to Go (2010) https://www.ncbi.nlm.nih.gov/pmc/articles/PMC6452141/

16. Hélène Huvenne, Béatrice Dubern, Karine Clément, Christine Poitou, *Rare Genetic Forms of Obesity: Clinical Approach and Current Treatments in 2016* (2016) https://www.ncbi.nlm.nih.gov/pmc/articles/PMC5644891/
17. "Despite the tremendous increase in our knowledge of the many genetic variants that differentiate the obese from the non-obese, we still do not understand how these genotypes translate into phenotypes in terms of eating behaviour or energy expenditure." – John R. Speakman, David A. Levitsky, David B. Allison, Molly S. Bray, John M. de Castro, Deborah J. Clegg, John C. Clapham, Abdul G. Dulloo, Laurence Gruer, Sally Haw, Johannes Hebebrand, Marion M. Hetherington, Susanne Higgs, Susan A. Jebb, Ruth J. F. Loos, Simon Luckman, Amy Luke, Vidya Mohammed-Ali, Stephen O'Rahilly, Mark Pereira, Louis Perusse, Tom N. Robinson, Barbara Rolls, Michael E. Symonds, Margriet S. Westerterp-Plantenga, *Set points, settling points and some alternative models: theoretical options to understand how genes and environments combine to regulate body adiposity* (2011) https://www.ncbi.nlm.nih.gov/pmc/articles/PMC3209643/
18. Veronique Beauloye, Gwenaelle Diene, Renske Kuppens, Francis Zech, Coralie Winandy, Catherine Molinas, Sandy Faye, Isabelle Kieffer, Dominique Beckers, Ricard Nergårdh, Berthold Hauffa, Christine Derycke, Patrick Delhanty, Anita Hokken-Koelega, Maithé Tauber, *High unacylated ghrelin levels support the concept of anorexia in infants with prader-willi syndrome* (2016) https://ojrd.biomedcentral.com/articles/10.1186/s13023-016-0440-0
19. Johannes Hebebrand, Anna-Lena Volckmar, Nadja Knoll, Anke Hinney, *Chipping Away the 'Missing Heritability': GIANT Steps Forward in the Molecular Elucidation of Obesity – but Still Lots to Go* (2010) https://www.ncbi.nlm.nih.gov/pmc/articles/PMC6452141/
20. Johannes Hebebrand, Anna-Lena Volckmar, Nadja Knoll, Anke Hinney, *Chipping Away the 'Missing Heritability': GIANT Steps Forward in the Molecular Elucidation of Obesity – but Still Lots to Go* (2010) https://www.ncbi.nlm.nih.gov/pmc/articles/PMC6452141/
21. Johannes Hebebrand, Anna-Lena Volckmar, Nadja Knoll, Anke Hinney, *Chipping Away the 'Missing Heritability': GIANT Steps Forward in the Molecular Elucidation of Obesity – but Still Lots to Go* (2010) https://www.ncbi.nlm.nih.gov/pmc/articles/PMC6452141/
22. D. Haslam, *Weight management in obesity – past and present* (2016) https://www.ncbi.nlm.nih.gov/pmc/articles/PMC4832440/
23. Martin Wainwright, *Bones reveal chubby monks aplenty* (2004) https://www.theguardian.com/uk/2004/jul/15/highereducation.artsandhumanities
24. Martin Davies, *The role of GABAA receptors in mediating the effects of alcohol in the central nervous system* (2003) https://www.ncbi.nlm.nih.gov/pmc/articles/PMC165791/

25. "The results of a large-scale adoption study in Denmark and of twin studies in the United States and Sweden are noteworthy in this regard (Stunkard 1991). The former study found a high correlation between the body weight of adoptees and those of their biological parents, coupled with little or no correlation between the weights of adoptees and those of their adoptive parents. The twin studies revealed quite high indices of heritability (0.75–0.80) for obesity in monozygotic pairs, even when the twins were raised apart under disparate conditions." – Richard E. Keesey, Matt D. Hirvonen, *Body Weight Set-Points: Determination and Adjustment* (1997) https://www.sciencedirect.com/science/article/pii/S0022316623015900
26. "The category of teenagers who play computer games four times a week or more (25.3% of the sample) is at increased risk of meal skipping; those who play more than four times a week are 10 times more likely weekly to skip a meal." – J. Van den Bulck, S. Eggermont, *Media use as a reason for meal skipping and fast eating in secondary school children* (2006) https://onlinelibrary.wiley.com/doi/abs/10.1111/j.1365-277X.2006.00683.x
27. Harvard Health Publishing, Howard E. LeWine, *Taking aim at belly fat* (2024) https://www.health.harvard.edu/staying-healthy/taking-aim-at-belly-fat
28. Michael Orthofer, Armand Valsesia, Reedik Mägi, Qiao-Ping Wang, Joanna Kaczanowska, Ivona Kozieradzki, Alexandra Leopoldi, Domagoj Cikes, Lydia M. Zopf, Evgenii O. Tretiakov, Egon Demetz, Richard Hilbe, Anna Boehm, Melita Ticevic, Margit Nõukas, Alexander Jais, Katrin Spirk, Teleri Clark, Sabine Amann, Maarja Lepamets, Christoph Neumayr, Cosmas Arnold, Zhengchao Dou, Volker Kuhn, Maria Novatchkova, Shane J.F. Cronin, Uwe J.F. Tietge, Simone Müller, J. Andrew Pospisilik, Vanja Nagy, Chi-Chung Hui, Jelena Lazovic, Harald Esterbauer, Astrid Hagelkruys, Ivan Tancevski, Florian W. Kiefer, Tibor Harkany, Wulf Haubensak, G. Gregory Neely, Andres Metspalu, Jorg Hager, Nele Gheldof, Josef M. Penninger, *Identification of ALK in Thinness* (2020) https://www.cell.com/cell/fulltext/S0092-8674(20)30497-9
29. NIH National Library of Medicine, *Congenital generalized lipodystrophy* (2019) https://ghr.nlm.nih.gov/condition/congenital-generalized-lipodystrophy
30. All3Media, *Raising Kids on Junk Food, Fast Food Baby* (2020) https://www.youtube.com/watch?v=B7Hh0PY1kks
31. "Far from being an insurmountable obstacle to the analysis of an organic system, a pathological disorder is often key to understanding it. We know of many cases in the history of physiology where a scientist became aware of an important organic system only after a pathological disturbance had caused its disease." – Konrad Lorenz, *Civilized Man's Eight Deadly Sins* (1974)
32. J.L Hornick, C Van Eenaeme, O Gérard, I Dufrasne, L Istasse, *Mechanisms of reduced and compensatory growth* (2000) https://www.sciencedirect.com/science/article/abs/pii/S0739724000000722
33. "Catch-up growth has been observed for many years (Reed 1921) in plants, in-vertebrates, and vertebrates, both in the laboratory and in the wild (Albon et al. 1987) and both in juveniles and in adults." – Marc Mangel, Stephan Munch, *A Life-History Perspective on Short- and Long-Term*

Consequences of Compensatory Growth (2006) https://www.researchgate.net/publication/7301777_A_Life-History_Perspective_on_Short-_and_Long-Term_Consequences_of_Compensatory_Growth

34. "Despite a significant amount of weight regain 6 years later, the mean RMR was 1,903 ± 466 kcal/day, which was not significantly different from the end of the competition..." – Erin Fothergill, Juen Guo, Lilian Howard, Jennifer C. Kerns, Nicolas D. Knuth, Robert Brychta, Kong Y. Chen, Monica C. Skarulis, Mary Walter, Peter J. Walter, Kevin D. Hall, *Persistent metabolic adaptation 6 years after "The Biggest Loser" competition* (2016) https://onlinelibrary.wiley.com/doi/full/10.1002/oby.21538
35. R L Weinsier 1, T R Nagy, G R Hunter, B E Darnell, D D Hensrud, H L Weiss, *Do adaptive changes in metabolic rate favor weight regain in weight-reduced individuals? An examination of the set-point theory* (2000) https://pubmed.ncbi.nlm.nih.gov/11063433/
36. "Frequent dieters (yo-yo) and women without a dietary history (non-yo-yo) were matched into the following groups: diet-exercise yo-yo (DE-Y), diet-exercise non-yo-yo (DE-NY), and diet-non-yo-yo group (D-NY). After 14 wk significant differences in weight loss and fat loss were revealed between D and DE groups but not between yo-yo and non-yo-yo dieters." – D van Dale, W H Saris, *Repetitive weight loss and weight regain: effects on weight reduction, resting metabolic rate, and lipolytic activity before and after exercise and/or diet treatment* (1989) https://pubmed.ncbi.nlm.nih.gov/2923073/
37. A Bosy-Westphal, B Schautz, M Lagerpusch, M Pourhassan, W Braun, K Goele, M Heller, C-C Glüer, M J Müller, *Effect of weight loss and regain on adipose tissue distribution, composition of lean mass and resting energy expenditure in young overweight and obese adults* (2013) https://pubmed.ncbi.nlm.nih.gov/23381557/
38. "Portion sizes began to grow in the 1970s, rose sharply in the 1980s, and have continued in parallel with increasing body weights." – Lisa R. Young, Marion Nestle, *The Contribution of Expanding Portion Sizes to the US Obesity Epidemic* (2002) https://www.ncbi.nlm.nih.gov/pmc/articles/PMC1447051/
39. "Restaurants are using larger dinner plates, bakers are selling larger muffin tins, pizzerias are using larger pans, and fast-food companies are using larger drink and french fry containers." – Lisa R. Young, Marion Nestle, *The Contribution of Expanding Portion Sizes to the US Obesity Epidemic* (2002) https://www.ncbi.nlm.nih.gov/pmc/articles/PMC1447051/
40. Buzzfeed Multiplayer, *McDonald's: 1955 Vs. Now* (2015) https://www.youtube.com/watch?v=oqI4rR6lXUo
41. Brian Wansink, James E Painter, Jill North, *Bottomless bowls: why visual cues of portion size may influence intake* (2005) https://pubmed.ncbi.nlm.nih.gov/15761167/
42. Stephanie M. Lee, *Here's How Cornell Scientist Brian Wansink Turned Shoddy Data Into Viral Studies About How We Eat* (2018) https://www.buzzfeednews.com/article/stephaniemlee/brian-wansink-cornell-p-hacking#.bmxLG1XPpN

43. Ellie Kincaid, *Cornell food marketing researcher who retired after misconduct finding is publishing again* (2022) https://retractionwatch.com/2022/05/31/cornell-food-marketing-researcher-who-retired-after-misconduct-finding-is-publishing-again/
44. C. Peter Herman, Janet Polivy, Lenny R. Vartanian, Patricia Pliner, *Are large portions responsible for the obesity epidemic?* (2016) https://www.sciencedirect.com/science/article/abs/pii/S0031938416300233
45. Eleni Mantzari, Gareth J Hollands, Rachel Pechey, Susan Jebb, Theresa M Marteau, *Perceived impact of smaller compared with larger-sized bottles of sugar-sweetened beverages on consumption: A qualitative analysis* (2018) https://www.ncbi.nlm.nih.gov/pubmed/28864259
46. M. M. Hetherington, P. Blundell-Birtill, *The portion size effect and overconsumption – towards downsizing solutions for children and adolescents* (2018) https://onlinelibrary.wiley.com/doi/full/10.1111/nbu.12307
47. Hollie A. Raynor, Colleen K. Kilanowski, Irina Esterlis, Leonard H. Epstein, *A cost-analysis of adopting a healthful diet in a family-based obesity treatment program* (2002) https://www.sciencedirect.com/science/article/abs/pii/S0002822302901483
48. "Dogs fed on demineralized food died in twenty-six to thirty days; whereas dogs completely deprived of all food lived for forty to sixty days." – Herbert M. Shelton, *The Science and Fine Art of Fasting* (1934)
49. "...rats deprived of all food and given a sweet saccharine solution to consume died significantly sooner than rats similarly deprived and given unflavored water to drink." – Stephen Woods, *The Eating Paradox: How We Tolerate Food* (1991) https://www.appstate.edu/~steelekm/classes/psy5150/Documents/Woods1991.pdf
50. Emily Tate Sullivan, *Some doctors slam anti-obesity device as 'medically sanctioned bulimia'* (2016) https://www.dispatch.com/story/lifestyle/health-fitness/2016/06/25/some-doctors-slam-anti-obesity/23848429007/
51. John E Pandolfino, Brintha Krishnamoorthy, Thomas J Lee, *Gastrointestinal Complications of Obesity Surgery* (2004) https://www.ncbi.nlm.nih.gov/pmc/articles/PMC1395777/
52. Anita Berg, *Untold stories of living with a bariatric body: long-term experiences of weight-loss surgery* (2019) https://onlinelibrary.wiley.com/doi/10.1111/1467-9566.12999
53. Anita Berg, *Untold stories of living with a bariatric body: long-term experiences of weight-loss surgery* (2019) https://onlinelibrary.wiley.com/doi/10.1111/1467-9566.12999
54. Anita Berg, *Untold stories of living with a bariatric body: long-term experiences of weight-loss surgery* (2019) https://onlinelibrary.wiley.com/doi/10.1111/1467-9566.12999
55. John E Pandolfino, Brintha Krishnamoorthy, Thomas J Lee, *Gastrointestinal Complications of Obesity Surgery* (2004) https://www.ncbi.nlm.nih.gov/pmc/articles/PMC1395777/
56. John E Pandolfino, Brintha Krishnamoorthy, Thomas J Lee, *Gastrointestinal Complications of Obesity Surgery* (2004) https://www.ncbi.nlm.nih.gov/pmc/

articles/PMC1395777/

57. "Metabolic bone disease is a well-documented long-term complication of obesity surgery. It is often undiagnosed, or misdiagnosed, because of lack of physician and patient awareness. Abnormalities in calcium and vitamin D metabolism begin shortly after gastrointestinal bypass operations; however, clinical and biochemical evidence of metabolic bone disease may not be detected until many years later." – Whitney S Goldner, Thomas M O'Dorisio, Joseph S Dillon, Edward E Mason, *Severe Metabolic Bone Disease as a Long-Term Complication of Obesity Surgery* (2002) https://link.springer.com/article/10.1381/096089202321019693
58. Reddit thread, *Wife wants gastric sleeve and I don't support it. Help me change my mind* (2023) https://www.reddit.com/r/loseit/comments/152gwvh/wife_wants_gastric_sleeve_and_i_dont_support_it/
59. "Weight regain is unfortunately a common phenomenon associated with all weight loss modalities including bariatric surgery." – Saketh R. Velapati, Meera Shah, Aravind R. Kuchkuntla, Barham Abu-dayyeh, Karen Grothe, Ryan T. Hurt, Manpreet S. Mundi, *Weight Regain After Bariatric Surgery: Prevalence, Etiology, and Treatment* (2018) https://link.springer.com/article/10.1007/s13668-018-0243-0
60. Pinterest-mom, reddit thread, *Just canceled my weight loss surgery 3 days before it was scheduled. I'm going to do this myself. Am I nuts??* (2020) https://www.reddit.com/r/loseit/comments/ixqirk/just_canceled_my_weight_loss_surgery_3_days/
61. Jacqueline Odom, Kerstyn C. Zalesin, Tamika L. Washington, Wendy W. Miller, Basil Hakmeh, Danielle L. Zaremba, Mohamed Altattan, Mamtha Balasubramaniam, Deborah S. Gibbs, Kevin R. Krause, David L. Chengelis, Barry A. Franklin, Peter A. McCullough, *Behavioral Predictors of Weight Regain after Bariatric Surgery* (2009) https://link.springer.com/article/10.1007/s11695-009-9895-6
62. John E Pandolfino, Brintha Krishnamoorthy, Thomas J Lee, *Gastrointestinal Complications of Obesity Surgery* (2004) https://www.ncbi.nlm.nih.gov/pmc/articles/PMC1395777/
63. Anita Berg, *Untold stories of living with a bariatric body: long-term experiences of weight-loss surgery* (2019) https://onlinelibrary.wiley.com/doi/10.1111/1467-9566.12999
64. R. John Rodgers, Matthias H. Tschöp, John P. H. Wilding, *Anti-obesity drugs: past, present and future* (2012) https://journals.biologists.com/dmm/article/5/5/621/3257/Anti-obesity-drugs-past-present-and-future
65. Timo D. Müller, Matthias Blüher, Matthias H. Tschöp, Richard D. DiMarchi, *Anti-obesity drug discovery: advances and challenges* (2021) https://www.nature.com/articles/s41573-021-00337-8
66. Chang Beom Lee, *Weight Loss Drugs Recently Approved by the FDA* (2013) https://synapse.koreamed.org/articles/1054901
67. Joram D. Mul,Denovan P. Begg, Jason G. Barrera, Bailing Li, Emily K. Matter, David A. D'Alessio, Stephen C. Woods, Randy J. Seeley, Darleen A. Sandoval, *High-fat diet changes the temporal profile of GLP-1 receptor-mediated*

hypophagia in rats (2013) https://journals.physiology.org/doi/full/10.1152/ajpregu.00588.2012

68. Kristin C. C. Petri, Steen H. Ingwersen, Anne Flint, Jeppe Zacho, Rune V. Overgaard, *Exposure-response analysis for evaluation of semaglutide dose levels in type 2 diabetes* (2018) https://dom-pubs.onlinelibrary.wiley.com/doi/full/10.1111/dom.13358
69. Chuanfeng Liu, Yuzhao Liu, Yu Xin, Yangang Wang, *Circadian secretion rhythm of GLP-1 and its influencing factors* (2022) https://www.frontiersin.org/articles/10.3389/fendo.2022.991397/full
70. L R Ranganath, J M Beety, L M Morgan, J W Wright, R Howland, V Marks, *Attenuated GLP-1 secretion in obesity: cause or consequence?* (1996) https://gut.bmj.com/content/gutjnl/38/6/916.full.pdf
71. Joaquín Santiago Galindo Muñoz, Diana Jiménez Rodríguez, Juan José Hernández Morante, *Diurnal rhythms of plasma GLP-1 levels in normal and overweight/obese subjects: lack of effect of weight loss* (2014) https://link.springer.com/article/10.1007/s13105-014-0375-7
72. OkDocument8476, Reddit thread, *I can eat whatever I want* (2023) https://www.reddit.com/r/Ozempic/comments/11gd8hh/i_can_eat_whatever_i_want/
73. "...my stomach for really the first time in my life felt full. Not the type of full that I feel sick if I eat anymore, just content and full. On the way home I almost broke down in tears thinking to myself "is this how normal people feel?"" – Nova-star561519, Reddit thread, *I almost broke down in tears after going out to eat with my fiancé* (2023) https://www.reddit.com/r/Ozempic/comments/11fb2fw/i_almost_broke_down_in_tears_after_going_out_to/
74. "It is suggested that up to 75% of secreted GLP-1 is degraded within the gut, with an additional 50% then degraded in the liver, before even entering the general circulation (Deacon et al., 1996). Within the circulation, GLP-1 binds and activates the GLP-1R expressed on various sites throughout the body." – Neil Tanday, Peter R. Flatt, Nigel Irwin, *Metabolic responses and benefits of glucagon-like peptide-1 (GLP-1) receptor ligands* (2021) https://bpspubs.onlinelibrary.wiley.com/doi/full/10.1111/bph.15485
75. "With 94% amino acid sequence homology to native GLP-1,4 semaglutide has three structural modifications that prolong its half-life to ~1 week, making it appropriate for once-weekly administration." – Kristin C. C. Petri, Steen H. Ingwersen, Anne Flint, Jeppe Zacho, Rune V. Overgaard, *Exposure-response analysis for evaluation of semaglutide dose levels in type 2 diabetes* (2018) https://dom-pubs.onlinelibrary.wiley.com/doi/full/10.1111/dom.13358
76. "Nausea occurred in 17.0%, diarrhea in 12.2% and vomiting in 6.4% of patients treated with semaglutide 0.5 mg. As for patients treated with semaglutide 1.0 mg, nausea occurred in 19.9%, diarrhea in 13.3% and vomiting in 8.4% of cases." – Kristin C. C. Petri, Steen H. Ingwersen, Anne Flint, Jeppe Zacho, Rune V. Overgaard, *Exposure-response analysis for evaluation of semaglutide dose levels in type 2 diabetes* (2018) https://dom-pubs.onlinelibrary.wiley.com/doi/full/10.1111/dom.13358
77. "Compared with placebo, liraglutide delayed gastric emptying of solids at 5 weeks (median 70 min [IQR 32 to 151] vs 4 min [-21 to 18]; p<0·0001) and 16

weeks (30·5 min [-11 to 54] vs -1 min [-19 to 7]; p=0·025)." – Houssam Halawi, Disha Khemani, Deborah Eckert, Jessica O'Neill, Hoda Kadouh, Karen Grothe, Matthew M Clark, Duane D Burton, Adrian Vella, Andres Acosta, Alan R Zinsmeister, Michael Camilleri, *Effects of liraglutide on weight, satiation, and gastric functions in obesity: a randomised, placebo-controlled pilot trial* (2017) https://pubmed.ncbi.nlm.nih.gov/28958851/

78. Girish P Joshi, *Anesthetic Considerations in Adult Patients on Glucagon-Like Peptide-1 Receptor Agonists: Gastrointestinal Focus* (2024) https://journals.lww.com/anesthesia-analgesia/fulltext/9900/anesthetic_considerations_in_adult_patients_on.653.aspx
79. Emily Cooke, *Can Ozempic and Wegovy cause 'stomach paralysis' and 'cyclic vomiting'?* (2023) https://www.livescience.com/health/medicine-drugs/can-ozempic-and-wegovy-cause-stomach-paralysis-and-cyclic-vomiting
80. Brenda Goodman, *They took blockbuster drugs for weight loss and diabetes. Now their stomachs are paralyzed* (2023) https://edition.cnn.com/2023/07/25/health/weight-loss-diabetes-drugs-gastroparesis/index.html
81. Michael A. Nauck, Guido Kemmeries, Jens J. Holst, Juris J. Meier, *Rapid Tachyphylaxis of the Glucagon-Like Peptide 1–Induced Deceleration of Gastric Emptying in Humans* (2011) https://diabetesjournals.org/diabetes/article/60/5/1561/33533/Rapid-Tachyphylaxis-of-the-Glucagon-Like-Peptide-1
82. Tuuli Sedman, Maarja Krass, Kertu Rünkorg, Eero Vasar, Vallo Volke, *Tolerance develops toward GLP-1 receptor agonists' glucose-lowering effect in mice* (2020) https://www.sciencedirect.com/science/article/abs/pii/S0014299920305355
83. N.M. Kushnarova, O.V. Zinych, V.V. Korpavchev, A.V. Kovalchuk, O.V. Prybyla, K.O. Shyshkan-Shishova, *Decrease in the efficacy of glucagon-like peptide-1 receptor agonists: what is the reason?* (2021) https://iej.zaslavsky.com.ua/index.php/journal/article/view/1134
84. Shu Meguro, Toshihide Kawai, Tomohiro Matsuhashi, Motoaki Sano, Keiichi Fukuda, Hiroshi Itoh, Yoshihiko Suzuki, *Basal-Supported Oral Therapy with Sitagliptin Counteracts Rebound Hyperglycemia Caused by GLP-1 Tachyphylaxis* (2014) https://www.ncbi.nlm.nih.gov/pmc/articles/PMC3967600/
85. Shu Meguro, Toshihide Kawai, Tomohiro Matsuhashi, Motoaki Sano, Keiichi Fukuda, Hiroshi Itoh, Yoshihiko Suzuki, *Basal-Supported Oral Therapy with Sitagliptin Counteracts Rebound Hyperglycemia Caused by GLP-1 Tachyphylaxis* (2014) https://www.ncbi.nlm.nih.gov/pmc/articles/PMC3967600/
86. "The increased pulse rate from baseline to end-of-trial compared with placebo has been seen previously with semaglutide8-11, 15, 16 and other GLP-1RAs,25 although there is no evidence of an increased cardiovascular risk." – Kristin C. C. Petri, Steen H. Ingwersen, Anne Flint, Jeppe Zacho, Rune V. Overgaard, *Exposure-response analysis for evaluation of semaglutide dose levels in type 2 diabetes* (2018) https://dom-pubs.onlinelibrary.wiley.com/doi/full/10.1111/dom.13358

87. "Rodent studies have indicated an increased risk of developing medullary thyroid carcinoma following treatment with GLP-1 RAs, but without existing confirmation of these results in humans (72,73)." – Kristin C. C. Petri, Steen H. Ingwersen, Anne Flint, Jeppe Zacho, Rune V. Overgaard, *Exposure-response analysis for evaluation of semaglutide dose levels in type 2 diabetes* (2018) https://dom-pubs.onlinelibrary.wiley.com/doi/full/10.1111/dom.13358
88. Anita Kabahizi, Briana Wallace, Linh Lieu, Dominic Chau, Yanbin Dong, Eun-Sang Hwang, Kevin W. Williams, *Glucagon-like peptide-1 (GLP-1) signalling in the brain: From neural circuits and metabolism to therapeutics* (2021) https://bpspubs.onlinelibrary.wiley.com/doi/full/10.1111/bph.15682
89. "The GLP-1 receptor is expressed throughout many regions of the brain including the brainstem, cerebellum, cerebral cortex, hippocampus, hypothalamus, substantia nigra and thalamus (Cork et al., 2015). As a result, GLP-1 receptors have important and potential pharmacologically exploitable effects within the CNS." – Neil Tanday, Peter R. Flatt, Nigel Irwin, *Metabolic responses and benefits of glucagon-like peptide-1 (GLP-1) receptor ligands* (2021) https://bpspubs.onlinelibrary.wiley.com/doi/full/10.1111/bph.15485
90. "Besides its appetite suppressing effect, GLP-1 acts on areas of the brain involved in stress response and emotion regulation. However, the role of GLP-1 in emotion and stress regulation, and whether it is a viable treatment for stress-induced compulsive overeating, has yet to be established." – Eva Guerrero-Hreins, Anthony P. Goldstone, Robyn M. Brown, Priya Sumithran, *The therapeutic potential of GLP-1 analogues for stress-related eating and role of GLP-1 in stress, emotion and mood: a review* (2021) https://www.sciencedirect.com/science/article/abs/pii/S0278584621000622
91. Katdicko, Reddit thread, *One year on and the colour is gone from life* (2023) https://www.reddit.com/r/Ozempic/comments/17exlil/one_year_on_and_the_colour_is_gone_from_life/
92. Clubmasterc, Reddit thread, *Why I Quit Ozempic (and don't regret it)* (2023) https://www.reddit.com/r/Ozempic/comments/1536c66/why_i_quit_ozempic_and_dont_regret_it/
93. Jens Juul Holst, quoted by Matt Reynolds, *What the Scientists Who Pioneered Weight-Loss Drugs Want You to Know* (2023) https://www.wired.com/story/obesity-drugs-researcher-interview-ozempic-wegovy/
94. Joram D. Mul,Denovan P. Begg, Jason G. Barrera, Bailing Li, Emily K. Matter, David A. D'Alessio, Stephen C. Woods, Randy J. Seeley, Darleen A. Sandoval, *High-fat diet changes the temporal profile of GLP-1 receptor-mediated hypophagia in rats* (2013) https://journals.physiology.org/doi/full/10.1152/ajpregu.00588.2012
95. Sinker12344, Reddit thread, *Ozempic tolerance* (2023) https://www.reddit.com/r/Ozempic/comments/15tzkwi/ozempic_tolerance/
96. KayCJones, Reddit thread, *Has anyone experienced tolerance?* (2022) https://www.reddit.com/r/Ozempic/comments/vwmqkq/has_anyone_experienced_tolerance/

97. John P. H. Wilding, Rachel L. Batterham, Melanie Davies, Luc F. Van Gaal, Kristian Kandler, Katerina Konakli, Ildiko Lingvay, Barbara M. McGowan, Tugce Kalayci Oral, Julio Rosenstock, Thomas A. Wadden, Sean Wharton, Koutaro Yokote, Robert F. Kushner, *Weight regain and cardiometabolic effects after withdrawal of semaglutide: The STEP 1 trial extension* (2022) https://dom-pubs.onlinelibrary.wiley.com/doi/10.1111/dom.14725
98. GreenFlatworm9675, *I now understand why people gain the weight back* (2023) https://www.reddit.com/r/Ozempic/comments/15lgnnc/i_now_understand_why_people_gain_the_weight_back/
99. R. John Rodgers, Matthias H. Tschöp, John P. H. Wilding, *Anti-obesity drugs: past, present and future* (2012) https://journals.biologists.com/dmm/article/5/5/621/3257/Anti-obesity-drugs-past-present-and-future
100. Timo D. Müller, Matthias Blüher, Matthias H. Tschöp, Richard D. DiMarchi, *Anti-obesity drug discovery: advances and challenges* (2021) https://www.nature.com/articles/s41573-021-00337-8
101. Calley Means, X status (2024) https://twitter.com/calleymeans/status/1755089152343760960
102. Anita Kabahizi, Briana Wallace, Linh Lieu, Dominic Chau, Yanbin Dong, Eun-Sang Hwang, Kevin W. Williams, *Glucagon-like peptide-1 (GLP-1) signalling in the brain: From neural circuits and metabolism to therapeutics* (2021) https://bpspubs.onlinelibrary.wiley.com/doi/full/10.1111/bph.15682
103. "...individuals with obesity who consumed higher levels of dietary added sugar had the lowest postprandial GLP-1 response." – Sabrina Jones, Shan Luo, Hilary M. Dorton, Alexandra G. Yunker, Brendan Angelo, Alexis Defendis, John R. Monterosso, Kathleen A. Page, *Obesity and Dietary Added Sugar Interact to Affect Postprandial GLP-1 and Its Relationship to Striatal Responses to Food Cues and Feeding Behavior* (2021) https://www.frontiersin.org/articles/10.3389/fendo.2021.638504/full
104. "...a disruption of diurnal GLP-1 levels in overweight/obese subjects, which worsen as body fat progresses." – Joaquín Santiago Galindo Muñoz, Diana Jiménez Rodríguez, Juan José Hernández Morante, *Diurnal rhythms of plasma GLP-1 levels in normal and overweight/obese subjects: lack of effect of weight loss* (2014) https://link.springer.com/article/10.1007/s13105-014-0375-7
105. "We found that the gut hormone GLP-1 and its receptor are present in taste buds and that GLP-1 signaling plays an important role in the modulation of sweet and umami taste." – Bronwen Martin, Cedrick D. Dotson, Yu-Kyong Shin, Sunggoan Ji, Daniel J. Drucker, Stuart Maudsley, Steven D. Munger, *Modulation of taste sensitivity by GLP-1 signaling in taste buds* (2013) https://www.ncbi.nlm.nih.gov/pmc/articles/PMC3731136/
106. Yu-Kyong Shin, Bronwen Martin, Erin Golden, Cedrick D. Dotson, Stuart Maudsley, Wook Kim, Hyeung-Jin Jang, Mark P. Mattson, Daniel J. Drucker, Josephine M. Egan, Steven D. Munger, *Modulation of taste sensitivity by GLP-1 signaling* (2008) https://onlinelibrary.wiley.com/doi/epdf/10.1111/j.1471-4159.2008.05397.x
107. A.M. Koball, M.R. Meers, A. Storfer-Isser, S.E. Domoff, D.R. Musher-Eizenman, *Eating when bored: Revision of the Emotional Eating Scale with a*

focus on boredom (2012) https://psycnet.apa.org/doiLanding?doi=10.1037%2Fa0025893

108. Edward E. Abramson, Shawn G. Stinson, *Boredom and eating in obese and non-obese individuals* (1977) https://www.sciencedirect.com/science/article/abs/pii/0306460377900156
109. Bruce K. Alexander, *Addiction: The View from Rat Park* (2010) https://www.brucekalexander.com/articles-speeches/rat-park/148-addiction-the-view-from-rat-park
110. "Stress is the nonspecific response of the body to any demand." – Hans Selye, *Stress in Health and Disease* (1976) https://www.sciencedirect.com/book/9780407985100/stress-in-health-and-disease
111. "It is difficult to see at first how such essentially different things as cold, heat, drugs, hormones, sorrow and joy could provoke an identical biological reaction. Nevertheless this is the case; it can now be demonstrated by highly objective, quantitative biochemical and morphologic parameters that certain reactions are totally nonspecific and common to all types of agents, whatever their superimposed effects may be." – Hans Selye, *Stress in Health and Disease* (1976) https://www.sciencedirect.com/book/9780407985100/stress-in-health-and-disease
112. Justin Faden, Douglas Leonard, John O'Reardon, Robin Hanson, *Obesity as a defense mechanism* (2013) https://www.ncbi.nlm.nih.gov/pmc/articles/PMC3537963/
113. "Others willfully put on weight to desexualize, in the hope that what happened to them as children will never happen again." – Olga Khazan, *The Second Assault* (2015) https://centerforhealthjournalism.org/our-work/reporting/second-assault
114. "Perceived burdensomeness significantly correlated with completer status and with more lethal means of suicide, even controlling for other relevant dimensions." – Thomas E. Joiner, Jeremy W. Pettit, Rheeda L. Walker, Zachary R. Voelz, Jacqueline Cruz, M. David Rudd, David Lester, *Perceived Burdensomeness And Suicidality: Two Studies On The Suicide Notes Of Those Attempting And Those Completing Suicide* (2005) https://guilfordjournals.com/doi/abs/10.1521/jscp.21.5.531.22624
115. Amanda J. Edmondson, Cathy A. Brennan, Allan O. House, *Non-suicidal reasons for self-harm: A systematic review of self-reported accounts* (2015) https://www.sciencedirect.com/science/article/pii/S0165032715307485
116. "Generally, Premack's analysis indicates that, like reinforcement, punishment is relative, not absolute. Even electric shock, which is usually viewed as an aversive stimulus or punisher, can function as reinforcement under appropriate conditions—as when a FI schedule of shock is superimposed on a schedule of food reinforcement for lever pressing or on a schedule of brain stimulation reinforcement in humans and other animals (Heath, 1963; Sidman, Brady, Boren, Conrad, & Schulman, 1955)." – W. David Pierce, Carl D. Cheney, *Behavior Analysis and Learning: A Biobehavioral Approach, Sixth Edition* (2017)

117. Amanda J. Edmondson, Cathy A. Brennan, Allan O. House, *Non-suicidal reasons for self-harm: A systematic review of self-reported accounts* (2015) https://www.sciencedirect.com/science/article/pii/S0165032715307485
118. Donald Hebb, *The Organization of Behavior: A Neuropsychological Theory* (1949)
119. Steven Slate, *Do Alcoholics Lose Control? The Results of Priming Dose Experiments Say NO* (2013) https://www.thecleanslate.org/do-alcoholics-lose-control-the-results-of-priming-dose-experiments-say-no/
120. Karen Dion, *My Sinclair Method Experience | Daily Drinker to Sobriety | Some Reflections* (2019) https://youtu.be/tCNs_mDY2Gc
121. James Olds, Peter Milner, *Positive reinforcement produced by electrical stimulation of septal area and other regions of rat brain* (1954) https://psycnet.apa.org/record/1955-06866-001
122. "Recent work on food use disorders has demonstrated that the same neurobiological pathways that are implicated in drug abuse also modulate food consumption. [...] Work presented in this review strongly supports the notion that food addiction is a real phenomenon." – Mark S. Gold, Damian M. Blumenthal, *Neurobiology of food addiction* (2010) https://pubmed.ncbi.nlm.nih.gov/20495452/
123. "Cigarettes cause about one death per million smoked with a latency of about 25 years..." – Robert N Proctor, *The shameful past: The history of the discovery of the cigarette–lung cancer link: evidentiary traditions, corporate denial, global toll* (2012) https://tobaccocontrol.bmj.com/content/21/2/87
124. W. David Pierce, Carl D. Cheney, *Behavior Analysis and Learning: A Biobehavioral Approach, Sixth Edition* (2017)
125. GBD 2017 Diet Collaborators, *Health effects of dietary risks in 195 countries, 1990–2017: a systematic analysis for the Global Burden of Disease Study 2017* (2019) https://www.thelancet.com/journals/lancet/article/PIIS0140-6736(19)30041-8/fulltext
126. Fulton Timm Crews, Charlotte Ann Boettiger, *Impulsivity, frontal lobes and risk for addiction* (2009) https://www.sciencedirect.com/science/article/pii/S0091305709001361
127. "Both obese rats and chronic drug users have low basal dopamine levels (Hamdi, Porter, & Prasad, 1992), experience periodic exaggerated dopamine release associated with either food (Fetissov et al., 2002) or drug intake (Worsley et al., 2000), and have reduced dopamine D2 receptor and increased D1 receptor expression (Fetissov et al., 2002). A number of addictive behaviors (alcoholism; cocaine, heroin, marijuana, and nicotine use; and glucose bingeing) have been associated with low expression or dysfunction of D2 receptors (Comings & Blum, 2000)." – Leonard H. Epstein, John J. Leddy, Jennifer L. Temple, Myles S. Faith, *Food Reinforcement and Eating: A Multilevel Analysis* (2007) https://www.ncbi.nlm.nih.gov/pmc/articles/PMC2219695/
128. Leonard H. Epstein, John J. Leddy, Jennifer L. Temple, Myles S. Faith, *Food Reinforcement and Eating: A Multilevel Analysis* (2007) https://www.ncbi.nlm.nih.gov/pmc/articles/PMC2219695/

129. Jakob Hohwy, *The hypothesis testing brain: Some philosophical applications* (2010) https://www.researchgate.net/publication/266447535_The_hypothesis_testing_brain_Some_philosophical_applications
130. "The idea is that the patient knows she had the intention to move, that she acted on the intention, probably she also knows that no-one physically pushed her around, and she knows how her body actually moved. The best explanation of the unusual experience, under these circumstances, is that some supernatural force, like a demon, initiated the movement. And this is then adopted as belief." – Jakob Hohwy, *The hypothesis testing brain: Some philosophical applications* (2010) https://www.researchgate.net/publication/266447535_The_hypothesis_testing_brain_Some_philosophical_applications
131. "...deeper studies of the logistic map and related maps have resulted in an equally surprising and profound positive result—the discovery of universal characteristics of chaotic systems." – Melanie Mitchell, *Complexity: A Guided Tour* (2011)
132. Melanie Mitchell, *Complexity: A Guided Tour* (2011)
133. "For many substance users, their substance use escalates after they go to treatment. Additionally, their binge usage becomes more frequent and their behavior in other areas may become more erratic." – Michelle L Dunbar, Steven Slate, Mark W Scheeren, *The Freedom Model for the Family* (2018)
134. "The relevant research shows most of those who meet the American Psychiatric Association's criteria for addiction quit using illegal drugs by about age 30, that they usually quit without professional help, and that the correlates of quitting include legal concerns, economic pressures, and the desire for respect, particularly from family members." – Gene M. Hayman, *Addiction and choice: theory and new data* (2013) https://www.ncbi.nlm.nih.gov/pmc/articles/PMC3644798/pdf/fpsyt-04-00031.pdf
135. Steven Slate, *Over 90% of addicts will recover even though less than 25% will get treatment* (2019) https://www.thecleanslate.org/over-90-percent-of-addicts-will-recover-even-though-less-than-25-will-get-treatment/
136. "Analyses were done for the sub-sample of individuals with lifetime history of abuse or dependence on sedatives (n = 402), tranquilizers (n = 372), opioids (n = 521), and stimulants (n = 765) at Wave 1 of the National Epidemiological Survey on Alcohol and Related Conditions (NESARC). Cumulative probability estimates and hazard ratios for remission from PDUD were obtained for the general population. Lifetime cumulative probability estimates of remission were above 96% for all substances assessed." – Carlos Blanco, Roberto Secades-Villa, Olaya García-Rodríguez, Marta Labrador-Mendez, Shuai Wang, Robert P. Schwartz, *Probability and predictors of remission from life-time prescription drug use disorders: Results from the National Epidemiologic Survey on Alcohol and Related Conditions* (2013) https://www.sciencedirect.com/science/article/abs/pii/S002239561200252X
137. Gene M. Heyman, Verna Mims, *What addicts can teach us about addiction: A natural history approach,* from *Addiction and Choice: Rethinking the relationship* (2016) https://geneheyman.com/wordpress/wp-content/uploads/2017/03/WhatAddictsCanTeachUs2016OUP.pdf

138. Gene M. Heyman, Verna Mims, *What addicts can teach us about addiction: A natural history approach,* from *Addiction and Choice: Rethinking the relationship* (2016) https://geneheyman.com/wordpress/wp-content/uploads/2017/03/WhatAddictsCanTeachUs2016OUP.pdf
139. "People who try to quit with the willpower method endure a constant conflict of will, a mental tug-of-war." – Allen Carr, *Stop Drinking Now: The original Easyway method* (2015)

11. The Right Mindset

1. National Institute on Alcohol Abuse and Alcoholism, US NIH, *Alcohol Facts and Statistics* (2023) https://www.niaaa.nih.gov/publications/brochures-and-fact-sheets/alcohol-facts-and-statistics
2. Bridget F. Grant, S. Patricia Chou, Tulshi D. Saha, *Prevalence of 12-Month Alcohol Use, High-Risk Drinking, and DSM-IV Alcohol Use Disorder in the United States, 2001-2002 to 2012-2013: Results From the National Epidemiologic Survey on Alcohol and Related Conditions* (2017) https://jamanetwork.com/journals/jamapsychiatry/fullarticle/2647079
3. Substance Abuse and Mental Health Services Administration, U.S. Department of Health & Human Services, *National Survey on Drug Use and Health* (2018) https://www.samhsa.gov/data/nsduh/reports-detailed-tables-2018-NSDUH
4. National Library of Medicine, US NIH, National Academy of Sciences, *Food Additives, Contaminants, Carcinogens, and Mutagens* (1983) https://www.ncbi.nlm.nih.gov/books/NBK216714/
5. M J Jarvis, M A Russell, C Feyerabend, *Absorption of nicotine and carbon monoxide from passive smoking under natural conditions of exposure* (1983) https://www.ncbi.nlm.nih.gov/pmc/articles/PMC459671/
6. Lotfi B. Merabet, Roy Hamilton, Gottfried Schlaug, Jascha D. Swisher, Elaine T. Kiriakopoulos, Naomi B. Pitskel, Thomas Kauffman, Alvaro Pascual-Leone, *Rapid and Reversible Recruitment of Early Visual Cortex for Touch* (2008) https://journals.plos.org/plosone/article?id=10.1371/journal.pone.0003046
7. Matthew Walker, *Why We Sleep* (2017)
8. Robert T. Mallet, Johannes Burtscher, Vincent Pialoux, Qadar Pasha, Yasmin Ahmad, Grégoire P. Millet, Martin Burtscher, *Molecular Mechanisms of High-Altitude Acclimatization* (2023) https://www.mdpi.com/1422-0067/24/2/1698
9. "One interesting property about taste bud cells is that they are constantly undergoing apoptosis and regeneration. The average lifespan of a taste bud cell has been estimated to be about 10 days." – Paul A.S. Breslin, Alan C. Spector, *Mammalian taste perception* (2008) https://www.cell.com/current-biology/fulltext/S0960-9822(07)02370-6
10. Gordon Shepherd, *Neurogastronomy: How the Brain Creates Flavor and Why It Matters* (2013)
11. Linda A. Barlow, Ophir D. Klein, *Developing and regenerating a sense of taste* (2015) https://www.ncbi.nlm.nih.gov/pmc/articles/PMC4435577/

12. "...you feel you've made a sacrifice. You force yourself into a self-imposed tantrum, like a child being deprived of its toys." – Allen Carr, *Stop Drinking Now: The original Easyway method* (2015)
13. "Birds were exposed to the schedule of reinforcement plus punishment at several levels of food deprivation. Recall that food deprivation is an establishing operation that should increase pecking of the key for food (and increase the reinforcement effectiveness of food). The animals were punished for responding at 60, 65, 70, 75, and 85% of free-feeding body weight. At 85% weight, punishment virtually stopped the birds' responding. However, at 60% weight the pigeons maintained a high, stable rate of response. [...] ...rate of response was ordered by level of deprivation—the less the deprivation for food (satiation), the more effective was punishment." – W. David Pierce, Carl D. Cheney, *Behavior Analysis and Learning: A Biobehavioral Approach, Sixth Edition* (2017)
14. "For a gambler, the sound of slot machines can be a potent trigger that sparks an intense wave of desire. For someone who rarely gambles, the jingles and chimes of the casino are just background noise. Cues are meaningless until they are interpreted." – James Clear, *Atomic Habits* (2018)
15. "The closest I can come to describing it is with metaphor, such as a switch being flipped, or a pivot point being reached." – Marc Lewis, quoted by Walter Armstrong, *Interview With an Addicted Brain* (2012) https://web.archive.org/web/20210309105318/https://www.thefix.com/content/interview-Marc-Lewis-addicted-brain8090

12. The Escape Method

1. M.A. Di Muro, C.E. La Rocca, H.E. Stanley, S. Havlin, L.A. Braunstein, *Recovery of Interdependent Networks* (2016) https://www.ncbi.nlm.nih.gov/pmc/articles/PMC4783785/
2. "One of the most common ways to change behavior–environment relationships is to have the person (or other organism) experience a period of deprivation or satiation. For example, a pigeon will peck a key for food only if it is deprived of food for some period of time. More specifically, the peck-for-food contingency depends on level of food deprivation. – W. David Pierce, Carl D. Cheney, *Behavior Analysis and Learning: A Biobehavioral Approach, Sixth Edition* (2017)
3. "If we reinforce a response in a group of organisms at the same level of deprivation and extinguish it in subgroups at different levels, we find that the number of responses in the extinction curve is a function of deprivation. The hungrier the organism, the more responses it will emit during extinction. If, on the other hand, we condition at different levels of deprivation and extinguish at the same level, we find, surprisingly enough, that the two extinction curves contain approximately the same number of responses. The effect of deprivation is felt during extinction, not during conditioning." – B.F. Skinner, *Science and Human Behavior* (1965)

4. Paul Jaminet, *Hunter-Gatherer Macronutrient Ratios: More Data* (2011) https://perfecthealthdiet.com/2011/02/hunter-gatherer-macronutrient-ratios-new-data/
5. Leah M. Kalm, Richard D. Semba, *They Starved So That Others Be Better Fed: Remembering Ancel Keys and the Minnesota Experiment* (2005) https://www.sciencedirect.com/science/article/pii/S002231662210249X
6. "The change does not happen instantly, however (Collier, 1982, 1989), and I suspect that the animal, as it adapts to consuming larger and larger meals, also learns to anticipate such meals by secreting more and more cephalic insulin and developing other adaptive responses. As long as the environment is perfectly predictable, large meals can be consumed and well tolerated. Cephalic insulin and other processes enable such consumption." – Stephen C. Woods, *The Eating Paradox* (1991) https://www.appstate.edu/~steelekm/classes/psy5150/Documents/Woods1991.pdf
7. Neil E. Rowland, *Order and disorder: Temporal organization of eating* (2012) https://www.ncbi.nlm.nih.gov/pmc/articles/PMC3424484/
8. Christopher Fairburn, *Overcoming Binge Eating, Second Edition* (2013)
9. C Lee, V D Longo, *Fasting vs dietary restriction in cellular protection and cancer treatment: from model organisms to patients* (2011) https://www.nature.com/articles/onc201191
10. Elizabeth F. Sutton, Robbie Beyl, Kate S. Early, William T. Cefalu, Eric Ravussin, Courtney M. Peterson, *Early Time-Restricted Feeding Improves Insulin Sensitivity, Blood Pressure, and Oxidative Stress Even without Weight Loss in Men with Prediabetes* (2018) https://www.sciencedirect.com/science/article/pii/S1550413118302535
11. Ameneh Madjd, Moira A. Taylor, Alireza Delavari, Reza Malekzadeh, Ian A. Macdonald, Hamid R. Farshchi, *Beneficial effect of high energy intake at lunch rather than dinner on weight loss in healthy obese women in a weight-loss program: a randomized clinical trial* (2016) https://ajcn.nutrition.org/article/S0002-9165(22)04622-6/pdf
12. M. Garaulet, P. Gómez-Abellán, J.J. Alburquerque-Béjar, Y-C. Lee, J.M. Ordovás, F.A.J.L. Scheer, *Timing of food intake predicts weight loss effectiveness* (2013) https://www.nature.com/articles/ijo2012229
13. Improvement Gnome, *Kidney Failure After 20 Day Water Fast* (2018) https://www.youtube.com/watch?v=FoxU6yJ3Vco
14. Herbert M. Shelton, *The Science and Fine Art of Fasting* (1934)
15. "The gut resets itself so that it produces digestive juice just before the food appears, and the liver clock resets to process nutrients that are absorbed in the gut." – Satchin Panda, *The Circadian Code* (2018)

Made in United States
Troutdale, OR
07/21/2025